Nursing Care of Children and Young People with Long-Term Conditions

Second Edition

*This book is dedicated to all children and young people
with long-term conditions and their families*

Nursing Care of Children and Young People with Long-Term Conditions

Second Edition

Edited by

MANDY BRIMBLE
RN, Dip. HE (Child), B.Sc. (Hons)
Community Health Studies (Public Health Nursing/
Health Visiting), Registered Nurse Prescriber, PGCE, M.Sc. Education
Senior Lecturer, Children and Young People's Nursing
School of Healthcare Sciences, Cardiff University, Cardiff, UK

PETER McNEE
RGN, RSCN, ENB (415), BA (Hons), PGCE, M.Sc.
Senior Lecturer, Children and Young People's Nursing
School of Healthcare Sciences, Cardiff University, Cardiff, UK

WILEY Blackwell

Registered Office(s)
John Wiley & Sons, Inc., 111 River Street, Hoboken, NJ 07030, USA
John Wiley & Sons Ltd, The Atrium, Southern Gate, Chichester, West Sussex, PO19 8SQ, UK

Editorial Office
9600 Garsington Road, Oxford, OX4 2DQ, UK

For details of our global editorial offices, customer services, and more information about Wiley products visit us at www.wiley.com.

Wiley also publishes its books in a variety of electronic formats and by print-on-demand. Some content that appears in standard print versions of this book may not be available in other formats.

Library of Congress Cataloging-in-Publication Data

Names: Brimble, Mandy, editor. | McNee, Peter, editor.
Title: Nursing care of children and young people with long term conditions /
    edited by Mandy Brimble, Peter McNee.
Other titles: Nursing care of children and young people with chronic illness
Description: Second edition. | Hoboken, NJ : Wiley-Blackwell, 2021. |
    Preceded by Nursing care of children and young people with chronic illness
    / edited by Fay Valentine, Lesley Lowes. 2007. | Includes bibliographical
    references and index. | Description based on print version record and CIP
    data provided by publisher; resource not viewed.
Identifiers: LCCN 2020024334 (print) | LCCN 2020024335 (ebook) |
    ISBN 9781119653165 (epub) | ISBN 9781119653158 (Adobe PDF) |
    ISBN 9781119653110 (paperback) | ISBN 9781119653110q(paperback) |
    ISBN 9781119653158q(Adobe PDF) | ISBN 9781119653165q(epub)
Subjects: | MESH: Chronic Disease–nursing | Long-Term Care–methods |
    Holistic Nursing | Patient Participation | Child | Adolescent
Classification: LCC RJ380 (ebook) | LCC RJ380 (print) | NLM WY 152.2 |
    DDC 618.92/044–dc23
LC record available at https://lccn.loc.gov/2020024334
LC record available at https://lccn.loc.gov/2020024335

Cover Design: Wiley
Cover Image: View Directly Below of Seven © Digital Vision/Getty Images, Group of children © momentimages/Getty Images, Portrait of smiling school kids © Inside Creative House/Shutterstock

Set in 10/12pt STIXTwoText by SPi Global, Pondicherry, India
Printed and bound by CPI Group (UK) Ltd, Croydon, CR0 4YY

10 9 8 7 6 5 4 3 2 1

Contents

Contributors

Angharad Dwynwen Barklam, RN(Child), BN (Child), Post Graduate Certificate in Education for Healthcare Professionals
Dwynwen is a Lectuer within the Children and Young People's Team at the School of Healthcare Sciences, Cardiff University. Prior to this she worked as a Practice Facilitator. Her role there comprised of training registered nurses to be mentors to student nurses and providing support to mentors when students are on placement. While working as a registered children's nurse, Dwynwen spent time working on the oncology unit and the medical unit in Noah's Ark Children's Hospital for Wales, where she had the opportunity to develop a keen interest in conditions within specialist fields such as oncology, gastro, neuro, respiratory, endocrine and metabolic as well as general medicine and safeguarding. Dwynwen is currently undertaking her Masters in Education for Healthcare Professionals.

Siân Bill, SRN, RN (Child), DNsg (CU), MN (Melb.), BN (Deakin), Grad. Dip. Adolescent Health (Melb.), Grad. Dip. Education & Training (Melb.), Grad. Dip. Nsg (Infant Child and Youth Health) (UWS)
Siân is a Lecturer within the Children and Young People's Team at the School of Heathcare Sciences, Cardiff University. Her main interests are in adolescent chronic illness, in particular cystic fibrosis, and in transitional care. Siân has worked extensively with young people in both the acute care and community setting. Sian has recently competed her Doctoral studies, which focused on the experiences of young people with cystic fibrosis and parents transitioning from child to adult healthcare services in Wales.

Mandy Brimble, RN, Dip. HE (Child), BSc (Hons) Community Health Studies (Public Health Nursing/Health Visiting), Registered Nurse Prescriber, PGCE, MSc Education
Mandy is a Senior Lecturer in the Children and Young People's Team, School of Healthcare Sciences, Cardiff University. She has worked as a children's nurse in general medicine, day surgery, at a special children's centre and as the research and education lead in a children's hospice. She has an interest in a wide range of medical and surgical conditions as well as a specific interest in all aspects of safeguarding children and young people. Her training and work as a health visitor has fostered a keen interest in public health and health promotion, particularly childhood accident prevention. Mandy is currently undertaking a Professional Doctorate. Her research project aims to explore long term relationships between children's nurses and parents in the hospice setting.

Dawn Daniel, RN (Child), BSc Community Health Studies (Children's Community Nursing), PGCE
Dawn is a Practice Development Nurse at Cwm Taf Morgannwg University Health Board. She has worked as a lecturer in children's nursing, children's nurse in children's surgery, children's high-dependency nursing and children's community nursing.

Dawn has an interest in children's community nursing and the care of children with long-term conditions. Dawn is currently studying an M.Sc. in Education at Cardiff University.

Jane Davies, RGN, RSCN, Dip. app SS (Open), BSc (Hons), PGCE, LLM, PhD
Dr Jane Davies is a Senior Lecturer in Children and Young People's Nursing, School of Healthcare Sciences, Cardiff University where she has held a number of senior roles. Jane has made a significant contribution to the development of simulated skills teaching in children and young people's nursing across the UK. Jane is a Florence Nightingale Scholar, has been awarded a visiting researcher residency at the Brocher Foundation, Geneva and was the recipient of a European Oncology Nursing Travel Award. Jane has recently completed a National Postdoctoral Fellowship awarded by RCBC Wales exploring the needs and role of partners when adolescents and young adults have cancer. Currently, her work involves a research grant from Tenovus Cancer Care, to find out more about the information needs of adolescents and young adults returning to work and education following cancer treatment.

Taryn Eccleston, RCN, BSc Nursing (Child), PGCertEd
Taryn is a children's nursing graduate from Swansea University. She started her career in a children's accident and emergency department in a major trauma centre in London before pursuing a career in critical care. During her time in paediatric intensive care she was privileged to work with and learn from children and families with long term conditions and continuing care needs. Many of these children and families required health education and clinical skills training, which ignited a passion that has greatly influenced her career. On her return to Wales Taryn worked primarily in nurse education as a Clinical Skills Tutor at Cardiff University before taking up her current post in neonatal intensive care.

Amie Hodges, MSc in Clinical Practice (Child), PGCE, BSc (Hons), Dip. Asthma, Dip. Allergy and Immunology, L/PE, RSCN, RGN, PhD
Dr Amie Hodges is a Senior Lecturer in the School of Healthcare Sciences, Cardiff University, she is a sociologist with a clinical background in both child and adult nursing. Amie's research interests focus around the sociology of health and illness; she uses participatory, visual and creative methods within her work with children, young people and families. Within her research she has used dramaturgy to explore the family-centred experiences of siblings living in the context of cystic fibrosis.

Professor Daniel Kelly, PhD, MSc, BSc, RN, PGCE, FRSA, FRCN
Professor Daniel Kelly has held the Royal College of Nursing Chair of Nursing Research at Cardiff University since 2011. His career has been spent mainly in cancer amd palliative care nursing and his Ph.D. was from London University on the impact of prostate cancer on men's lives. His research interests are primarily qualitative, with topics having included cancer and palliative care experiences, cancer in early life, clinical safety and leadership. He has produced over 165 journal publications, 15 book chapters and two books, and has generated over £3M in research income. He was awarded a Fellowship of the Royal College of Nursing of the UK in 2016 for research and international work and was President of the European Oncology Nursing Society between 2015–17. He is a member of the Executive Board of the European Cancer Organisation. He is also a Visiting Professor in Nursing Studies at Edinburgh University and Honorary Professor at the Centre for Targeted Intervention in the Division of Surgery at UCL. He has recently been appointed a Trustee of St Christopher's Hospice in London.

Peter McNee, RGN, RSCN, ENB (415), BA (Hons), PGCE, MSc
Peter is a Senior Lecturer in the Children and Young People's Team, School of Healthcare Sciences, Cardiff University. His clinical background is predominantly within paediatric critical care. His main areas of teaching include the acquisition of clinical skills,
paediatric critical care, safeguarding and acute clinical care. Peter is in the final year of
a Ph.D. using a narrative approach to exploring fathers' experiences when their child is
born with congenital heart disease.

Martina Nathan, RSCN, RGN, BSc Professional Practice, PGCE,
MSc Advanced Practice (Education)
Martina is a Lecturer in the School of Healthcare Sciences, Cardiff University. Her
clinical background is predominantly within acute paediatric oncology. She has worked
in Ireland, Singapore and Wales. Her main areas of interest are children's and young
people's cancer care, higher education and recruitment to undergraduate nursing programmes.

Melda Price, MSc, BSc (Hons), RGN, RSCN, PGCHPE, Dip. DN
Until very recently, Melda was a Lecturer in Children's Nursing in the School of Healthcare Sciences, Cardiff University, having served children's nursing education for 18
years. This followed a 20-year clinical career in primary, secondary and tertiary children's nursing settings. Her teaching expertise was in the care of children with long-
term and complex conditions in the community, with an emphasis on interprofessional
collaboration in care. Her research interests are the continuing care needs of children
and young people with chronic illness and complex needs, and their families; the developing role of the community children's nurse and their interprofessional working and
care management of children with life-limiting and life-threatening conditions.

Sian Thomas, RGN, RSCN, MSc
Sian is Consultant Nurse in Child Health at Aneurin Bevan University Health Board.
Prior to this Sian was Senior Nurse at the Community Childrens' Nursing Service. Her
specialist clinical and research interests are children with complex health needs and
the use of blended diets. She was RCN Wales Nurse of the Year in 2016 for her work
in supporting a child with complex health to receive a blended diet. In 2019, she was
awarded a Florence Nightingale Foundation Travel Scholarship to explore the use of
blended diets in the USA.

Julia Tod, RGN, RM, RSCN, ENB405/998, BSc (Hons) Psychology,
MSc (Health Psychology), PGCE
Julia's clinical nursing practice was mainly in neonatal care in North and South Wales,
Glasgow and Nottingham. She is currently a Nurse Lecturer and Programme Manager
at Cardiff University. Her areas of interest include childhood bereavement and health
behaviour of young carers.

Introduction

Mandy Brimble and Peter McNee

Currently, there are limited books available which analyse the context, theory and practice of nursing children and young people with long-term conditions. This second edition provides a comprehensive and fully updated resource for nursing students and post-registration children's nurses on assessing health needs and delivering care and services holistically within and across a variety of care settings in order to meet the changing needs of children and young people with long-term conditions and their families.

Although each chapter can be read independently, the book is designed to provide a comprehensive insight into the changing health care needs of children and young people with long-term conditions and the implications for delivering nursing care and services to children and young people of several age groups, cultural backgrounds, with differing conditions and in a variety of care settings.

In each of the chapters, individualised case studies and reader activities are used to apply theoretical principles and current evidence to nursing practice. In addition, readers are able to gain a greater understanding of the clinical conditions featured in the case studies, both in relation to development issues and associated care needs.

Chapter 1 revisits the aetiology of long-term illness, examining the genetic basis of children and young people's long-term conditions and certain disabilities as a consequence of hereditary influence, providing an overview of chromosomal anomalies and genetic pathways of inheritance. The latter half of this chapter explores the differing onsets of long-term conditions, considering prenatal, neonatal and late onset, and their implications for practitioners and care delivery.

Chapter 2 examines some of the current political, economic and social policies that are shaping the context and service delivery for children and young people with long-term illness, and the issues and challenges these bring to managers, practitioners and service users. Particular points discussed include workforce changes, patient engagement and commissioning. Examples of service models and nursing roles are analysed to apply these issues and challenges to nursing practice and demonstrate the changing boundaries of clinical practice, multidisciplinary working and service delivery.

Chapter 3 provides a theoretical basis for the impact of long-term illness on the child and parents, examining in detail some classic and contemporary theories relating to grief, loss, coping and adaptation. Suggestions are made concerning effective care strategies and practices to support and help parents adapt to their child's diagnosis of long-term illness. A clinical case scenario of a girl with type 1 diabetes is used to apply the key principles outlined in the chapter.

Chapter 4 is new for this second edition and specifically examines the impact of having a sibling with a long term condition. Contemporary thinking on the rights and needs of siblings is addressed together with impact of becoming a carer for a member of your family. A case study is used to examine these issues in relation to a baby with cystic fibrosis.

Chapter 5 explores these issues further by examining the particular care needs of a girl with eczema, focusing on the implications for children, young people and their families in their adaptation to long-term illness and addressing the practical implications of assessing and meeting their physical, psychological and social needs. Interesting discussions include issues around ethnicity, culture, spirituality, social isolation and the use of complementary therapies.

Chapter 6 provides insights into the general principles for the need to inform, educate and promote health to children and young people with long-term conditions and their families as an effective means of empowering them to be 'experts' in their care. Using an asthma case scenario, challenges that may arise due to the receptiveness of children, young people and their families, or their intellectual or resource ability to change behaviour, are considered.

Chapter 7 reviews ethical, legal and professional aspects of nursing children and young people with long-term conditions. Scenarios from other chapters are analysed within a framework of ethical principles to identify potential ethical debates and difficult decision-making that practitioners may encounter. The ethical discussions are applied to the practice situation.

Chapter 8 presents a partnership approach between theory and practice, examining changing service boundaries, nursing roles and relationships with parents in the provision of continuing care for children and young people with long-term conditions and their families in the community. To explore this from a practice perspective, multidisciplinary working, discharge planning and respite care are considered using the case scenario of a Welsh-speaking rurally isolated family with a child with the neuromuscular disorder of Batten's disease. The contemporary issue of blended diet administration via gastrostomy is covered in this chapter.

Chapter 9 recognises the importance of acute emergency care, resulting from illness or an unrelated admission, for children and young people with a long-term illness, and the need to ensure effective services and communication processes. Using an oncological haematological condition, current debates and care practices are explored including the need for alternative admission settings.

The last two chapters of the book are especially devoted to teenagers, an increasingly important issue for nurses to consider due to the increasing life expectancy of children with long-term conditions. Chapter 10 provides a critical analysis of the impact of long-term illness upon development transitions of adolescence and the possible health associated risks and longer-term consequences of these. The implications for practitioners in particular focus on communication, body image, compliance and resilience. Chapter 11 builds upon some of the themes raised in Chapter 10 by exploring further a number of aspects of adolescent development in relation to the planning and delivery of effective transition from child to adult services.

This edited book brings together contributions from a team of experienced academics and lecturers in the Children and Young People's Team at the School of Healthcare Sciences, Cardiff University, practitioners, a practice educator and a nurse consultant.

CHAPTER 1

The Definition and Aetiology of Long-Term Conditions

Siân Bill and Angharad Dwynwen Barklam

Introduction

The intention of this chapter is to help the reader further develop their knowledge and understanding of the genetic basis of children and young people's long-term conditions and certain disabilities as a consequence of hereditary influences. Following an overview of chromosomal anomalies, genetic pathways of inheritance will be defined and illustrated via examples of both sex-linked and autosomal recessive and dominant disorders. This chapter does not intend to provide an in-depth critique on the current ethical debates, research and practice controversies surrounding genetic engineering and modification. For this the reader is guided to websites such as www.bionews.org.uk.

The latter half of the chapter focuses on examining the differing onsets of long-term conditions, considering prenatal, neonatal and late onset. To provide the reader with a practice focus, case studies will be used as examples to examine the professional and care implications of nursing children, young people and their families whose long-term conditions have been diagnosed at various stages of their development. To allow these issues to be further developed and explored, the same case studies will be used in subsequent chapters.

Aim of the chapter

To enhance the genetic knowledge and understanding of nurses, including the aetiology of long-term conditions in children, and to examine how this genetic competence can be implemented in their practice to:

- Lead to a reduced risk of conditions occurring, or a reduction in severity for those where a condition has been identified.

Nursing Care of Children and Young People with Long-Term Conditions, Second Edition.
Edited by Mandy Brimble and Peter McNee.
© 2021 John Wiley & Sons Ltd. Published 2021 by John Wiley & Sons Ltd.

- Enable them to fully participate in the relevant debates and ethical discussions that can have implications for children, young people and their families.

Intended learning outcomes

- To examine the hereditary influences upon the genetic basis of long-term conditions in childhood
- To determine patterns of genetic inheritance
- To investigate the origins of long-term conditions
- To explore the role of the children's nurse during the period leading to, and at the time of, diagnosis

Genetic knowledge

This chapter is written on the assumption that the reader comprehends the basic foundations and principles of genetics. These being: the biology of chromosomes, the structure and role of deoxyribonucleic acid (DNA) in coding genetic information, its ability to replicate and the mechanisms for protein synthesis. In particular, knowledge of the nitrogenous bases and the mechanisms of transcription and translation are required. A good grasp of the cell cycle and its governing control system, along with knowledge of the distinct stages of mitosis and the two divisions, 1 and 2, of meiosis and their resulting products, is also assumed. It is important that the reader has knowledge and understanding of these basic units relating to normal DNA development and of the processes undertaken for the production of sperm and oocytes. Without this knowledge, the reader may find it difficult to comprehend how DNA mutations can cause disease and how errors within the processes of mitosis and meiosis can result in chromosomal abnormalities.

Test your knowledge

- What are the two major phases of a somatic cell cycle?
- What are the four stages of mitosis?
- What are the subdivisions of meiosis 1?
- What are the products of meiosis 2?
- What are the three parts of a DNA nucleotide?
- What are the four nitrogenous bases in DNA?
- In what way does RNA differ from DNA?
- Cells contain three different kinds of RNA. What are they and what is their function in carrying out the instructions encoded in DNA?
- Do you understand the following terms? Haploid and diploid germ cell, homologous chromosomes, allele, heterozygosity and homozygosity?

If the reader wishes to refresh their knowledge on these areas following this test, they are advised to refer to a nursing anatomy and physiology text such as *Wong's Nursing Care of Children* (Hockenberry *et al.*, 2019) or Brown (2011) *Introduction to Genetics: A Molecular Approach*. Additionally, the CPD article by Davies and Meimaridou (2020) would be a valuable learning resource.

The need for genetic knowledge

Several authors have argued that children's nurses increasingly need genetic/genomic knowledge to maintain currency of practice (Skirton *et al.*, 2010; Botkin *et al.*, 2015; Prows, 2019). This is regarded as essential if they are to provide appropriate information and advice to families and be able to engage in policy decisions and relevant genetic debates. The genetics White Paper *Our Inheritance, Our Future* (DoH, 2003) supports this premise, emphasising that education for health professionals is vital to enable advances in genetics to be translated and applied to everyday clinical practice. In response, a genetics educational framework was developed for nurses and midwives by an expert panel and endorsed by the Nursing and Midwifery Council (NMC) (Kirk *et al.*, 2013). Since the implementation of the framework in 2003, advances in genetics/genomic has been far more significant than predicted (House of Lords Science and Technology Committee, 2009). The House of Lords Inquiry into genomic medicine (2009) foresaw that as the requests for genetic testing would increase, so would the need for education and training in genetics and genomics across the breadth of the health care professions. The Inquiry urged the NMC to set standards on genetic and genomics across the nursing curriculum for both pre-registration and post-registration education. However, the NMC fell short of this recommendation in their revised pre-registration nurse training requirements in 2010 (Kirk *et al.*, 2013). It was therefore seen as timely to review the framework (Kirk *et al.*, 2013). Following the inquiry, the Human Genomics Strategy Group (HGSG) was established in 2010. In their report (2012), they continue to emphasise the vital importance of genomic education so that health care professionals can respond to new challenges. A review of training and education included the establishment of Health Education England, who developed core educational standards for genomics which evolve in response to advances made within the field, as well as monitor outcomes. They predict that genomics will have some degree of impact on almost every role in all clinical fields. Therefore, there is a requirement to build an awareness, knowledge and understanding of genomics across the whole of the NHS. The Progress Educational Trust (PET) have also produced a guide to genetics and epigenetics, which provides a good basic overview of genetics (Pembrey, 2012).

For children's nurses, this genetic education would be required to impart several key areas of practice when delivering care and education to children and young people with long-term conditions and their families. Sex education and genetic advice may be required for the teenager with a genetic long-term condition, for example sickle cell anaemia, who may be considering commencing a sexual relationship. Alternatively, parents may require support, advice and guidance following the diagnosis of their child with a genetic disorder. Parents who already have a child with a genetic condition and are considering future pregnancies may also require genetic counselling and advice.

If children's nurses are to deliver sensitive, informed, evidence-based information, education and support to children, young people and their families, they must ensure that they have a current knowledge base upon which to draw. They must also be professionally aware of their limitations in this field and have a good knowledge of, and guide their patients to, local resources and expertise. This could be a hospital's local genetic department or a genetic specialist nurse.

The ethical, legal and social implications in the screening, testing and recording of genetic information

Along with technological advances, our enhanced knowledge and understanding of the human genome and the role of genes in body processes has enabled the mechanisms for genetic screening and testing to be realised for a number of genetic disorders. This new ability to predict the potential for, or to identify, disease-related genes in individuals long before they can be clinically detected, has brought both positive advantages and some practice challenges. For example, knowing from birth that a child has Duchenne muscular dystrophy provides the opportunity for prophylactic treatment regimes and health education strategies to commence immediately. This potentially reduces the complications that can negatively impact upon a child's quality of life. However, this new knowledge has also resulted in some ethical dilemmas and debates that need to be considered; for example, issues such as consent, confidentiality, and the management of situations where the child or young person, their family and the professional's views are not in unison.

Other areas of debate and controversy include who should be tested? What should be the availability of testing? Is mandatory prenatal testing and neonatal screening required or ethical? What are the predictive values of the genetic test and the appropriateness of testing for diseases where there is no treatment or intervention available, as in the case of Huntington's chorea? For those children and families that are tested, there are concerns about possible stigmatisation or discrimination (Williams *et al.*, 2010; Prows, 2019; World Health Organization, 2019) and the role of family counselling within this process (Craufurd *et al.*, 2015; Henneman *et al.*, 2016). A document published by the European Society of Human Genetics recommends that psychosocial support and information should be given pre and post screening and post-screening counselling should be available to all carrier couples (Hennman *et al.*, 2016). Prows (2019) suggests that the most important area for nursing practice is conveying clear information and teaching, making them a valuable resource to help families make the best decision and to reduce anxiety. Ashtiani *et al.* (2014) support this point when discussing parents' experience of receiving their child's diagnosis. In their study, parental experiences were far more positive when they felt that they had active participation in discussions rather than the medical team being dominant and using jargon-heavy language. They required sufficient emotional support and counselling as well as being provided with hope and perspective and a clear plan for follow-ups. It is also suggested that the emotional impact of a diagnosis was less significant when parents were prepared for the diagnosis and they were better able to receive and retain the information without feeling overwhelmed.

This chapter, however, wishes only to draw the reader's attention to these growing ethical dilemmas and the legal and social issues related to genetic screening and the identification of a genetic disease. Although there is no absolute guide to good action, there are frameworks and models for resolving ethical decision-making. For further information regarding these ethical frameworks, the reader is directed to Chapter 7, where ethical frameworks are used to guide the reader through decisions.

🔑 Key points

Children's nurses need genetic competence to implement this knowledge and understanding into their practice in order to:

- Lead to a reduction of risk of conditions occurring, or a reduction in severity for those where a condition has been identified.
- Enable them to fully participate in the relevant debates and ethical discussions that can have implications for children, young people and their families.

The determinants of genetic disease

Due to the intricate nature of DNA formation that occurs during embryological and foetal development, chance mutations or damage can easily alter DNA, producing abnormal sequences of base molecules. There are natural processes within the cell to monitor, recognise and repair defects produced in DNA base sequencing. However, if these internal mechanisms do not detect or repair this damage, expression of the dysfunctional gene can either cause a congenital problem in that child or become part of the genome to be passed on to future generations (hereditary).

Environmental insults to DNA material caused by chemical (carcinogenic), physical (heat) and ionising radiation (X-ray) processes may also produce damage to the genetic material (Martin and Fry, 2018). Damage to somatic cells by radiation, carcinogenic chemicals and ultraviolet light may cause mutations, particularly in cells that are constantly regenerating, and can lead to tumour growth in that individual (Parsa, 2012). However, damage to the sex cells that go on to produce the gametes for fertilisation means that the mutation will not affect the individual but could be passed on to future generations.

The term 'multifactorial inheritance' is used to describe the origin of diseases where there are multiple genetic and environmental factors involved in determining the phenotype, such as leukaemia, where there is familial clustering, and asthma. Some writers believe, however, that the environment has a role to play in all genetic conditions. Although most diseases are influenced by a genetic/genomic predisposition, they can be activated, modified or suppressed by environmental factors (Prows, 2019).

Later in the chapter, prenatal onsets of genetic disorders are discussed in more detail including potential permanent effects caused to the developing foetus by the prenatal intrauterine environment.

🕐 **Time out**

- Before you get to that section write a list of teratogens – agents that cause birth defects.

Chromosomal abnormalities

In humans, each cell, except the germ cells (ova in girls, sperm in boys), contains 46 chromosomes, which are further classified as 22 pairs of autosomes and one pair of sex chromosomes (XX in girls, XY in boys). Located throughout the chromosome are genes, intricate chemical units made up of DNA. As chromosomes are inherited from both parents, individuals have a copy of genes from both the maternal and paternal line. In homologous chromosomes, each gene sequence inherited from the father will have a corresponding gene sequence inherited from the mother (Coleman, 2015). Depending on inheritance factors, the gene sequences may be identical or different.

Chromosomes are numbered according to size and centromere position. Chromosome number 1, for instance, is the largest pair of chromosomes and number 22 the smallest pair of autosomes. The centromere, a constriction on the chromosome either in the centre or close to one end, divides the chromosome into a shorter arm (p) and a longer arm (q). The relative centromeric position allows the morphological classification of chromosomes: metacentric (p and q in equal lengths), submetacentric (q slightly greater than p), acrocentric (q much greater than p), or telocentric (the centromere terminal).

Where a chromosomal anomaly is detected, it can be present in all or just a certain set of cells within the body, demonstrating what is termed a 'mosaic pattern'. Chromosomal anomalies are usually categorised into three discrete areas:

1. Numerical abnormalities, where there is an excess or deficit in the normal complement of 46 chromosomes.
2. Structural abnormalities of the chromosomes.
3. Uniparental disomy, caused through non-disjunction of a chromosome pair.

Numerical abnormalities

If a haploid gamete or a diploid cell lacks the expected number of chromosomes, aneuploidy exists. Monosomy is the term used to depict where there is a deficit in the expected chromosomal numbers. Although autosomal monosomy is usually lethal (e.g. 45XY) in Turner syndrome, monosomy (45X) is not always lethal.

The term 'trisomy' identifies the presence of an additional chromosome. Autosomal trisomy usually occurs as a result of meiotic non-disjunction, with the most common autosomal trisomy being Trisomy 21 (Down syndrome). Other common trisomy syndromes include Trisomy 18 (Edwards syndrome) and Trisomy 13 (Patau syndrome). The term 'polysomy' is frequently applied if the additional chromosome is a sex chromosome, for example 47XXY (Klinefelter syndrome).

The most common reason for abnormalities in chromosome number is a process called non-disjunction during cell division. Non-disjunction is a failure of separation of the homologous chromosomes during meiosis 1, or of sister chromosomes during meiosis 2. If non-disjunction occurs at meiosis 1, the gamete will have too few chromosomes, or too many if non-disjunction occurs at meiosis 2. Non-disjunction can involve both autosomes and sex chromosomes.

Translocations

Translocations are structural abnormalities where one or more chromosomes break and there is an exchange of genetic material between two or more chromosomes. Translocations are classified into two main types: a Reciprocal translocation and a Robertsonian translocation. In a Reciprocal translocation, the broken fragments of two different chromosomes exchange places. A Robertsonian translocation, however, occurs in acrocentric chromosomes where the centromere is situated near one end, with one arm much longer than the other. Acrocentric chromosomes are Group D (13, 14 and 15) and Group G (21, 22). In these translocations two whole chromosomes merge together through the fusion of their centromeres. One of the most important Robertsonian translocations involves chromosomes 14 and 21.

Translocations are important in heredity, disability and long-term conditions depending on whether they are balanced or unbalanced. Where infants are phenotypically normal and the translocation is referred to as balanced, it is assumed that during the translocation no genetic material was lost or gained and infants are not themselves affected. However, as they are carriers, in adulthood they should carefully consider their decision to have children, as their children could inherit what is termed an unbalanced form of the translocation. However, if infants are phenotypically abnormal, an unbalanced arrangement, either deficiency or duplication of genetic material, is assumed and the translocation is referred to as unbalanced (Chen et al., 2011; Chang et al., 2013). The degree of disability for a child will depend upon which chromosomes are affected and the extent of genetic material lost or gained. There will, unfortunately though, always be some degree of disability in an unbalanced translocation.

Deletions and duplications

Partial chromosome abnormalities involve a deletion (missing) or duplication (extra) segment of a chromosome. A classic deletion syndrome is Cri du chat, where there is a deletion of the short arm of chromosome 5. Contiguous gene syndrome has been used to identify smaller sections of chromosome abnormalities, such as microdeletions and microduplications (Prows, 2019). The end result is an altered, normal gene dosage, which leads to a specific and complex phenotype that, in some cases, is recognised as a generic syndrome (Strachan et al., 2014; Pereira and Marion, 2018). Some major contiguous gene syndromes include DiGeorge syndrome and Prader-Willi syndrome, both occurring as a result of microdeletions. DiGeorge syndrome involves chromosome 22 and children with this syndrome tend to have cardiac defects, learning difficulties, feeding and speech problems due to a cleft palate or weakness of the palate. Other medical problems can be kidney abnormalities, poor immune systems and neurological and endocrine abnormalities. Prader-Willi syndrome involves a microdeletion on chromosome 15. Classic features of this syndrome include floppy muscles and, initially, poor feeding and weight gain. However, by 3 years of age, children with Prader-Willi syndrome develop large appetites and suffer from obesity. There is also associated pubertal delay along with learning and behavioural challenges.

Chromosomal nomenclature

At a certain stage during cell division, chromosomes form into visible structures and can be detected by photography, producing a picture known as an ideogram.

This picture represents the complete diploid number of chromosomes in a cell called the karyotype.

An official chromosomal nomenclature exists (McGowan-Jordan *et al.*, 2016) and designates the chromosomal complement in the following manner:

- The total number of chromosomes (e.g. 45, 46 or 47).
- A comma.
- The sex chromosome complement (XX in normal females; XY in normal males).
- The specific abnormality, if any.

A + or − sign indicates the addition or absence of autosomes in a complement. This is followed by the specific chromosome responsible.

Examples of official nomenclature include:

46, XY	Normal male karyotype
46, XX	Normal female karyotype
45, X	Monosomy X
47, XXX	Polysomy X
47, XXY	Polysomy X
47, XY+21	Trisomy 21 Down syndrome
46, XX, Sp-	Cri du chat syndrome (caused by a deletion on the short arm of chromosome S)

Single gene (Mendelian) disorders

Single gene disorders occur as a result of a mutation or defect, usually involving only a single genetic locus, rather than a partial or total chromosomal abnormality. These disorders normally follow a simple, definite inheritance pattern. However, the transmission of mutant genes within families is dependent upon whether the gene is dominant or recessive in nature and also whether the mutant gene is located on an autosome or sex chromosome. This leads to the possibility of five transmission patterns:

- autosomal dominant
- autosomal recessive
- X-linked dominant
- X-linked recessive
- Y-linked.

If the homologous chromosomes contain both dominant genes, then the genotype is homozygous dominant and if both are recessive genes, homozygous recessive. If both dominant and recessive genes are present, then the genotype is heterozygous for that trait. This is illustrated in Punnet squares 1 and 2. Mendelian patterns of inheritance are illustrated in Punnet squares 3–12.

Punnet squares 1 and 2.

Example of homozygous and heterozygous gamete

Father has brown eyes with homozygous dominant gamete (BB), and mother has blue eyes with homozygous recessive gamete (bb).

		FATHER	
		B	B
MOTHER	b	Bb	Bb
	b	Bb	Bb

All offspring will have brown eyes and be heterozygous (Bb) for that trait.

If that child, when an adult, has a child with a partner who has blue eyes with homozygous recessive gamete (bb)

		Child now Adult	
		B	b
PARTNER	b	Bb	bb
	b	Bb	bb

then there will be a 50% chance of the offspring having brown eyes and being heterozygous (Bb) for that trait and a 50% chance their child will have blue eyes and be homozygous recessive.

Autosomal recessive inheritance

A large proportion of genetic diseases appear to be inherited in a recessive manner. Consequently, for the gene mutation to be expressed, the offspring must be homozygous recessive for that trait. The heterozygous offspring will be carriers for that gene mutation, with the ability to transfer it to their own children. Examples of autosomal recessive disorders include cystic fibrosis, thalassaemia, sickle cell anaemia and phenylketonuria.

Test your knowledge

With autosomal recessive cystic fibrosis, if one parent has cystic fibrosis and has a child with an adult who is heterozygous for the affected mutant cystic fibrosis gene, what is the percentage chance that their offspring will:

- Be carriers of the cystic fibrosis disease?
- Have cystic fibrosis disease or that their children will be normal?

Punnet squares 3–5.

If the father is heterozygous for the mutant gene cystic fibrosis (Cc) and the mother is homozygous normal (cc)

		FATHER	
		C	c
MOTHER	c	cC	cc
	c	cC	cc

then there will be a 50% chance of the offspring having heterozygous (Cc) and being carriers for cystic fibrosis.

If the father is heterozygous for the mutant gene cystic fibrosis (Cc) and the mother is heterozygous for the mutant gene cystic fibrosis (Cc)

		FATHER	
		C	c
MOTHER	C	CC	Cc
	c	Cc	cc

then there will be a 50% chance of the offspring having heterozygous (Cc) and being carriers for cystic fibrosis, a 25% chance their child will be homozygous normal (cc) and a 25% chance that they will have cystic fibrosis and be homozygous (CC).

		FATHER	
		C	C
MOTHER	c	cC	cC
	c	cC	cC

If a parent who has cystic fibrosis, and is therefore homozygous for the mutant affected gene, has a child with an unaffected homozygous adult, their offspring will all be carriers.

For all Punnet square examples, C is the defective mutant cystic fibrosis gene.

Autosomal dominant inheritance

As illustrated by the two Punnet squares, in autosomal dominant inheritance, all affected individuals have an affected parent and there are no carriers. Diseases that have this inheritance pattern include Marfan syndrome, myotonic dystrophy, achondroplasia, neurofibromatosis and Noonan syndrome. If a parent is heterozygous affected with, for example, myotonic dystrophy, then there is a 50% chance that their offspring will have myotonic dystrophy (Punnet 6). If both parents are heterozygous affected with the dominant mutant myotonic dystrophy, then there is a 25% chance that their offspring will be normal, a 50% chance that they will have myotonic dystrophy (heterozygous expressed) and a 25% chance that they will have myotonic dystrophy (homozygous expressed), although generally the foetus is non-viable (Punnet 7).

Punnet squares 6 and 7.

EXAMPLE 6			
		FATHER	
		M	m
MOTHER	m	mM	mm
	m	mM	mm

EXAMPLE 7			
		FATHER	
		M	m
MOTHER	M	MM	Mm
	m	mM	mm

For both Punnet square examples, M is the defective mutant haemophilia A gene.

X-linked recessive inheritance

As illustrated by the three Punnet squares, in X-linked recessive inheritance, males are principally affected. Haemophilia A and B and Duchenne muscular dystrophy are the more commonly known diseases that have this inheritance. If the father, for example, has haemophilia A, then his sons will be normal and his daughters will be carriers of the haemophilia trait (Punnet 8). If the mother is a carrier of the recessive mutant haemophilia gene, then half the daughters will be carriers and half the boys will have haemophilia A (Punnet 9).

Test your knowledge

With sex-linked recessive haemophilia A, if the father has haemophilia A and the mother is a carrier for the defective mutant haemophilia gene, what is the percentage chance that their sons and daughters will:

- Be carriers of haemophilia A?
- Have haemophilia A?
- Be normal?

Punnet squares 8–10.

EXAMPLE 8

		FATHER	
		א	Y
MOTHER	X	א X	XY
	X	א X	XY

EXAMPLE 9

		FATHER	
		X	Y
MOTHER	א	א X	א Y
	X	XX	XY

EXAMPLE 10

		FATHER	
		X	Y
MOTHER	א	א X	א Y
	א	א X	א Y

If the mother has the disease, because the mutant recessive gene is located on both the mother's X chromosomes then all boys (46, XY) will express the mutation as they have no other X chromosome to challenge it.

For all three Punnet square examples, **א** is the defective mutant haemophilia A gene.

X-linked dominant inheritance

As illustrated by the two Punnet squares 11 and 12, in linked dominant inheritance, all affected individuals have an affected parent and there are no carriers. A disease that has this inheritance pattern is Fragile X syndrome. If the father is affected, that is has Fragile X syndrome, then his sons will be normal and his daughters will have Fragile X syndrome (although generally more mildly) (Punnet 11). If the mother has Fragile X syndrome, then half the daughters will have Fragile X syndrome and half the boys will have Fragile X syndrome (Punnet 12).

Inherited variations

Not all diseases, however, follow the traditional patterns of inheritance. This can involve either single genes or the whole chromosome. Some diseases can express both dominant and recessive inheritance patterns, for example osteogenesis imperfecta, commonly known as brittle bone disease. Osteogenesis imperfecta is caused by an abnormality in the maturation of collagen protein, resulting in skeletal alterations such as bone fragility and low bone mass, along with connective tissue manifestations such as hyperlaxity of ligaments and skin. Arising from both autosomal dominant and recessive forms of inheritance, or as a consequence of a spontaneous mutation, osteogenesis imperfecta has clinical features and diagnosis types ranging from mild to severe forms including perinatal lethality. The condition often leads to an increased likelihood of bone fractures, hearing impairment, loose teeth, shortness in stature and bruising. The presence of blue or grey sclera is a controversial diagnostic feature in the infant age range as it can be found in healthy individuals (Fahiminiya *et al.*, 2013; Forlino and Marini, 2016). Table 1.1 illustrates chronic childhood conditions and their inheritance patterns.

Punnet squares 11 and 12.

EXAMPLE 11				
		FATHER		
		ꭓ	Y	
MOTHER	X	ꭓ X	XY	
	X	ꭓ X	XY	

EXAMPLE 12				
		FATHER		
		X	Y	
MOTHER	ꭓ	ꭓ X	ꭓ Y	
	X	XX	ꭓ Y	

For both Punnet square examples, ꭓ is the defective mutant Fragile X gene.

TABLE 1.1   Patterns of inheritance.

Patterns of inheritance	
Autosomal dominant	**Autosomal recessive**
Achondroplasia	Cystic fibrosis
Huntington's chorea	Congenital adrenal hypoplasia
Myotonic dystrophy	Osteogenesis imperfecta
Marfan syndrome	Phenylketonuria
Neurofibromatosis	Sickle cell disease
Noonan syndrome	Thalassaemia
Ostetogenesis imperfecta	Wilson disease
Spherocytosis	
Sex-linked dominant	**Sex-linked recessive**
Fragile X syndrome	Duchenne muscular dystrophy
	Haemophilia A and B
	Hunter disease
	Multifactorial
Neural tube defects	Cardiac defects
Cleft lip/and or palate	Renal agenesis
Pyloric stenosis	Congenital dislocation of the hip
Hypospadias	Talipes

Source: Adapted from Wong, 1999.

Test your knowledge

1. Using nomenclature, how would the following be described in a cyto-genic report?

    a. A normal male chromosome arrangement.
    b. A chromosomal arrangement indicative of Turner syndrome.
    c. A chromosomal arrangement of Edwards syndrome.
    d. A chromosomal arrangement where there is a microdeletion on the short arm of chromosome S.

2. Describe the change to the normal human chromosome pattern designated by the following:

    a. 47, XY +18
    b. 48, XXXX

3. What are the three main areas of chromosomal anomalies?
4. Where is the centromere positioned in acrocentric chromosomes?
5. Name three antenatal screening techniques.
6. Identify three important reasons why children's nurses need knowledge of genetics.

As highlighted at the beginning of this chapter, knowledge and understanding of genetics is important to children's nurses, with the HGSG Report (2012) emphasising that genetic knowledge is important for health professionals at all levels. With advances in scientific findings within the field of genetics, nurses are likely to become increasingly involved in the delivery of advice and support for children, young people and their families affected by genetic deviations (Skirton *et al.*, 2010; HGSG, 2012; Metcalfe, 2018). Information related to the genetic basis of a child's condition needs to be given sensitively, requiring the nurse to have the necessary knowledge to be able to access relevant information and direct children, young people and families to appropriate sources. (See the list of websites at the end of the chapter.) This chapter will now explore the study of the causes or origins of disease or long-term conditions, defined as aetiology, of which genetics is just one aspect.

The aetiology of many long-term conditions such as cystic fibrosis (CF) or Duchenne muscular dystrophy (DMD) can be relatively simple to explain or, as in the case of type 1 diabetes or eczema, may involve complex factors that may not reflect the expression of severity of a child's condition. As previously described in this chapter, although CF results from a single gene mutation, there is multisystem involvement for the child. The aetiology of type 1 diabetes or eczema cannot be explained in such simple genetic terms. When a child has type 1 diabetes, just one cell type within the pancreas malfunctions at diagnosis or, in the case of eczema, just the skin is affected. There may be a genetic influence relating to the chronic condition, but other factors can be involved in the onset of disease. Aetiological factors can include diet, lifestyle, infection, aberrations in foetal developmental or a chronic condition being part of another syndrome. For example, epilepsy can be part of Fragile X syndrome or a metabolic disorder. (See www.epilepsy.org.uk for a list of conditions where epilepsy can be a feature.) A chronic condition can manifest itself at any time during childhood, from the antenatal period to 18 years of age, and into adulthood. The genetic condition, Huntington's chorea, normally manifests in adulthood and is rarely seen in childhood. Although multifactorial conditions, such as coronary heart disease, are identified in adulthood, early risk factors for cardiac disease are now being identified in pre-adolescent children (Truong *et al.*, 2012), particularly in children classed as obese. In Chapter 6, the implications of obesity in children and young people with long-term conditions are discussed. Via various screening programmes, the identification of long-term conditions in children begins as early as the prenatal period and continues throughout childhood.

Antenatal period

Using improved antenatal screening techniques, many conditions are identified before the baby is born, leading to a long-term conditions diagnosis. Problems that can be identified in the foetus include congenital heart defects (CHDs), Fragile X and osteogenesis imperfecta.

 Time out

Suggest some of the antenatal screening procedures that may be employed to identify specific long-term conditions.

Response

- Ultrasonography to identify:
    - organ and bone structure
    - size of foetus
- Chorionic villus sampling to identify:
    - genetic or chromosomal abnormalities
- Amniocentesis to identify:
    - genetic or chromosomal abnormalities

 # Case study 1.1

An ultrasound examination has identified a congenital heart defect in a foetus at 18 weeks gestation. What information could be gained from parents that may reveal the aetiology of this condition? Consider your response in relation to pre-pregnancy issues and factors during pregnancy. You may consider elements from a family history that may reveal important information leading to possible identification of aetiology for the heart condition.

Development of the heart during the foetal period is very complex and can be arrested or altered by several factors. Impairment may occur as a result of teratogenic influences such as infection or drugs taken by the mother during the first trimester of pregnancy. Drugs used in the treatment of epilepsy are known to cross the placenta (Wlodarczyk *et al.*, 2012; Eadie, 2016) and increase the risk of CHD in the foetus. The contraction of an infection such as rubella by the mother is known to increase the risk of CHD (Ziwei *et al.*, 2019). In addition to infection, if the mother has a chronic condition, the risks increase for CHD in the child. A mother who has diabetes preconceptually has an increased risk of 3.6% for the child developing CHD compared to non-diabetic mothers (Øyen *et al.*, 2016). The mechanism that leads to an alteration of foetal heart development has not yet been determined. A heart condition may not be present in isolation but be part of a broader syndrome such as Triploidy, Trisomies 13, 18 and 21, Noonan syndrome or DiGeorge syndrome (Stroll *et al.*, 2015). A family history can reveal other family members with different syndromes or heart defects and small chromosomal deletions or translocations have been implicated. Studies also reveal an increased occurrence of CHD during foetal development where a parent has defective heart valves (Ellesøe *et al.*, 2018). Both autosomal recessive and dominant inheritance have been implicated.

🌐 Case study 1.2

During an ultrasound antenatal scan, it is noted that the skeletal system of the foetus does not appear completely normal. The limbs are shorter than average and bowed. The foetus also has a degree of scoliosis. From what condition may the foetus be suffering?

There is a wide range of differential diagnoses that could be suggested (Krakow, 2015) and the presence or absence of fractures would be significant. In the absence of fractures, it is possible that the child will have one of the dwarfing syndromes such as achondroplasia or thanatophoric dysplasia, both of autosomal dominant aetiology. If there are fractures seen on the scan, osteogenesis imperfecta (OI) is more likely to be suggested. Again, this condition, which was discussed earlier, has both autosomal recessive and dominant forms.

It is not always possible to reach a diagnosis until further investigations such as genetic testing via amniocentesis or chorionic villus sample are carried out. Although the aetiology of these conditions is known to be genetic, both achondroplasia and type 2 OI have been noted to result from new mutations in most cases (Donnelly *et al.*, 2010; Sillence, 2013; Shirley & Ain, 2013), and in some cases of OI, it has been found that a parent has cell mosaicism. If a parent is known to have a chronic skeletal condition such as OI, genetic analysis can be carried out earlier in pregnancy by chorionic villus sampling.

Time out

Using Punnet squares, estimate the risk for the children in the following situations:

1. The mother has achondroplasia and the father does not.
2. The father is heterozygous for osteogenesis imperfecta (OI) and the mother is genetically normal for OI (does not carry the OI gene).

Response

1. In this example the father is heterozygous for osteogenesis imperfecta and the mother does not have the condition. Because the condition is autosomal dominant, the risk is that 50% of the children will have the condition.

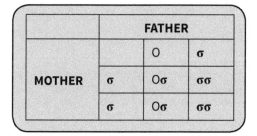

2. Again, because achondroplasia is autosomal dominant, if the mother has the condition and the father does not, 50% of the children are at risk of inheriting the condition.

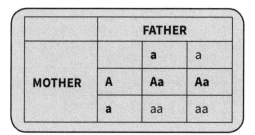

Both amniocentesis and chorionic villus sampling can be used for other genetic and chromosomal problems

The neonatal period

During the first 28 days of life (the neonatal period), many long-term conditions can be diagnosed either following direct observation of the infant, or as a result of signs that are characteristic of certain physiological problems. When problems are suspected, further investigations need to be carried out to confirm a diagnosis. For instance, CHDs that have not been identified earlier may be suspected if the child is cyanosed and has tachypnoea. A neonate may have seizures or unexplained hypoglycaemia, which could indicate a diagnosis of a metabolic or endocrine disorder.

During the neonatal period, a range of long-term conditions can be identified by a heel prick test. This is carried out by allowing large drops of blood to drop from the baby's heel onto a prepared absorbent paper, which is then left to dry before laboratory testing. This is sometimes called the PKU test (from phenylketonuria, the condition for which the test was originally devised), or the Guthrie test (from the name of the scientist who developed the test for PKU in the 1960s). The test was expanded in 2015 (Department of Health, 2015) to include four additional rare long-term conditions to the original five it tested for (https://www.gov.uk/government/news/newborn-babies-screened-for-more-rare-conditions).

🕐 Time out

Identify the long-term conditions that can be diagnosed by the heel prick test carried out within the first week of life. Suggest the aetiology of these.

Response

Phenylketonuria	Autosomal recessive
Duchenne muscular dystrophy	X-linked recessive
Hypothyroidism	Multifactorial
Cystic fibrosis	Autosomal recessive
Sickle cell disease	Autosomal recessive
Thalassaemia	Autosomal recessive
Galactosaemia and other metabolic disorders	Usually autosomal recessive

---

Identification of these conditions would not have occurred until the post-neonatal age prior to this test being carried out. Diagnosis would have been made as symptoms arose and/or the child's physical health deteriorated. There would be a deterioration of cognitive and mental health development in a child who has phenylketonuria or hypothyroidism. The aetiology of PKU is autosomal recessive inheritance (Hafid & Christodoulou, 2015) whereas that of hypothyroidism has multiple origins, although genetic origins have been identified in about 15–20% of instances (Grasberger & Refetoff, 2011). According to Tobias *et al.* (2011), 1:3000–4000 cases of hypothyroidism are congenital. In a comprehensive update of childhood hypothyroidism, Peters *et al.* (2018) explain the pathology that results in the condition. Agenesis, dysplasia or absence of the thyroid gland occurring as an aberration of foetal development, result in reduced or absent secretion of thyroid hormones. A lack of production of these hormones may also result from a defect of other body systems that normally would, through their release of enzymes or hormones, maintain or stimulate thyroid function. One example of this would be a defective pituitary gland that produces the thyroid stimulating hormone, an essential hormone for normal functioning of the thyroid gland. Although PKU and congenital hypothyroidism are relatively uncommon in the UK, 1:10 000 and 1:2000 births respectively (Barber, 2017; Knowles *et al.*, 2018), nurses may be involved with the family at the time of diagnosis. Due to the absence of any indication of a problem during the neonatal period, families can experience a range of emotions on being told of the diagnosis. Chapter 3 examines theories of grief and loss and models of adaptation associated with families following the diagnosis of their child with a long-term condition.

Post-neonatal period

More commonly, conditions are diagnosed after the first month of life, even though their origins may be present earlier. A number of neuro/musculo/skeletal problems can develop, such as Duchenne muscular dystrophy, which is well recognised as an X-linked recessive genetic disorder. Signs of the disorder will not be evident until the child is aged 2–4 years, when physical development milestones are not achieved and the child begins to lose motor ability. (See Chapter 8 for a more detailed discussion of a child with a neuromotor disability, the resulting physical and psychosocial effects, and the required associated care management pathway.) Other conditions identified after the first month of life include epilepsy, type 1 diabetes and juvenile arthritis.

🕒 **Time out**

- Identify factors that may influence the onset of epilepsy. You need to consider issues such as environmental, genetic, medical history and trauma.

Epilepsy can develop at any age, with most diagnoses being made after the neonatal period and before the age of 20 years, often causing distress for the children, young people and their families. A diagnosis of epilepsy is only made following two or more seizures and many children suffer one isolated seizure. Studies of aetiology of this condition suggest neuropathological origins. This could be an insult by an infection, such as encephalitis or meningitis, or as a result of a tumour or trauma caused during delivery or an accident. However, children who exhibit the same disease process do not necessarily develop epilepsy, or, if epilepsy does develop, the same phenotypical epilepsy. It has also been noted that epilepsy can develop following complex febrile convulsions (Rubenstein & Levy, 2019) and that febrile seizures may be a marker of a child's seizure threshold (Sharawat *et al.*, 2016). As with cardiac malformations, epilepsy can be a feature of a more complex syndrome (see www.ilae.org), which would lead to the child requiring more complex care. As a single disorder, one of the features of epilepsy is the unpredictable nature of its expression. A child may have seizures infrequently and/or irregularly, and the expression of the epilepsy may be shown by a child having different types of seizure: complex and/or partial.

Other aetiological factors are known and studies have suggested a genetic influence to the development of the condition, although this is not always conclusive. A definite genetic aetiology for epilepsy, where there is no other identified pathology, accounts for at least 40% of sufferers (Guerrini & Noebels, 2014). Investigations into twin studies have confirmed a genetic link (Vadlamudi *et al.*, 2014). Twin studies have shown higher concordance rates for epilepsy in monozygotic twins compared to dizygotic twins; and in dizygotic twins, the likelihood of both developing epilepsy is higher than for the general population (Corey *et al.*, 2011; Koeleman, 2018). Identifying epilepsy via genetic screening would be a complex process, as mutations have been identified on several chromosomes. There are also complexities in relation to genotype and phenotype with this condition, where the same phenotype expressed in two people has been found to have different genotypes (Helbig & Tayoun, 2016).

⊛ Case study 1.3

A 5-year-old boy has been diagnosed with type 1 diabetes. The parents do not know of any close relatives who have the condition. What information could you give when the parents ask what has caused this?

Even greater complexity in aetiology has been highlighted for type 1 diabetes. A number of nutritional influences have been documented in studies involving children with type 1 diabetes, including failure to breastfeed or short duration of breastfeeding and the early introduction of cow's milk and food containing gluten, although results remain inconclusive (Lamb *et al.*, 2015; Nucci *et al.*, 2015). The mechanism that initiates the auto-immune process of destruction of beta cells in the pancreas, and the reason why some children develop the condition and others do not, is not understood. Protective genes have been identified to prevent this process, but other gene mutations are known to influence the onset (Kozhakhmetova & Gillespie, 2016). As with epilepsy, these are not single gene mutations, but loci are found on a number of chromosomes, although most closely associated with HLA genes that lie on the short arm of chromosome 6 (Steck & Rewers, 2011; Bilous & Donnelly, 2010). Twin studies show a much lower concordance in comparison with those that investigate epilepsy prevalence, with views that genetic risk factors are stimulated by environmental influences (Bilous & Donnelly, 2010). People who have migrated from an area of low to an area of high incidence for type 1 diabetes seem to adopt the same level of risk as the population to which they move (Bilous & Donnelly, 2010). This may be the result of contact with resident viruses that are thought to play a role in the aetiology of type 1 diabetes, particularly in children (Bilous & Donnelly, 2010). Viruses that have been implicated as a result of infection in children and timing of onset of diabetes are enteroviruses, pertussis and rubella. A number of studies have also shown a link between maternal viral infection during pregnancy and childhood onset of type 1 diabetes (Bilous & Donnelly, 2010).

Researchers are challenged in identifying risk factors for diabetes as the incidence is increasing, which cannot be explained through genetic aetiology. Single gene, recessive or dominant conditions, or sex-linked conditions follow the same inheritance patterns over time, and the incidence remains relatively unchanged, such as with cystic fibrosis or achondroplasia. Vaccines are now used to prevent pertussis and rubella in most of the population, thus potentially decreasing the prevalence of type 1 diabetes as a result of this risk factor.

Challenges are also evident in identifying aetiology of allergic conditions affecting this age group. Again, there appear to be genetic influences, but these are not straightforward and the research is sometimes conflicting. Much of the litera-ture discusses more than one allergic condition, including food allergies, asthma, eczema and/or allergic rhinitis (hay fever). Those affected children whose parent/s had allergic conditions were at greater risk, although this inheritance pattern was not always strong. Links between atopic disease and T helper cell function and IgE productions have been identified (Holloway *et al.*, 2010; McFadden *et al.*, 2015; Ortiz & Barnes, 2015). Infections in childhood have been implicated in these conditions although aetiological explanations are complex, particularly for asthma and allergic rhinitis. Busse *et al.* (2010) suggest there is protection against the development of non-atopic asthma and allergy, but atopic asthma is triggered following respiratory infections in childhood (Rantala *et al.*, 2011). Exposure to older siblings has been found to reduce the risk of developing asthma, eczema and allergic rhinitis, except early onset asthma (before the age of 2 years) (Miller *et al.*, 2014; Strachan *et al.*, 2015). Perhaps having older siblings provided an early and constant exposure to a wide variety of organisms, somehow protecting susceptible genes from being over-stimulated, leading to allergic disease. Mukherjee and Zhang (2011) suggest that a child may have genes that are susceptible to interaction with environmental triggers, with a number of triggers being recognised to exacerbate allergic long-term condi-tions. However, the onset of the disease process is not fully understood (Busse *et al.*, 2010; WHO, 2017). Reactions are seen in a child following ingestion of certain foods to which the child is sensitive and links have been found between food allergies and asthma (Foong *et al.*, 2017), with increasing severity of the condition when a child consumes particular foods. Unfortunately, whether the food allergy or the asthma appears first is not stated. Dietary intake can also be seen to influence atopic eczema, but it is not suggested that this is a cause of eczema (Fleischer *et al.*, 2011; Lyons *et al.*, 2015).

Most cases of eczema are seen in the first three months of life, and food allergies by 12 months of age. Other factors are known to influence expression of the disease, which affects around 15–20% of children (Nutten, 2015). Multiple causes are suggested, including several from the environment. A reverse class gra-dient is seen with a higher prevalence amongst children from more advantaged backgrounds, which may reflect environmental factors such as dietary intake and pollution (Taylor-Robinson *et al.*, 2015). This may also be related to the increased incidence among people migrating from a low prevalence area to a geographical area of higher prevalence.

Although it is well known that eczema and asthma affect children, it is not com-monly recognised that chronic arthritis can affect those under the age of 18 years. Many consider that this group of long-term conditions only affect older people (Arthritis Research UK, 2012), but there are a number of arthritic conditions that are seen in children of all ages. It is a complex group of conditions affecting the joints, causing pain, swelling and restricted movement for the child.

🕐 **Time out**

- Access the Arthritis Society website http://www.arthritis.ca/types and identify the different types of arthritis that may be seen in childhood.

The variety, expression and types of conditions are also reflected in the range of aetiologies, which are still not fully understood (Rigante *et al.*, 2015). Auto-immune processes are evident and infections have been implicated. Arthritis has been seen following a number of viral and bacterial infections, as discussed in Ellis *et al.*'s review of research studies (2010). The rubella virus has been isolated from affected joints when neither natural infection nor vaccination has occurred. Seasonal variation of onset has been noted that may be linked with infections, which themselves may predominate at different times of the year (Joo *et al.*, 2019). In addition, there are genetic origins to juvenile chronic arthritis, with gene mutations identified on several chromosomes (Wong *et al.*, 2017).

As most children and young people will be cared for at home, children's nurses may see few children and young people admitted to hospital with arthritis. This may result in nurses having limited knowledge and understanding of juvenile arthritis, thus leading to difficulties in the nursing care of these children and families. With about 1 child per 1000 being affected (James & Wedderburn, 2016), it is likely that at some time during their practice, many children's nurses will be involved in the nursing care of these children and young people, and their families. Parents may be shocked to learn of their child's diagnosis (refer to Chapter 3 for family response to recent diagnosis of their child with a long-term conditions) and it is important that nurses are able to offer advice, and have an understanding of psychological and practical issues related to the care of the child. It is suggested that following initial diagnosis parents and children may need longer appointment times, in comparison with adults, to discuss some of these issues with a clinical nurse specialist (Arthritis and Musculoskeletal Alliance, 2010). Parents and children will need information, and children's nurses need to have knowledge of the problem and be able to suggest sources of information for parents and for the patient, such as the websites referenced at the end of this chapter.

Adolescent period

Some conditions, the aetiology of which have already been discussed, may begin or be first diagnosed at almost any time during childhood, such as epilepsy, type 1 diabetes, allergic conditions or arthritis. Other chronic problems are more commonly first seen during adolescence or early adulthood, although these can occasionally occur before the teenage years. One group of long-term conditions with a peak diagnostic age of 15–30 years (Lemmens *et al.*, 2014) is irritable or inflammatory bowel disease (IBD), with the two most common being identified as Crohn's disease (CD) and ulcerative colitis (UC). The molecular origins of this group of conditions remain largely unknown, but significant research has identified complex factors that appear to contribute to their development. A number of research studies focus on Crohn's disease and ulcerative colitis, showing some similarities but considerable differences between aetiological elements. It is suggested by Salim and Söderholm (2011) that an abnormality in the function of the gut barrier, when one or more of these elements is present, or increased gut permeability, may predispose the individual to IBD (Papamichael *et al.*, 2014; Michielan & D'Incà, 2015).

In a comprehensive literature review of the genetic basis of CD and UC, Gordon *et al.* (2015) identified research showing monozygotic twin concordance of 20–55%, and dizygotic twin concordance of 0–3.6%, for CD, with only 6.3–17% and 0–6.3% respectively for UC. They report gene mutations on a range of chromosomes for the two conditions, some of which are common to both. Another factor that may suggest a genetic link is the increased risk between certain population groups, for example among Ashkenazi Jews (Schiff *et al.*, 2018). This may also suggest links to lifestyle factors common to groups, which may increase the risk of developing IDB. Dietary intake has been considered as an influence in the deterioration of UC and thus may also trigger the onset. A high intake of meat, meat products and fat has been linked to relapses of UC and processed foods have also been shown to be detrimental to UC (Wu *et al.*, 2013; Rashvand *et al.*, 2015). Smoking is another lifestyle factor that may reduce deterioration in UC, but certainly does cause deterioration in CD (Lunney *et al.*, 2015). Smoking, therefore, may have some influence in the onset of CD, particularly as its onset coincides with the time when many young people begin smoking. This emphasises the importance of the role of the children's nurse in giving advice to young people on the many risks to their health of continued smoking. Alternatively, children's nurses could be challenged in their ability to give health promotion advice in relation to smoking if a young person has UC, when the condition is less severe among smokers.

In addition to these factors, infection has been implicated as contributing to IBD with mycoplasms and helicobacter being identified in patients (Navaneethan *et al.*, 2010; Papamichael *et al.*, 2014). Measles has also been implicated as a contributing factor to CD in numerous studies; however, this remains contentious, with a research studies such as Polymeros *et al.* (2014), unable to confirm a link.

Conclusion

As initially discussed at the start of this chapter, the need for children's nurses to have genetic knowledge, including the understanding of aetiology of long-term conditions in children, is an important element of their practice. Several examples were given where there are opportunities for introducing strategies in care management to lead to a reduced risk of conditions occurring, or a reduction in severity for those where a condition has been identified. Examples given earlier related to advice for a young person or parents considering further pregnancies. When a known genetic cause for a long-term condition is identified, such as an autosomal recessive (e.g. CF or phenylketonuria) or dominant gene mutation (e.g. osteogenesis imperfecta or achondroplasia), children's nurses can become involved in genetic advice, which can help couples come to decisions about future pregnancies. Indeed, it may be the young person who is embarking on a sexual relationship and seeks help about future children. These decisions are not easy and may be more difficult if a sporadic gene mutation is identified. Alternatively, if someone has a genetic condition and that person is considering parenthood, advice can be given regarding pregnancy and risk factors. Risk factors include the mother's health during pregnancy if she is the one with the condition.

In relation to conditions where lifestyle has an impact, nurses, health visitors and midwives can advise families, including the child who has the long-term condition, on ways to make lifestyle changes where this would be advantageous to the child or young person's well-being. Children's nurses or school nurses could implement strategies that target children and/or parents to develop healthy lifestyles. This can lead to a reduced risk of some long-term conditions such as type 2 diabetes.

Specialist nurses are in the best position to address psychological aspects of care and provide a range of information. Following diagnosis is a time when families, including the child if he or she is old enough to understand, need information relating to the condition. Also, support is needed, which may be nursing, medical, social or psychological. This support can be more comprehensive if the nurse has a good knowledge base of the aetiology of the condition. Support for families is an important aspect of care that can influence the long-term psychological outcome for the child or young person with a long-term condition (Straus & Baird, 2018).

With advances in genetics and the increasing impetus for the development of strategies to ameliorate or cure long-term conditions with genetic origins, it is becoming increasingly important that nurses develop competence in the area of genetics. They will need not only to give appropriate information in an understandable way to those who need the help, whatever their culture, but also to be aware of other multidisciplinary agencies or support networks to which young people and/or parents can be referred for counselling (Skirton *et al.*, 2010; Rowland & Metcalfe, 2013). Due to genetics being of high media and public interest, particularly in relation to the complexities and ethical issues surrounding cloning, the manipulation of genes through gene therapy and the uncertainties of the long-term outcomes, it is essential that nurses caring for children and young people develop their genetic knowledge and understanding. They must, along with other professionals, be able to fully participate in the relevant debates and ethical discussions that can have implications for children, young people and their families.

🔑 Key points

- Developing genetic knowledge and competence is essential for children's nurses and children's nursing.
- A chronic condition can manifest itself at any time during childhood, from the antenatal period to 18 years of age, and into adulthood.

Useful websites

Antenatal screening resources
www.arc-uk.org
https://www.gov.uk/topic/population-screening-programmes/newborn-blood-spot

Arthritis
http://www.arthritis-ca/about-arthritis-types-(a-z)

Bio-News: latest genetic information
www.bionews.org.uk

British Society of Genetic Medicine
www.bsgm.org.uk

Contact a family for background information on a wide range of long-term conditions
www.contact.org.uk

Genetics home reference which gives basic information on genetics
www.ghr.nlm.nim.gov

Genetic Alliance: national alliance of 200 organisations that support children, families and individuals affected by genetic disorders.
www.genetcalliance.org.uk

Gene Sense, giving information on science, ethics and practice issues using case studies
www.genesense.org.uk

Muscular Dystrophy
www.musculardystrophyuk.org

International Society for Nurses in Genetics
www.isong.org

The Cambridge Genetics Knowledge Park, Public Health Foundation
www.phgfoundation.org

The Child Growth Foundation
www.childgrowthfoundation.org

The Turner Syndrome Support Society
www.tss.org.uk

The Wales Gene Park
www.walesgenepark.cardiff.ac.uk

The Wellcome Trust for information on genetics, ethics and the Human Genome Project
http://www.abeldenger.org/wecom-to-wellcome-trust-huma-genome/

UK National Screening Committee
http://www.gov.uk/government/groups/uk-national-screening-committee-uk-nsc

References

Arthritis and Musculoskeletal Alliance (2010) *Standards of Care for Children and Young People with Juvenile Idiopathic Arthritis*. London, ARMA.

Arthritis Research UK (2012) *Understanding Arthritis: A Parliamentary Guide to Musculoskeletal Health*. Chesterfield, Arthritis Research UK.

Ashtiani, S., Makel, N., Carrion, P., *et al.* (2014) Parents' experiences of receiving their child's genetic diagnosis: a qualitative study to inform clinical genetics practice. *American Journal of Medical Genetics*, **164A** (6), 1496–1502. https://doi:10.1002/ajmg.a.36525.

Barber, C. (2017) Rare health conditions 4: acromegaly, Usher syndrome, phenylketonuria (PKU). *British Journal of Healthcare Assistants*, **11** (9), 430–433.

Bilous, R. & Donnelly, R. (2010) Introduction to diabetes. In: *Handbook of Diabetes* (fourth edition). Oxford, Wiley-Blackwell.

Botkin, J.R., Belmont, J.W., Berg, J.S., *et al.* (2015) Points to consider: ethical, legal, and psychosocial implications of genetic testing in children and adolescents. *The American Journal of Human Genetics*, **97** (3), 6–21. http//dx.doi.org/10.1016j.ajhg.2015.05.022.

Brown, T. (2011) *Introduction to Genetics: a Molecular Approach*. London, Garland Science.

Busse, W.W., Lemaske Jr, R.F. & Gern, J.E. (2010) The role of viral respiratory infections in asthma and asthma exacerbations. *Lancet*, **376** (9743), 826–834. https://doi:10.1016/S0140-6736(10)61380-3.

Chang, Y.-W., Wang, P.-H., Li, W.H., *et al.* (2013) Balanced and unbalanced reciprocal translocation: An overview of 30-year experience in a single tertiary medical center in Taiwan. *Journal of the Chinese Medical Association*, 76 (3), 153–157. http://dx.doi.org/10.10/16/j.jcma.2012.11.002.

Chen, C.-P., Wu, P.-C., Lin, C.-J., *et al.* (2011) Unbalanced reciprocal translocations at amniocentesis. *Taiwanese Journal of Obstetrics & Gynecology*, 50 (2011), 4–57.

Corey, L.A., Pellock, J.M., Kjeldsen, M.J., *et al.* (2011) Importance of genetic factors in the occurrence of epilepsy syndrome type: a twin study. *Epilepsy Research*, **97** (1–2), 103–11. https://doi:10.1016/j.eplepsyres.2011.07.018.

Coleman, A.M. (2015) *A Dictionary of Psychology* (fourth edition). Oxford, Oxford University Press.

Craufurd, D., MacLeod, R., Frontali, M., *et al.* (2015) Diagnostic testing for Huntington's disease. *Practical Neurology*, **15** (1), 80–84. http://dx.doi.org/10.1136/practneurol-2013-000790.

Davies, K. & Meimaridou, E. (2020) Biological basis of child health 1: understanding the cell and genetics. *Nursing Children and Young People*, **32** (3), 25–34.

Department of Health (2003) *Our Inheritance, Our Future. Realising the Potential of Genetics in the NHS*. London, The Stationery Office.

Department of Health (2015) Newborn babies screened for more rare conditions. https://www.gov.uk/government/news/newborn-babies-screened-for-more-rare-conditions Accessed 2/2/20.

Donnelly, D.E., McConnell, V., Paterson, A., *et al.* (2010) The prevalence of thanatophoric dysplasia and lethal osteogenesis imperfecta type II in Northern Ireland – a complete population study. *Ulster Medical Journal*, **79** (3), 114–118.

Eadie, M.J. (2016) Antiepileptic drug safety in pregnancy: possible dangers for the pregnant woman and her foetus. *The Pharmaceutical Journal and Clinical Pharmacist*, **8** (1). http://doi:10.1211/CP.2016.20200320

Ellesøe, S.G., Workman, C.T., Bouvagnet, P., et al. (2018) Familial co-occurrence of congenital heart defects follows distinct patterns. *European Heart Journal*, **39**, 1015–1022. http://doi:10.1093/eurheartj/ehx314.

Ellis, J.A., Munro, J.E. & Ponsonby, A.-L. (2010) Possible environmental determinants of juvenile idiopathic arthritis. *Rheumatology*, **49**, 411–425. http://doi:10.1093/rheumatology/kep383.

Fahiminiya, S., Majewski, J., Mort, J., *et al.* (2013) Mutations in WNT1 are a cause of osteogenesis imperfecta. *Journal of Medical Genetics*, **50**, 345–348. http://doi:10.1136/jmedgenet-2013-101567.

Fleischer, D.M., Bock, S.A., Spears, G.C., *et al.* (2011) Oral Food Challenges in Children with a Diagnosis of Food Allergy. *The Journal of Pediatrics*, **158** (4), 578–583. http://doi:1016/j.jpeds.2010.09.027.

Foong, R.-X., du Toit, G., & Fox, A.T. (2017) Asthma, food allergy, and how they relate to each other. *Frontiers in Pediatrics*, **5**, 89. http://doi:10.3389/fped.2017.00089.

Forlino, A. & Marini, J.C. (2016) Osteogenesis Imperfecta. *The Lancet*, **387**, 1657–1671. http://dx.doi.org/10.1016/S0140-6736(15)00728-x.

Gordon, H., Moller, F.T., Andersen, V., *et al.* (2015) Heritability in inflammatory bowel disease: from the first twin study to genome-wide association studies. *Inflammatory Bowel Disease*, **21** (6), 1428–1434. http://doi:10/1097/MIB.0000000000000393.

Grasberger, H. & Refetoff, S. (2011) Genetic causes of congenital hypothyroidism due to dyshormonogenesis. *Current Opinion in Pediatrics*, **23** (4): 421–428. http://doi:10.1097/MOP.0b013e32834726a4.

Guerrini, R. & Noebels, J. (2014) How can advances in epilepsy genetics lead to better treatments and cures? *Advances in Experimental Medicine and Biology*, **813**, 309–317. http://doi: 10.1007/978-94-017-8914-1_25.

Hafid, N.A. & Christodoulou, J. (2015) Phenylketonuria: a review of current and future treatments. *Translational Pediatrics*, 4 (**4**), 304–317. http;//doi:10.3978/j.issn.2224-4336.2015.10.07.

Helbig, I. & Tayoun, A.N.A. (2016) Understanding genotypes and phenotypes epileptic encephalopathies. *Molecular Syndromology*, **7**, 172–181. http://doi: 10.1159/000448530.

Henneman, L., Borry, P., Chokoshvili, D., *et al.* (2016) Responsible implementation of expanded carrier screening. *European Journal of Human Genetics*, **24**, e1-e12. http://doi: 10.1038/ejhg.2015.271.

Hockenberry, M.J., Wilson, D. & Rogers, C.C. (eds) (2019) *Wong's Nursing Care of Infants and Children (eleventh edition)*. St. Louis, Elsevier.

Holloway, J.W., Yang, I.A. & Holgate, S.T. (2010) Genetics of allergic disease. *Journal of Allergy Clinical Immunology*, **125** (2), 581. http://doi:10.1016/j.jaci.2009.10.071.

House of Lords Science and Technology Committee (2009) *Genomic Medicine*. London, The Stationary Office Ltd.

Human Genomic Strategic Group (2012) Building on our Inheritance. *Genomic Technology in Healthcare*. https://www.gov.uk/government/publications/genomic-technology-in-healthcare-building-on-our-inheritance Accessed 22/06/20.

James, R.A. & Wedderburn, L.R. (2016) Modern management of juvenile idiopathic arthritis. *The Journal of Prescribing and Medicine Management*, 27 (6), 37–43. http://doi.org/10.1002/psb.1472.

Joo, Y.B., Lim, Y. H., Kim, K.J., *et al.* (2019) Respiratory viral infections and the risk of rheumatoid arthritis. *Arthritis Research and Therapy*, **21**, 199. http://doi:10.1186/s13075-019-1977-9.

Kirk, M., Tonkin, E. & Skirton, H. (2013) An iterative consensus-building approach to revising a genetics/genomics competency framework for nurse education in the UK. *Journal of Advanced Nursing*, **70** (2), 405–420.

Knowles, R.L., Oerton, J., Cheetham, T., *et al.* (2018) Newborn screening for primary congenital hypothyroidism: estimating test performance at different TSH thresholds. *Journal of Clinical Endocrinology and Metabolism*, **103** (10), 3720–3728. doi:10.1210/jc.2018-00658.

Koeleman, B.P.C. (2018) What do genetic studies tell us about the heritable basis of common epilepsy? *Neuroscience Letters*, **667**, 10–16. https://doi.org/10/1016/j.neulet.2017.03.042.

Kozhakhmetova, A. & Gillespie, K.M. (2016) Type 1 diabetes: current perspectives. In: *Type-1 Diabetes. Methods in Molecular Biology* (ed. K. Gillespie), pp. 1–12. New York, Humana Press.

Krakow, D. (2015). Skeletal dysplasias. *Clinics in Perinatology*, 42 (2), 301–19. http://doi:10.1016/j.clp.2015.03.003.

Lamb, M.M., Miller, M., Seifert, J.A., *et al.* (2015) The effect of childhood cow's milk intake and HLA-DR genotype on risk of islet autoimmunity and type 1 diabetes: the diabetes autoimmunity study in the young. *Pediatric Diabetes*, **16** (1), 31–38. http://doi: 10.1111/pedi.12115.

Lemmens, B., De Hertogh, G. & Sagaert, X. (2014) Inflammatory bowel disease. In: *Pathobiology of Human Disease. A Dynamic Encyclopedia of Disease Mechanism* (eds L. McManus & R. Mitchel), pp. 1297–1394. Amsterdam: Academic Press. http://dx.doi.org/10.1016/B978-0-12-386456-7.03806-5.

Lunney, P.C., Kariyawasam, V.C., Wang, R.R., *et al.* (2015) Smoking prevalence and its influence on disease course and surgery in Crohn's disease and ulcerative colitis. *Alimentary Pharmacology and Therapeutics*, **42**, 61–70. http://doi:10.1111/apt.13239.

Lyons, J.J., Milner, J.D. & Stone K.D. (2015) Atopic dermatitis in children: clinical features, pathophysiology, *and treatment. Immunology and Allergy Clinics of North America*, **35** (1), 161–83. http://doi:10.1016/j.iac.2014.09.008.

Martin, E.M. & Fry, R.C. (2018) Environmental influences on the epigenome: exposure-associated DNA methylation in human populations. *Annual Review of Public Health*, **39**, 309–333. https://doi.org/10.1146/annurev-publhealth040617-014629.

McFadden, J.P., Thyssen, J.P., Basketter, D.A., *et al.* (2015) T helper cell 2 immune skewing in pregnancy/early life: chemical exposure and the development of atopic disease and allergy. *British Journal of Dermatology*, **172**, 584–591. https://doi.org/10.1111/bjd.13497.

McGowan-Jordan, J., Simons, A. & Schmid, M. (eds) (2016) *ISCN 2016: An International System for Human Cytogenomic Nomenclature*. Basel: Karger.

Metcalfe, A. (2018). Sharing genetic risk information: implications for family nurses across the life span. *Journal of Family Nursing*, **24** (1), 86–105. https://doi.org/10.1177/1074840718755401.

Michielan, A. & D'Incà, R. (2015) Intestinal permeability in inflammatory bowel disease: pathogenesis, clinical evaluation and therapy of leaky gut. *Mediators of Inflammation*. http://doi.org/10.1155/2015/628157

Miller, E.K., Avila, P.C., Khan, Y.W., *et al.* (2014) Wheezing exacerbation in early childhood: evaluation, treatment, and recent advances relevant to the genesis of asthma. *The Journal of Allergy and Clinical Immunology: In Practice*, **2** (5), 537–543. http://doi:10.1016/j.jaip.2014.06.02.

Mukherjee, A.B. & Zhang, Z. (2011) Allergic asthma: influence of genetic and environmental factors. *The Journal of Biological Chemistry*, **286** (38), 32883–32889. http://doi: 10.1074/jbc.R110.197046.

Navaneethan, U., Venkatesh, P.G.K. & Shen, B. (2010). Clostridium difficile infection and inflammatory bowel disease: understanding the evolving relationship. *World Journal of Gastroenterology*, **16** (39), 4892–4904. http://doi:10.3748/wjg.v16.i39.4892.

Nucci, A.M., Virtanen, S.M. & Becker, D.J. (2015) Infant feeding and timing of complementary foods in the development of type 1 diabetes. *Annals of Nutrition and Metabolism*, **66** (1), 8–16. http://doi:10.1007/s11892-015-0628-z.

Nutten, S. (2015) Atopic dermatitis: global epidemiology and risk factors. *Current Diabetes Reports*, **15** (9), 1–6.

Ortiz, R.A. & Barnes, K.C. (2015) Genetics of allergic diseases. *Immunology and Allergy Clinics of North America*, **35** (1), 19–44. http://doi:10.1016/j.iac.2014.09.014.

Øyen, N., Diaz, L.J., Leirgul, E., *et al.* (2016) Prepregnancy diabetes and offspring risk of congenital heart disease. *Circulation*, **133** (23), 2243–2253. http://doi: 10.1161/CIRCULATIONAHA.115.017465.

Papamichael, K., Konstantopoulos, P. & Mantzaris, G.J. (2014) Helicobacter pylori infection and inflammatory bowel disease: is there a link? *World Journal of Gastroenterology*, **20** (21), 6374–6385. http://doi:10.3748/wjg.v20.i21.6374.

Parsa, N. (2012) Environmental factors inducing human cancers. *Iranian Journal of Public Health*, **41** (11), 1–9.

Pembrey, M. (2012) *The Introduction to the Genetics and Epigenetics of Human Disease*. London, Progress Educational Trust.

Pereira, C. & Marion, R. (2018) Contiguous gene syndromes. *Pediatrics in Review*, **9** (1), 46–49. https://doi.org/10.1542/pir.2016-0073.

Peters, C. van Trotsenberg, A.S.P., & Schoenmakers, N. (2018) Diagnosis of endocrine disease: congenital hypothyroidism: update and perspectives. *European Journal of Endocrinology*, **179** (6), 297–317. https://doi.org/10.1530/EJE-18-0383.

Polymeros, D., Tsiamoulos, Z.P., Koutsoumpas, A.L., *et al.* (2014) Bioinformatic and immunological analysis reveals lack of support for measles virus related mimicry in crohn's disease. *Bio Medical Central Medicine*, **12** (139), 1–10.

Prows, C.A. (2019) Hereditary influences on health promotion of the child and family. In: *Wong's Nursing Care of Infants and Children (eleventh edition)*, (eds M.J. Hockenberry, D. Wilson & C.C. Rogers), pp. 41–79. St. Louis, Elsevier.

Rantala, A., Jaakkola, J.J.K., & Jaakkola, M.S. (2011) Respiratory infections precede adult-onset asthma. *PLoS ONE*, **6** (12), 27912. http://doi:10.1371/journal.pone.0027912.

Rashvand, S., Somi, M.H., Rashidkhani, B., *et al.* (2015) Dietary protein intakes and risk of ulcerative colitis. *Medical Journal of the Islamic Republic of Iran*, **29** (253), 1–7.

Rigante, D., Bosco, A., & Esposito, S. (2015) The etiology of juvenile idiopathic arthritis. *Clinical Reviews in Allergy & Immunology*, **49** (2), 253–261.

Rowland, E. & Metcalfe, A. (2013) Communicating inherited genetic risk between parent and child: a meta-thematic synthesis. *International Journal of Nursing Studies*, **50**, 870–880. http://dx.doi.org/10.1016/j.ijnurstu.2012.09.002.

Rubenstein, S. & Levy, A. (2019) Seizures in childhood: aetiology, diagnosis, treatment, and what the future may hold. *European Medical Journal*, **7** (1), 62–70.

Salim, S.Y. & Söderholm, J.D. (2011) Importance of disrupted intestinal barrier in inflammatory bowel disease. *Inflammatory Bowel Disease*, **17** (1), 362–381. http://doi:10.1002/ibd.21403.

Schiff, E.R., Frampton, M., Semplici, F., *et al.* (2018) A new look at familial risk of inflammatory bowel disease in the Ashkenazi Jewish population. *Digestive Diseases and Sciences*, **63**, 3049–3057. https://doi.org/10.1007/s10620-018-5219-9.

Sharawat, I.K., Singh, J., Dawman, L., *et al.* (2016) Evaluation of risk factors associated with first episode febrile seizure. *Journal of Clinical and Diagnostic Research*, **10** (5), 10–13. http://doi:10.7860/JCDR/2016/18635.7853

Shirley, E.D. & Ain, M.C. (2013) Achondroplasty. In: *Brenner's Encyclopedia of Genetics* (second edition), (eds S. Maloym & K. Hughes), pp. 4–6. Cambridge, Massachusetts, Academic Press.

Sillence D.O. (2013) Osteogenesis Imperfecta. In: *Brenner's Encyclopedia of Genetics (second edition)*, (eds S. Maloym & K. Hughes), pp. 191–196. Cambridge, Massachusetts, Academic Press.

Skirton, H., Lewis, C., Kent, A. & Coviello, D.A. (2010) Genetic education and the challenge of genomic medicine: development of core competences to support preparation of health professionals in Europe. *European Journal of Human Genetics*, **18**, 972–977. https://doi.org/10.1038/ejhg.2010.64.

Steck, A.K. & Rewers, M.J. (2011) Genetics of type 1 diabetes. *Clinical Chemistry*, **57** (2), 176–185.

Strachan, D.P., Aït-Khaled, N., Foliaki, S., *et al.* (2015) Siblings, asthma, rhinoconjunctivitis and eczema: a worldwide perspective from the international study of asthma and allergies in childhood. *Clinical & Experimental Allergy*, **45**, 126–136. http://doi:10.1111/cea.12349.

Strachan, T., Goodship, J. & Chinnery P.F. (2014) *Genetics and Genomics in Medicine*. New York, Garland Science

Straus, E. & Baird, J. (2018) Clinical guidelines for support of families of children with long term conditions. *Journal of Pediatric Nursing*, **43**, 136. https://doi.org/10.1016/j.pedn.2018.09.013.

Stroll, C., Dott, B., Alembik, Y., *et al.* (2015) Associated noncardiac congenital anomalies among cases with congenital heart defects. *European Journal of Medical Genetics*, **58**, 75–85. http://doi:10.1016/j.ejmg.2014.12.002

Taylor-Robinson, D.C., Williams, H., Pearce, A., *et al.* (2015) Do early-life exposures explain why more advantaged children get eczema? Findings from the U.*K. millennium cohort study. British Journal of Dermatology*, **174**, 569–578. http://doi:10.1111/bjd.14310.

Tobias, E.S., Connor, J.M. & Ferguson-Smith, M.A. (2011) *Essential Medical Genetics* (sixth edition). Chichester, Wiley-Blackwell.

Truong, U.T., Maahs, D.M. & Daniels, S.R. (2012) Cardiovascular disease in children and adolescents with diabetes: where are we, and where are we going? *Diabetes Technology and Therapeutics*, **14** (1), 1–21. http://doi:10.1089/dia.2012.0018.

Vadlamudi, L., Milne, R.L., Lawrence, K., *et al.* (2014) Genetics of epilepsy. The testimony of twins in the molecular era. *Neurology*, **83** (12), 1042–1048. https://doi.org/10.1212/WNL.0000000000000790.

Williams, J.K., Erwin, C., Juhl, A.R., *et al.* (2010) In their own words: reports of stigma and genetic discrimination by people at risk for Huntington disease in the International RESPOND-HD study. *American Journal of Medical Genetics. Part B, Neuropsychiatric Genetics: The Official Publication of the International Society of Psychiatric Genetics*, **153B** (6), 1150–1159. http://doi:10.1002/ajmg.b.31080.

Wlodarczyk, B.J., Palacios, A.M., George, T.M., *et al.* (2012) Antiepileptic drugs and pregnancy outcomes. *American Journal of Medical Genetics A*, **158A** (8), 2071–2090. http://doi:10.1002/ajmg.a.35438.

Wong, L., Jiang, K., Chen, Y., *et al.* (2017) Genetic insight into juvenile idiopathy arthritis derived from deep whole genome sequencing. *Nature Scientific Reports*, **7** 2657. https://doi.org/10.1038/s41598-017-02966-9.

World Health Organization (2017) Asthma. https://www.who.int/news-room/fact-sheets/detail/asthma Accessed 9/11/19.

World Health Organization (2019) Human Genomics in Global Health. https://who.int/genomics/elsi/gentesting/em Accessed 9/11/19.

Wu, G.D., Bushmanc, F.D. & Lewis, J.D. (2013) Diet, the human gut microbiota and IBD. *Anaerobe*, **24**, 117–120. https://doi.org/10.1016/j.anaerobe.2013.03.011.

Ziwei, Y., Wang, L., Yang, T., *et al.* (2019) Maternal viral infection and risk of fetal congenital heart diseases: a meta-analysis of observational studies. *Journal of the American Heart Association*, **8** (9). https://doi.org/10.1161/JAHA.118.011264.

CHAPTER 2

Context of Care and Service Delivery

Peter McNee

Introduction

The purpose of this chapter is to explore some of the current political, economic and social policies that are shaping the context of nursing practice and service delivery for children and young people with long-term illnesses. To analyse these external change drivers, examples of service models and nursing roles will be used, demonstrating their influence upon the shifting boundaries of clinical practice and service delivery.

The chapter intends to raise awareness of the issues and challenges that managers, practitioners and service users face as a consequence of these external influences impacting upon their service. An in-depth discussion on the complexities and contentions surrounding the multitude of, and sometimes radical, service delivery models utilised within health care is not within the scope of this chapter, although some of these and the current dialogues surrounding advancing nursing practice will be touched upon in this and subsequent chapters.

Aim of the chapter

To raise awareness and knowledge about the external political, social and economic drivers that are influencing how services for children and young people with long-term illness are developing, along with the resulting implications and opportunities for children's nurses.

Intended learning outcomes

- To analyse current political, economic and social policies that are impacting upon service and practice delivery for children and young people with long-term illnesses and their families

Nursing Care of Children and Young People with Long-Term Conditions, Second Edition.
Edited by Mandy Brimble and Peter McNee.
© 2021 John Wiley & Sons Ltd. Published 2021 by John Wiley & Sons Ltd.

- To examine current and future service models and the workforce required for them to be delivered in partnership with children and young people with long-term illnesses and their families
- To explore the complexities surrounding shifting health and social care workforce role boundaries, associated competencies and their impact upon service users, professionals and managers

Context of change

In relation to the provision of health care services for children and young people with long-term illnesses, several external change drivers have been influencing the development and shaping the context of nursing practice for this client group and their families. These external drivers stem from political, economic and social sources and are creating the imperative for health care leaders, managers and professional organisations to review children and young people's journeys through the health care system, reconsider the workforce required for their delivery, examine how the NHS can be more responsive to patients' needs through effective commissioning processes, and implement strategies that enhance cross-organisational boundary and multidisciplinary partnership working.

To realise a long-term vision of an NHS that is patient led, equitable, responsive and at the same time sustainable within the current and future economic and political environments, various governments over the last 20 years have strongly influenced the introduction of some key changes. These include introducing patient choice into models of service provision, strengthening governance and accountability arrangements, relinquishing control to more local-based health care services and encouraging patients to be fully 'engaged' as partners in their health care. This at a time when devolution has meant that there are divergent funding streams, health care policy and commissioning leading to similar but not identical service delivery across the four home nations.

Key political strategies to achieve this have been the development of foundation trusts, Clinical Commissioning groups, practice-based primary-led commissioning, payment by results and longer term integrated health and social care strategies (Wanless, 2002; Audit Commission, 2004; Department of Health, Social Services and Public Safety Northern Ireland (DHSSPSNI) 2005; Foundation Trust Network, 2005; Scottish Executive, 2005; NHS Scotland, 2010; Department of Health Northern Ireland, 2016; Welsh Government, 2019; and NHS England, 2019).

Political influences

The health care and well-being of society has been the focus of increased governmental and public attention in the UK. This interest was partly driven by the visibility of several high-profile public enquiries involving the deaths of children and young people. These reviews made transparent to the public some of the deficits of maintaining a consistently high quality and safe service within the current health care system. These safety risks and quality issues have been attributed to poor partnership working and ineffective communication networks between professional groups and agencies responsible for safeguarding and delivering services to children and young people, thereby leading to fragmentation and critical incidents. Other contributing factors include the inadequate supervision and monitoring of professional practice (Kennedy *et al.*, 2001; Laming, 2003; Laming, 2009; Munro, 2011), poor leadership, accountability and governance (Kennedy *et al.*, 2001; Redfern *et al.*, 2001; Laming, 2009; Munro, 2011; DOH UK, 2012; Francis, 2013), along with a lack of involving parents in the decision-making process. The outcomes from these reviews and, in light of them, mounting public pressure, have encouraged health care policies and recommendations for children and young people's services to be designed and delivered around their needs, and to safeguard them (NHS, 2019).

Key policy initiatives have included England's 10-year *Children's Workforce Strategy* programme (DfES, 2005) devised to implement *Every Child Matters* (DfES, 2003), and to reiterate the government's commitment to supporting and safeguarding children. England and Wales produced their *National Service Frameworks for Children, Young People and Maternity Services* (DoHUK, 2004; WAG, 2005a). These were substantial policies which were designed to transform services. In recent years, this policy has been built upon and developed further. Current policy and strategies include Department of Health Northern Ireland (2016) *A Strategy for Paediatric Healthcare Services Provided in Hospitals and in the Community* – this will span 10 years from 2016–2026. Welsh Government (2018) *A Healthier Wales: Our Plan for Health and Social Care* aims to provide seamless local health and social care closer to home, this approach also appears in the NHS long-term plan for England (NHS, 2019).

In response to the aforementioned key government and subsequent policy documents, some founding principles for children and young people's health care services have been agreed by various professional bodies, voluntary and parent groups and children's welfare organisations. These have been incorporated into national policy and numerous Royal College of Paediatrics and Child Health (RCPCH) and Royal College of Nursing (RCN) guidance and standard setting documents. These include:

- Better communication and coordination of children and young people's health and social care services.
- Child and family empowerment.
- Services closer to the child's home.
- Children only being admitted to hospital if medically required to do so.
- The importance of considering developmental issues with the provision of age appropriate services.
- Increasing emphasis upon preventative health and health promotion strategies (DoH UK, 2011; RCN, 2014; RCPCH, 2018a; RCPCH, 2019).

These approaches are immediately recognisable within the NHS long-term plan (2019) and equivalent devolved administration policy and legislation (The Scottish Government, 2016).

Economic influences

With increasing medical technological advances, particularly in neonatal care, along with enhanced care-giving practices and new medical treatments, children and young people with long-term illnesses are living longer, requiring more complex and continuing care needs to be addressed into adulthood. Meeting these needs is often dependent on interventions and equipment that in the past would have required the child or young person to be hospitalised. Today they are often provided in the local community or the child's home environment, resulting in the traditional boundaries of health care provision shifting from the acute care setting to one provided nearer to, and often by, the family within community and primary care settings (Hinde *et al.*, 2016). It is suggested that, when cared for at home, children with complex and continuing health needs have improved physical, psychosocial and development outcomes (Hewitt-Taylor, 2005; DoH UK, 2011; RCN, 2020), and that this service delivery mode is a more cost-effective choice for the NHS. A report by DoH, UK (2011) *NHS at Home: Community Children's Nursing Services* found that the community children's nursing services in Lambeth, Lewisham and Southwark provided care at home with a cost of 30–50% less than that provided in hospital. Consequently, this delivery mode is an appealing choice for government and health care managers who are trying to deliver quality effective services within the financial constraints of a climate of rising health care costs. On the whole, government policy has been to increase NHS funding, but with the financial crisis this has been a challenge. It could be argued, though, that this NHS cost saving may be transferred to the family if the appropriate support services are not instigated, including financial benefits, psychosocial and educational support, or adaptations to the family home.

Social influences

To address the problems of an increasing number of children and young people with long-term illnesses and complex health care needs, government task forces, health care managers and professional bodies have had to examine alternative service delivery models. Models advocated are those that emphasise an integrated approach between health, social care and education services and collaborative working with the voluntary and independent sector. The aim is that partnership working between these services will ensure a holistic approach, taking into account the child, young person and families' physical, developmental, social and psychological needs (DoH UK, 2011; WG, 2019; NHS, 2019).

Often compounding some of the needs of children and young people with long-term illness and their families is the increasing evidence of the impact of poverty and social exclusion upon their health and welfare (Marmot, 2010; Pillas *et al.*, 2014; Wickham *et al.*, 2016). These include the ability to access services, the financial hardship associated with parents having to give up employment to care for their child with the added difficulty of navigating the benefits system, poor public transport links, housing issues and the ability to provide adequate nutritional support. Recent government health and social care policies have attempted to recognise service poverty, where improving public services could play a key role in breaking cycles of poverty along with influencing the development of services closer to the patient's home.

Clinical networks and locally based commissioning arrangements exist in some format in the four UK countries and are both being pursued in the hope that they will minimise constraints that can affect equity and access to services. Possible constraints could be geographical location, the level of local funding, or the availability of professional expertise, new medical technologies and treatments (RCPCH, 2012).

Managed clinical networks and locally based commissioning are to be discussed in more detail in the following section.

Considering the external influences so far discussed, it is essential that health care services are sufficiently flexible to enable a responsive approach to meet the frequently complex individual needs of children and young people and consider these in relation to their level of independence, maturity, social circumstances and the features of their long-term illness process.

New models of service delivery

As previously intimated, new ways of delivering services have had to be examined in order to meet the government's health service plans and agendas and thus implement key policy and service provision.

Service models that have been developed have tended to provide more integrated, community and ambulatory care facilities and the reconfiguration of specialised tertiary services onto one site within a locality through the establishment of managed clinical networks. These models aim to facilitate earlier discharge from hospital, prevent admissions, support parents as experts in the care of their child or adolescent with a long-term illness, while at the same time ensure safe services through centralising specialised resources. Managed clinical networks are seen by government and professional bodies as a method of enhancing service provision through better commissioning and delivery of services for those children who require treatment and care across a range of professional groups and organisational boundaries.

The generally accepted definition of managed clinical networks was published by the Scottish Office in 1999 and then used within the National Service Framework programmes. They have been defined as: 'Linked groups of health professionals and organisations from primary, secondary and tertiary care, and social services and other services working in a coordinated manner' (DoH UK, 2004); and 'Managed local networks are fundamentally about enabling services to be formed or linked across boundaries (whether physical or financial) with the overall aim to ensure an optimal patient journey through and across services' (DoH UK, 2005). This very much mirrors the patterns of service provision that we see today, with some specialist treatment such as cardiac surgery and burns being delivered in a smaller number of hospitals across the UK (RCPCH, 2012).

Managed clinical networks are viewed as enabling the concentration of health professionals with specialist skills. They have also encouraged service leads and NHS modernisation teams to reconsider how they best use professional roles and competencies to allocate staff in the right place at the right time and with the necessary competencies to meet children, young people and families' needs within a modernised patient-led NHS. However, these are not without controversy, with families having to travel some distance to access some specialist services – for example, cardiac surgery for children and young people is not provided in Wales – and ongoing proposals to reconfigure services for paediatric cardiac surgery across the UK (NHS, 2010; NSCG, 2010).

Managed clinical networks define and support several ideal pathways of care for children and young people with particular health problems, spanning not only primary, secondary and tertiary care, but also local authority and voluntary sector-based services. They provide a guide for professionals on the optimal care required for that particular problem, identifying the standards, resources and quality improvement processes (RCPCH, 2012). An example could be a managed clinical network for children and young people with respiratory disorders, which could support an asthma, chronic lung and cystic fibrosis pathway of care. Another example could be a managed clinical network for cancer, incorporating pathways of care for leukaemias, solid tumours, haemoglobinopathies and lymphomas. Key within these pathways is the competence of professionals and the communication networks with the child, young person and family.

To support children and young people in the community, several service models have been developed to meet local needs. These include hospital-based outreach services, community-based in-reach services, the employment of specialist nurses who practise across community and acute sectors, and hospital at home or ambulatory care teams (Whiting, 2004). The RCN (2020) in their guidance *Futureproofing Community Children's Nursing* provide a range of examples of current and innovative practice in the provision of services to children and young people. One such example is the Evelina London Children's at Home and Community Nursing Service. This is a seven-day integrated approach where the team operate from both hospital and community and are able to respond to a referral and review the child or young person at home within three hours of discharge. The service aims to reduce bed stay, admissions to hospital and attendance at the emergency department. This and other approaches demonstrate improved patient experiences and flow.

🕐 **Time out**

- Consider some of the children and young people you have met with long-term illnesses while out on community placements.
- What type of service models did they experience?
- What were the key elements of this service?

Overall, the literature supports the existence of multiagency working but, where this is implemented, least common is a model that delivers this through an identified contact person, except in the case of key workers for children with disabilities (Greco & Sloper, 2004; Noyes *et al.*, 2014). Generally, though, there are few sound evaluative studies demonstrating outcomes of multiagency working for service users.

It must be remembered, though, that one professional discipline does not have the sole responsibility of delivering the new service models. To ensure a holistic child and family focused approach, care based upon the best current evidence must be delivered throughout the child and young person's health care pathway by multidisciplinary teams including all relevant specialist staff (McNamara & Goodger, 2017). This requires a flexible and needs-led approach rather than one based on professional boundaries. Membership and governance of these teams must be explicit and include clearly defined responsibility for clinical leadership and management

Modernising workforce

To achieve real change for children and young people, it will be a necessary to focus on staff groups such as nursing or health care support workers and develop an overall workforce strategy that considers cross-professional and service sector roles. This will require a collective will to change, partnership working, shared accountability and major workforce changes between health care settings, social care and education sectors (Ham *et al.*, 2018). Applying these issues to children and young people with long-term illnesses, such a cross-sector role could be an adolescent transitional care practitioner who would work across adult and children's health care services and in partnership with health, social care and educational sectors. This role could facilitate a coordinated and planned transition programme for young people from child to adult services and enable their physical, psychosocial and educational or employment needs to be incorporated within this plan. Recent examples of the modernisation agenda has been the introduction of the nurse associate role which developed out of *Health Education England's Shape of Caring* review (2015). These roles are now established with the NMC (2018) publishing standards for proficiency for nursing associates.

(🕐) **Time out**

- Can you think of any other potential roles that could be developed that would facilitate more effective services to be delivered for children and young people with long-term illnesses across organisations and different health care sectors?
- Compare your thoughts to some potential roles identified at the end of this chapter.

Over the last few years, children and young people's health care services have witnessed an increasing number of condition-specific specialist/advanced practitioner/consultant nurse positions. Roles such as advanced nurse practitioner have been somewhat controversial, differ from one region to another in terms of job titles, role descriptors, areas of accountability, qualifications, competencies required to fulfil the role and pay and employment conditions (RCN, 2014). Frequently, these positions incorporate extended roles that have traditionally been those of junior medical doctors. This could include nurse-led outpatient clinics, baseline assessments, reviewing treatment programmes, prescribing medicines, providing valuable health education, family support services, undertaking research, influencing policy agendas and delivering specialist staff education and training programmes (NHS Scotland, 2010; NLIAH Wales, 2010). The RCN (2014) have produced useful guidance and a role framework for preparing children and young people's nurses for future advanced and specialist roles. These included examples of current practice including a consultant nurse in acute care and a specialist diabetes advanced nurse practitioner. However, professional nursing bodies have expressed caution regarding the professional regulation of these advanced roles (NMC, 2007; RCN, 2017). In its evaluation of post-registration standards of proficiency for specialist community public health nurses and the standards for specialist education and practice standards, the NMC (2019) have highlighted the need to examine the advanced practitioner role.

A key concern is the need to ensure that these roles are redesigned based upon quality improvement strategies and meeting the child, young person and families' needs rather than just taking on an area of responsibility or practice that is no longer deemed an important aspect of another profession's role. To safeguard children and young people and professionals, these advanced roles need to be supported by protocols, clear guidelines, agreed accountability structures and supervision networks. Rolfe (2014) found that there is some variability in practice standards, role and competence of those employed as advanced nurse practitioners.

A useful illustration of a consultant nurse role is a children and young person's consultant oncology nurse, whose role and responsibilities will include elements of delivering expert clinical practice, professional leadership, developing education programmes and support systems, scholarly activity and consultancy work across professional and organisational boundaries. Extended advanced elements of the role could include the ordering and interpreting of appropriate screening, laboratory and other diagnostic tests, and administering timely supportive treatment regimens according to agreed protocols. However, when new roles are planned, often challenging traditional working patterns and role boundaries, a strategic approach is required. This strategy would need to be based upon robust systems and frameworks that support enhanced quality and effectiveness of services so that professionals, children, young people and their families can clearly identify the longer-term advantages.

Increasing patient expectations and engagement

So far, this chapter has illustrated that an intricate range of services are required for children and young people with long-term and complex illnesses. The underpinning rationale for this is sustained continued care provision, which often involves many disciplines and professional staff crossing organisational and institutional boundaries. Integrated pathways incorporating processes for referral, assessment, service delivery and review, which also give young people and families a central role in planning services, are essential.

Policies and guidance highlight the importance of involving service users in their health care practice (NHS, 2019). Involvement also includes evaluating existing and new service developments. As children and young people's views about their own needs may not be the same as those of their parents or adult proxies, there has been increasing interest regarding how they can be consulted (Whiting *et al.*, 2018), including the provision of children's advocacy services to enable children and young people to complain and give suggestions for service improvement and the development of NHS Youth Boards (NHS England, 2018).

A study by Whiting *et al.* (2018) examined the role of members of the NHS England Youth Forum. This research utilised an evaluative mixed-methods approach with data collected using activity logs, a questionnaire and semi-structured interviews. A range of themes were identified from the study including motivation, commitment and knowledge expertise from NHS staff. The study concluded by identifying the rapid expansion and success of the forum alongside the commitment that the young people have to their role and the positive impact that this initiative has on service provision.

Parents, whose child or young person requires ongoing medical or technological interventions within the community or family home environment, often have to deliver some care practices that traditionally would have been carried out by children's nurses or health care support workers (Lenehan, 2017). Supporting parents to perform these care practices, cope with the demands of administering treatments, provide 24-hour care and deal with general aspects of parenting and family life can be challenging. Alternative models of health care delivery services that strengthen community provision, and a review of the type of staff needed and the associated role competencies, are required. Methods of actively engaging children, young people and their families in services and treatment options requires highly tuned communication skills and an understanding that these parents often have increased knowledge and skills (McCann *et al.*, 2012).

Parents of children and young people with long-term conditions and complex health needs are often very knowledgeable about their child's condition and the practicalities of managing their child's symptoms, care and treatment choices. These 'expert parents' can be assertive and may challenge professional views regarding treatment options and care strategies (Shaw & Barker, 2004). Health care professionals must work in partnership with children, young people and parents to negotiate new roles and responsibilities to take on supportive and educative roles (Carter *et al.*, 2014). These new roles in the community and family home require specific competencies to be developed. The nature of the relationship has changed regarding the power equation in the familiarity of the environment and also the knowledge base in relation to some rarer long-term medical conditions. Parental role transfer and the implications for nursing skill development will be expanded upon later in the chapter.

⏲ Time out

- Reflecting on the parents of children and young people with long-term illnesses that you have met in practice, what skills:
- Did these parents undertake that normally would have been done by a nurse?
- Did the nurses need to support these parents?
- Compare your thoughts with the section on parental needs later on in this chapter.

Locally based commissioning

Planning, commissioning and funding all aspects of care for children and young people across the whole health care system should be coordinated to ensure that there is an appropriate balance of service provision and allocation of resources to address local social, economic and environmental factors that affect people's health and well-being (WG, 2019; NHS, 2019).

There have been changes to the mechanisms for funding and commissioning health care services to encourage more integrated local needs-based commissioning and increasing accountability and governance of health care expenditure (WG, 2019; NHS, 2019). New commissioning organisations and processes, which vary across the four countries in the UK, all have elements that strengthen the governance and accountability arrangements of clinicians and managers over budgets, achieving national and local health performance targets, such as equity, efficiency and cost containment, alongside facilitating meaningful engagement of children, young people and their families to ensure responsiveness to their needs. These drivers have produced an opportunity to reconfigure services to develop sustainable models of provision, with integrated approaches to care delivery that are often community-based alternatives to hospital care.

Challenges for the commissioning bodies include delivering the right commissioning models within an overall context of community engagement and partnership working. They need to address health inequalities, meet national priorities and performance targets, determine clinical service models and ensure patient choice. Consider, for instance, a children's diabetes service that has to meet the needs of a local population that geographically encapsulates both a densely populated city and a rural community. Effective access and equity of services for all children and young people with diabetes would require the development of services within the city and locally in the rural areas (RCPCH, 2018b). Delivery of care closer to home can result, for example, in reduced travelling costs, less disruption to family life, reduced school absences, sibling social and family participation and less employment time loss. Furthermore, there could be the added advantage of children, young people and families developing increased confidence in local services. Unfortunately, the costs incurred by increasing the provision of local services and the provision of appropriate support to families and carers closer to home have not been addressed; for example, the continuing development of children's community nursing teams.

The remainder of this chapter will consider some of the implications of the political, social and economic drivers upon service from a practice context. It will particularly highlight the impact on the roles of parents and nurses, and service challenges that need to be addressed to support these changes.

Staffing implications

As intimated earlier, due to advances in treatment and innovative life-promoting technologies, children whose conditions would have been deemed incompatible with life are now surviving and are able to be cared for at home (Hewitt-Taylor, 2005; WG, 2012; RCN, 2020). This shift towards the provision of home care raises a number of issues for those tasked with providing that care. One of the key debates for home care concerns who should deliver it. A number of reports have identified the need for wider service provision that crosses traditional organisational boundaries (DoH UK, 2004; DoH UK, 2011; WG, 2012). Children with long-term illness and complex health needs often require skilled intervention, and it has often fallen on parents to provide home care with little or no preparation or training; however, their expertise and competence to manage care and treatment is increasingly recognised (Vickers *et al.*, 2007).

Staff education and competence

Key to providing the appropriate care to meet and support children and young people's needs in both home and hospital environments is the effective education and training of staff involved in the delivery of this provision. Children who require advanced technological support, including those requiring long-term ventilation, often experience difficulty in having those needs met. This group of children with long-term illness can often have protracted periods of hospitalisation due to a lack of collaboration between the acute and community settings, greater parental stress and financial burdens (Noyes, 2002; Darvill *et al.*, 2009). This requires services to be established and presents nurses with the opportunity to develop roles that can facilitate well planned, coordinated transitional programmes from hospital to home environments.

Margolan *et al.* (2004) found four consistent causes for delayed discharge: the provision of health authority funding, the need to employ community carers, adaptation of the child's home and the purchase of equipment and consumables in order to provide and establish a safe home care environment. It was also clear from this study that parents often felt excluded from the discharge process and confused by the input from a variety of health and social care organisations.

To facilitate a seamless transition from hospital to home, there is a need for a coordinated approach across organisational boundaries, with perhaps an identified named nurse commissioning the whole process. With such a current ad hoc approach to discharge planning, it would be appropriate for nursing staff to develop guidelines and protocols concerning the purchase of equipment and consumables and the maintenance of ordering systems. Management plans should also be in place, which identify the various components of the commissioning process from home adaptation to the recruitment and training of carers. Margolan *et al.* (2004) highlight the need for children to be nursed in an appropriate environment, including high dependency units and transitional care beds, to avoid the stress of children's intensive care units. While barriers exist across organisational boundaries, the commissioning process of services for children requiring long-term ventilation will remain unwieldy, failing to meet the most basic and essential needs of the child.

Glendinning and Kirk (2000) found a number of issues regarding the organisation and the commissioning of care that impacted heavily on parents. The study involved interviewing 24 parents whose children had long-term health needs, and identified that parents often assumed primary responsibility for their child's care to ensure a more rapid discharge from the hospital setting. This can be seen to exploit the parental role if adequate service provision is not available. It is estimated that there are up to 6000 technology-dependent children living in the UK, and the cost of equipment and, in some cases, ventilatory support, is approximately £130 000 per annum per child (Glendinning & Kirk, 2000). Their study also identified that parents increasingly found their homes loaded with technology, with the focus on technical proficiency rather than the psychological aspects of undertaking often distressing procedures on their own children. In this area, where ongoing care is required over a 24-hour period, parents are expected to perform what would be traditionally understood as nursing interventions, including suctioning, tracheostomy care and the setting up of intravenous infusions. To try to meet these needs, a number of roles have been developed, including the key worker role, which will be discussed later on in the chapter. Nurses undertaking coordinating roles need to assist in the establishment of multidisciplinary care management pathways, which identify professional roles and responsibilities within the process and provision of appropriate resources to individual children and young people.

Hewitt-Taylor (2005) undertook a pilot study to ascertain the training needs of staff involved in the care of children and young people with long-term illness. A wide range of educational and training needs were identified as important, including the knowledge and skills related to invasive therapies such as assisted ventilation and tracheostomy care. To be effective, planned education and training needs have to be targeted to ensure that they meet the needs of both qualified and unqualified nurses, as they are the professionals delivering care outside the hospital environment (Robinson & Jackson, 1999). Much of the input is focused on the acquisition of clinical knowledge and skills but it is equally important to ensure that there is equivalent attention paid to the psychological and developmental needs of the children. This would suggest that there is a role for shared education between children's nurses, mental health nurses and professionals working within child psychology teams. It must be ensured that care is delivered holistically so that all the health and social care needs of the family are met (Hewitt-Taylor, 2005).

Reflection

Reflecting on the parents of children and young people with long-term illnesses that you have met in practice what:

- Impact did their child's long-term illness have upon them?
- Strategies were used by professionals to minimise these impacts?
- Roles and services could be provided to help support children and young people in their homes?

Meeting parental needs

The diagnosis of a long-term illness is a life-changing event for the family concerned. Moore *et al.* (2010) described parents as experiencing a significant impact on their lives when caring for a child with continuing or complex needs. The parents often experience a significant change in their role because they have to become primary care-givers in order to meet their child's needs; this has a physical, psychological, emotional, spiritual and environmental impact (Moore *et al.*, 2010). Parents often become dependent on the provision of home carers to meet the ongoing needs of their children. Margolan *et al.* (2004) found wide variations between the recruitment and ongoing training of carers, with some organisations having no specific training programmes available. Only one service was identified that provided ongoing training of home carers, where families' needs were regularly reviewed with input increased or decreased as the needs of the child and family changed. This type of responsive service provision ought to be the norm not the exception, with other service providers and commissioning bodies taking note of best practice to further develop their own services. The process of transition and adaptation can cause an inordinate amount of stress on the whole family, which requires health care professionals to be aware of the individual and holistic needs of all members of the family group. It is essential that children's nurses are educationally prepared to deliver this kind of responsive service through post-registration education and supervision by management teams.

Effective communication is essential if service provision is to meet the holistic needs of families coping with a child with an ongoing long-term illness (Carter *et al.*, 2014). Various authors have identified parental needs as the desire for normality and certainty, particularly around the diagnosis and ongoing management of disease processes, the need for information and the need for a sense of partnership with members of the multidisciplinary team involved in the provision of services and care delivery (Fisher, 2001; WG, 2012). This partnership approach has to be established across a range of health care and social settings including the educational environment. Perhaps one reason why service provision is fragmented, and at times uncoordinated, is a lack of recognition of the role of children's community nurses. The work undertaken by community teams is often hidden as it is not high on the political agenda in comparison to the provision of acute services. Carter *et al.* (2014) recognise that this issue impacts on the role and development of services within the home care environment. Much of the work undertaken by community workers is not wholly transparent. Byrne (2003) found that a variety of nursing strategies are employed to meet the needs of children and young people with complex needs; but much of this work was not evidenced in documentation, such as assessment charts, as it focused on psychological and social care, an area that is often undervalued and immeasurable. A clear gap emerges between documentation and the scope of nursing within the home environment. Nurses have developed and combined a range of skills that focus on empowerment, physical assessment and care, teaching and providing effective guidance and support to families (WG, 2012; RCN, 2020). To provide community care, families will require a broad range of nursing input from both qualified nurses and unqualified carers.

Reflection

Reflect upon the children and young people with long-term and complex illness within the community. What differing skills and knowledge do you require to meet their needs in this environment, as opposed to providing care for them in the acute setting? Consider the following to guide your thoughts:

- Professional responsibility and accountability.
- Parents as experts in the care of their own child.
- Resource issues.
- The environment of care.

It is important to establish the correct skill mix and division of labour to ensure that care needs are fully met. To achieve this, community teams need to collaborate and ensure that all team members have access to ongoing training and development to fulfil the required roles. When establishing community teams, educational programmes need to be developed to ensure that a broad range of knowledge and skills are taught to the participants. With the varied skill mix in some community teams, the topics taught have to meet the needs of both trained and untrained nurses (Hewitt-Taylor, 2005; Price, 2018; RCN, 2020). The delivery of nursing care to children in their own homes requires a comprehensive level of knowledge and skill acquisition. The ability to meet care needs through a combination of nursing and parentally delivered care will remain problematic while commissioning and funding deficits remain. The skills and knowledge required for effective delivery of care to children and young people in the community setting should include:

- Sound interpersonal skills in order to develop good working relationships with families and professionals.

- Knowledge of ethics and the law to advocate on behalf of children, young people and their families.
- A thorough knowledge of both statutory and voluntary provision.
- The ability to provide holistic care, including meeting the physical, social, emotional and psychological needs of those in their care.

It is of paramount importance that nurses establish an evidence base for the effectiveness of community-based care for the needs of children and young people with long-term illness to be met. Home nursing care delivery needs to be both identifiable and measurable for the development of best practice, clear and consistent discharge planning and the commissioning of services.

Innovative practices – new roles

A variety of strategies and schemes have been developed to support children and young people and their families in their home, including telemedicine, which will be discussed later in the chapter. A range of professionals will be involved in care delivery. It is envisaged that there will be a growth in the development of roles such as consultant nurses, key workers and the further development and enhancement of children's community nursing teams to meet the needs of children, young people and their families (DoH UK, 2004; WAG, 2005a,b; Davies and Bodycombe-James, 2017). What is required to take these services forward is nurse leadership in the development and provision of care packages. The recognition and development of the role of the children's nurse, not only in delivering but commissioning services, has been clearly recognised (WAG, 2004; DOH UK, 2011; WG, 2012). Increasing integration and commissioning of services is seen as a way of ensuring quality of care and reducing duplication in the assessment and sometimes delivery of services. The role of the consultant nurse in the community setting is intended to ensure clear lines of care provision and communication. Caerphilly Local Health Board (LHB) in Wales established the role of the children's community nurse consultant in delivering coordinated care to children and young people with ongoing and complex needs. This followed on from the 2005 partnership strategy for health, social care and well-being (Caerphilly LHB, 2005), which sought to plan, administer and deliver a range of services across the health and social care arena. This approach to coordination across traditional boundaries is intended to provide targeted and cost-effective services to children, young people and their families in a range of settings and circumstances.

🕐 **Time out**

Consider the role of the nurse in the provision of care to children and young people with a long-term illness in the community setting:

- How do health and social care influences affect the provision of care?
- How could new nursing roles such as a consultant nurse improve this situation?

Telemedicine

Telemedicine has been seen as an opportunity for parents to opt for more care to be provided for children and young people in their own homes. Telemedicine has been defined as: 'The use of information and communication technology to deliver health or social care in new ways on a person-to-person basis, where those people are physically apart' (TEIS UK, 2004).

In the past, this has served to combat issues around geographical distance and the high cost of bringing children and young people to regional centres for consultation. Guest *et al.* (2005) highlighted the benefits of telemedicine for a specific group of neurologically impaired children, but potentially this has far-reaching implications for a range of children with long-term illness and severe disability. Clear benefits arise from this technology, including the ability of children and families to access information about their condition, treatment options and hold consultations with health care professionals (Bacigalupe, 2011).

This approach to care delivery could have a much broader application, particularly when providing care for technology-dependent children. This group of children often experience delays in the discharge process while services are configured to meet their needs (Wang & Barnard, 2004). For children requiring long-term ventilation, telemedicine offers the possibility of real-time support, which is important for both parents and carers (Edwards *et al.*, 2004). The benefits of such technology are clear, but it is important that clear policies are developed to ensure appropriate children and young people access this provision. Guidelines also need to be developed for practitioners to ensure safe practice and accountability, alongside appropriate education and skills development (Smith & Stoner, 2011; RCPCH, 2015; RCN, 2020).

Key worker role

Fragmented service provision and a lack of coordination between professional disciplines, agencies and health care settings has often been raised as an issue for the parents of children and young people living with a long-term illness (National Collaborating Centre for Cancer, 2005; Noyes *et al.*, 2014). Within the NHS, over recent years, a number of nursing roles have been established, which are often disease orientated; for example, clinical nurse specialists in oncology, cystic fibrosis and diabetes. A number of outreach and specialist services have made some impact on providing services that are across organisational boundaries, particularly from tertiary centres, but this type of service has been hampered at times by organisational culture and economic factors – something integrated health and social care policy is attempting to address (WG, 2019; NHS, 2019). Noyes *et al.* (2014) identified the benefits of the key worker role as being more effective communication, greater accessibility of information and support for families, advocacy for the child and the focused coordination of services.

🕒 **Time out**

- What type of roles and responsibilities do you think a key worker might have to undertake to ensure the delivery of a coordinated package of care?

Various reports outline the role of a key worker, particularly regarding services for children and young people with complex health care needs or oncological conditions where there may be shared health care between tertiary and secondary organisations, often in different health authorities. This role includes the coordinated provision of information, the provision of care and treatment plans and communication with members of the wider multidisciplinary team to ensure effective and timely interventions appropriate to the care of the child or young person concerned (McGirr & Richardson-Reed, 2018). It has been found that a number of titles are used to describe the key worker role, including care coordinator, lead professional, family support worker and link worker (Greco & Sloper, 2004; Noyes *et al.*, 2014; Scottish Government, 2016), which has led to some confusion in attempting to identify the prerequisites of the role and its potential boundaries.

As far back as the Warnock committee report (Department of Education and Science, 1978), it was recognised that there was a need for an identified professional to whom parents could turn for advice and support in accessing services. A number of authors have identified the benefits of the key worker role for families as: the reduction of multiple visits by numerous professionals, an improvement in communication between the hospital and community settings and less confusion about the role boundaries of the multitude of professionals involved in the care of a single child and family. Difficulties in advancing the key worker role are often related to a lack of detailed action plans, a lack of commitment and the existence of territorialism by a number of agencies, poor communication and a lack of access to a designated budget – which is partially being addressed with the move to integrated health and social care (NHS, 2019). Many care coordination schemes are established on short-term funding, and joint funding by statutory agencies remains uncommon (Greco & Sloper, 2004). What is not clear is how widespread key worker roles and care coordination services are within the UK. The key worker type role affords the child and family the opportunity for some continuity of care and integration of the primary, secondary and tertiary roles. This role encompasses health, social care and education.

National and devolved government have recognised the importance of this expansive role (DoH UK, 2013; Scottish Government, 2016). To be successful, key workers need to be able to span all agencies involved in the care and treatment of children and young people living with a long-term illness. This role, from a nursing perspective, involves the care and support of the individual family concerned and may involve teaching new clinical skills, case management between clinical settings and the coordination of future treatment and care. The key worker needs to be accessible to both the families and other professionals (Noyes *et al.*, 2014). Walker (2012) found evidence of good practice within integrated care which was partly due to most initiatives having all three statutory agencies of health, social care and education involved in establishing schemes.

Role diversification is becoming more prevalent within a range of clinical settings; traditional nursing roles are evolving, leading to opportunities for both qualified and unqualified nurses. The development of the role of the registered nurse has led to an expansion in the role of the health care support worker, who will continue to provide basic nursing care and perhaps more complex procedures in both acute and community settings. Within nursing, as previously discussed, there are huge opportunities for nurses to take lead roles in assessing, delivering, coordinating and evaluating packages of care and their effectiveness. Nurses now face the challenge of taking the key worker role forward in order to meet the complex health needs of children and young people with long-term illness.

Mental health issues

Crenna-Jennings and Hutchinson (2020) found that national estimates projected that up to 1.25 million children and young people in the UK have a diagnosable mental illness (NHS Digital, 2018). It has long been recognised that child and adult mental health services have been under resourced and unable to meet demand with only a third of children with a diagnosable condition accessing treatment (Crenna-Jennings & Hutchinson, 2020). Children and young people living with a long-term illness will, over time, experience a range of physical, psychological and emotional issues that may impact on their sense of worth and mental well-being. Although medical advances have increased survivability, the challenges of living with a long-term illness through adolescence and into adulthood remain. Children and young people with long-term illness experience a range of issues that impact on the development and maintenance of this health dimension (NHS Digital, 2015). Bazalgette *et al.* (2015) found that the incidence of mental health issues rises significantly in mid to late adolescence. To attempt to meet these needs, it is important that, as children's nurses, we recognise the limitations of our skills and knowledge and refer on, when necessary, to specialist services. A possible solution in attempting to meet the holistic needs of children, young people and families is to increase interprofessional collaboration. It is important that children's nurses share their knowledge and skills and, where deficits are identified, appropriate professional involvement should be encouraged.

In attempting to meet the mental health needs of children and young people, it would be appropriate for children's nurse managers to employ mental health nurses within community nursing teams. This is by no means a unique situation as we have seen mental health nurses employed on adolescent units and children's nurses employed in child and adolescent mental health settings. LeBovidge *et al.* (2005) examined adjustment to chronic illness in 75 children and young people aged 8–18 years with chronic arthritis. The data were collected using a questionnaire which examined attitudes towards illness, depressive symptoms and anxiety. A range of psychosocial stressors was experienced, which impacted on day-to-day living and the individual mental health of the children concerned. Parents of the children also completed a measure of psychosocial adjustment. From this study, it became clear that health care professionals and others involved in the care, support and treatment of this specific group of children needed to develop interventions in order to assist children and young people to come to terms with their illness and develop coping mechanisms. Only with the appointment of nurses with the appropriate skills, or by establishing multidisciplinary teams, will these needs be met. Children's nurses are in a position to recognise mental health issues in this vulnerable group, but they may feel that they lack the knowledge and experience in order to manage care. Appropriate and early referral is important, as is recognition of the limitation of one's own practice (RCN, 2014).

Multiagency working

The impact of long-term illness upon children and young people in relation to their physical, social and psychological well-being emphasises the importance of children's nurses being able to work in partnership with other members of the multidisciplinary team. This would help ensure that all aspects of children and young people's needs are met to minimise the risk of complications occurring, such as behavioural problems, depression, non-compliance or poor educational attainment. King *et al.* (2006) highlight the use of a multidisciplinary approach in attempting to meet the educational needs of children with sickle cell anaemia and cerebral infarcts. In this study, the multidisciplinary team included a nurse practitioner, social worker, neurologist and neuropsychologist, among others. Their role was aimed at reducing absenteeism and lost education by providing home tutoring and ensuring that educational environments were geared for children's needs when they were in school. The role of the nurse was to provide ongoing care in both the acute and ambulatory setting. What is important is that this type of coordinated approach to care delivery is being established and used across a wide range of settings so that children and young people have full access to education, health and social care.

Multidisciplinary team (MDT)/ Interprofessional working (IPW)

MDT or IPW centres on the working relationships between a range of professionals from a wide variety of agencies including health, social care and education (SCIE, 2009). This may entail developing close working relationships with groups of professionals whose working methods are relatively unknown to nurses. In terms of mental health, joint appointments and commissioning of posts appears to be the most effective way forward. For service provision to be holistic, children's community nursing teams must have a varied skill mix, with nurses able to meet the wide range of complex health needs, not just physical needs but also mental health and educational needs.

A number of high-profile reports and recommendations have recognised gaps in service delivery and fragmentation of services. This has contributed to a lack of workforce planning and poor integration of services (DoH UK, 2004; WG, 2019; NHS, 2019). Danvers *et al.* (2003) found a number of issues that impact on the role and function of the MDT. These included a lack of standardised documentation, tension between services providing input to the same child and family and a lack of coordinated shared education and training. The establishment of Diana children's community teams provided nurse-led services aimed at establishing high-quality seamless services focusing on supporting children with life-threatening or life-limiting illnesses, which in turn has led to an increase in multiprofessional collaboration and partnership across agencies (Danvers *et al.,* 2003). Problems around effective interprofessional working have been identified since the NHS was introduced (Atwal & Caldwell, 2005).

MDT/ IPW working is a key aspect of effective health care delivery, with teams varying in composition, leadership styles and culture. This variation can have a profound impact upon the clinical effectiveness of service delivery and ultimately on the management of care for the individual child and family. Gaps and omissions in services and the fragmented approach to care delivery is a government priority that is clearly identified throughout the various policies. The benefits of MDT/IPW working have been clearly identified. These included improved planning, clinical effectiveness, avoidance of duplication and fragmentation of services and the provision of holistic care which is coordinated to meet the child's ongoing needs (Doyle, 2008; Kings Fund, 2011). An effective MDT approach can lead to the eradication of dysfunctional professional barriers, which have impacted on the service provision and ultimately the quality of care. Danvers *et al.* (2003) identify various positive examples within multiprofessional collaborative approaches, including the development of joint visiting and a palliative care pathway. The value of developing a pathway that can be used by the wider team has clear benefits to the care and treatment of children and young people with a range of life-limiting or threatening conditions, particularly in ensuring that the holistic needs of the individual service user are met by the wider agencies involved in care provision.

 Time out

Reflecting on the parents of children and young people with long-term illnesses that you have met in practice, can you:

- Identify key members of the MDT and their roles within the acute or community setting?
- Identify barriers that may have impacted on effective MDT working?

Nursing implications, challenges and opportunities in MDT/IPW working

Some challenges that have been identified in relation to effective multidisciplinary working include duplication of care, clinical risk, organisation logistics in the provision of effective working between agencies and the management of resources (Doyle, 2008; Pollard *et al.*, 2010; Collier, 2013). However, within this collaborative approach there are clear opportunities for the children's nurse to develop shared policies and standards, thereby avoiding duplication and confusion around referral processes and appropriate access to professional care. To establish the cost effectiveness and validity of a multi-agency approach, different service delivery models and partnership approaches need to be evaluated. This would appear to be a good opportunity to embed and justify the role of a children's community nurse consultant across the UK, presenting the evidence base for this approach to the delivery of care to those with the most complex health care needs. Within this MDT/IPW approach, opportunities will present themselves for the integration of interprofessional research and education and also the potential for children's nurses to expand their roles and skills.

Conclusion

This chapter has considered the political, social and economic influences on service provision. To meet the future physical and psychosocial health care needs of children and young people with long-term illnesses and their families, it is apparent that policy-makers, commissioners and deliverers of children and young people's health, social and education services must work together to remove some of the real and potential barriers of dysfunctional professional boundaries, organisational infrastructures, unresponsive commissioning processes and outdated routine practices. There is a need to ensure integration and coordination of care within primary, secondary and tertiary care settings and between the voluntary sector, health, social care and educational organisations.

This requires coordinated planning, commissioning and funding arrangements. However, this breaking down of barriers and the building of effective partnership working arrangements will require children, young people and their families to be truly 'engaged' in shaping new services and working practices. This chapter has also examined some of the implications for children's nurses of increasing integration of services, changing role boundaries and practice settings along with an increasing engagement with children, young people and their families.

Acknowledgement

I acknowledge the contribution of Fay Valentine with whom I jointly authored the previous version of this chapter (Valentine & McNee, 2007).

Useful websites

Audit Commission
https://www.gov.uk/government/organisations/audit-commission

Department of Health
https://www.health-ni.gov.uk/

Department for Education
www.dfes.gov.uk

Kings Fund
www.kingsfund.org.uk

NICE
www.nice.org.uk

RCN
www.rcn.org.uk

RCPCH
https://www.rcpch.ac.uk/

Scottish Government
https://www.gov.scot/

Welsh Government
https://gov.wales/

References

Atwal, A. & Caldwell, K. (2005) Do all health and social care professionals interact equally: a study of interactions in multidisciplinary teams in the United Kingdom. *Scandinavian Journal of Caring Science*, **19**, 268–273.

Audit Commission (2004) Payment by Results: Key Risks and Questions to Consider for Trust and PCT Managers and Non-executives. London, Audit Commission.

Bacigalupe, G. (2011) Is there a role for social technologies in collaborative healthcare. *Families, Systems and Health: The Journal of Collaborative Family Health Care*, **29**, 1–14.

Bazalgette, L., Rahilly, T. & Trevely, G. (2015) Achieving Emotional Wellbeing for Looked After Children: A Whole System Approach. London, NSPCC.

Byrne, M.W. (2003) Culture-derived strategies of a paediatric home-care nursing speciality team. *International Nursing Review*, **50**, 34–43.

Caerphilly Local Health Board (2005) A Partnership Strategy for Health, Social Care and Well-being in Caerphilly County Borough. Caerphilly, Caerphilly Local Health Board.

Carter, B., Bray, L., Dickinson, A., *et al.* (2014) *Child-Centred Nursing: Promoting Critical Thinking*. London, Sage.

Collier, S. (2013) Preparation for professional practice. In: *Essential Nursing Care for Children and Young People: Theory, Policy and Practice* (ed. C. Thurston). Abingdon, Routledge.

Crenna-Jennings, W. & Hutchinson, J. (2020) Access to child and adolescent mental health services in 2019. Education Policy Institute. https://epi.org.uk/wp-content/uploads/2020/01/Access-to-CAMHS-in-2019_EPI.pdf Accessed 31/01/20.

Danvers, L., Freshwater, D., Cheater, F., *et al.* (2003) Providing a seamless service for children with life-limiting illness: experiences and recommendations of professional staff at the Diana Princess of Wales Children's Community Service. *Journal of Clinical Nursing*, **12**, 351–359.

Darvill, J., Harington, A. & Donovan, J. (2009). Caring for ventilated children at home: the child's perspective. *Neonatal, Paediatric and Child Health Nursing*, **12** (3), 9–13.

Davies, R. & Bodycombe, J.M. (2017) Community children's nursing. In: *Children and Young Peoples Nursing: Principles for Practice* (eds A. Davies & R. Davies) pp. 183–197. Hampshire, CRC Press.

Department of Education and Science (1978) Special Educational Needs: Report of the Committee of Enquiry into the Education of Handicapped Children and Young People. The Warnock Report. London, HMSO.

Department for Education and Skills (2003) Every Child Matters. London, Department for Education and Skills.

Department for Education and Skills (2005) Children's Workforce Strategy: A Strategy to Build a World-class Workforce for Children and Young People: *Every Child Matters: Change for Children*. London, Department for Education and Skills.

Department of Health, Northern Ireland (2016) Providing High Quality Healthcare for Children and Young People: A Strategy for Paediatric Healthcare Services Provided in Hospitals and in the Community. Belfast, Department of Health.

Department of Health, UK (2004) National Service Framework for Children, Young People and Maternity Services: Standard 8. Disabled Children and Young People and those with Complex Health Needs. London, The Stationery Office.

Department of Health, UK (2005) A Guide to Promote a Shared Understanding of the Benefits of Local Managed Networks. London, Department of Health.

Department of Health, UK (2011) NHS at Home: Community Children's Nursing Services. London, Department of Health UK.

Department of Health, UK (2012). Winterbourne View. https://www.gov.uk/government/publications/winterbourne-view-hospital-department-of-health-review-and-response Accessed 31/01/20.

Department of Health, UK (2013) Integrated Care: Our Shared Commitment. London, Department of Health UK.

Department of Health, Social Services and Public Safety Northern Ireland (2005) A Healthier Future: A Twenty-year Vision for Health and Well-being in Northern Ireland. Belfast, Department of Health, Social Services and Public Safety Northern Ireland.

Doyle, J. (2008) Barriers and facilitators of multidisciplinary team working: a review. *Paediatric Nursing*, **20** (2), 26–29.

Edwards, E.A., O'Toole, M. & Wallis, C. (2004) Sending children home on tracheostomy dependent ventilation: pitfalls and outcomes. *Archives of Disease in Childhood*, **89**, 251–255.

Fisher, H.R. (2001) The needs of parents with chronically sick children: a literature review. *Journal of Advanced Nursing*, **36** (4), 600–607.

Foundation Trust Network (2005) Foundation Trusts: Future Thinking, Challenges and Change. London, The NHS Confederation Publications.

Francis, R. (2013) Report of the Mid Staffordshire NHS Foundation Trust Public Inquiry. London, The Stationery Office.

Glendinning, C. & Kirk, S. (2000) High tech care: high skilled parents. *Paediatric Nursing*, **12** (6), 25–27.

Greco, V. & Sloper, P. (2004) Care coordination and key worker schemes for disabled children: results of a UK wide survey. *Child, Care, Health and Development*, **30**, 13–20.

Guest, A., Rittey, C. & O'Brien, K. (2005) Telemedicine: helping neurologically impaired children to stay at home. *Paediatric Nursing*, **17** (2), 20–22.

Ham, C., Charles, A. & Wellings, D. (2018) Shared responsibility for health: the cultural change we need. London, The King's Fund. https://www.kingsfund.org.uk/publications/shared-responsibility-health Accessed 31/1/2020.

Health Education England (2015) Raising the Bar: Shape of Caring A Review of the Future Education and Training of Registered Nurses and Care Assistants. London, Health Education England.

Hewitt-Taylor, J. (2005) Caring for children with complex needs: staff education and training. *Journal of Child Health Care*, **9** (1), 72–86.

Hinde, S., Allgar, V., Richardson, G., *et al.* (2016) An evaluation of the costs and consequences of children's community nursing teams. *Journal of Evaluation in Clinical Practice*, **23** (4), 767–772.

Kennedy, I., Howard, R., Jarman, B., *et al.* (2001) Learning from Bristol: The Report of the Public Inquiry into Children's Heart Surgery at the Bristol Royal Infirmary 1984–1995. Norwich, The Stationery Office.

King, A., Herron, S., Mckinstry, R., *et al.* (2006) A multidisciplinary health care team's efforts to improve educational attainment in children with sickle cell anaemia and cerebral infarcts. *Journal of School Health*, **76**, 33–37.

Kings Fund (2011) Case Management: What It Is and How It Can Best Be Implemented? London: The Kings Fund.

Laming, W.H. (2003) The Victoria Climbie Inquiry – Report of an Inquiry by Lord Laming Presented to Parliament by the Secretary of State for Health and the Secretary of State for the Home Department by Command of Her Majesty. Norwich, The Stationery Office.

Laming, The Lord (2009) The Laming Report. The Protection of Children in England: A Progress Report. London, The Stationery Office.

LeBovidge, J.S., Lavigne, J.V. & Miller, M.L. (2005) Adjustment to chronic arthritis of childhood: the roles of illness related stress and attitude towards illness. *Journal of Pediatric Psychology*, **30** (3), 273–286.

Lenehan, C. (2017). These are our children. London, Council for Disabled Children. https://www.ncb.org.uk/sites/default/files/field/attachment/These%20are%20Our%20CHildren_Lenehan_Review_Report.pdf Accessed 31/01/20.

Margolan, H., Fraser, J. & Lenton, S. (2004) Parental experiences of services when their child requires long-term ventilation. Implications for commissioning and providing services. *Child: Care, Health and Development*, **30** (3), 257–264.

Marmot, M. (2010) A review of health inequalities in England. www.instituteofhealthequity.org Accessed 31/01/20.

McCann, D., Bull, R. & Wizenberg, T. (2012) The daily patterns of time use for parents of children with complex needs: a systematic review. *Journal of Child Health Care*, **16** (1), 26–52.

McGirr, D. & Richardson-Reed, S. (2018) Interprofessional working with children and young people. In: *Essentials of Nursing Children and Young People* (eds J. Price & O. Mc Alinden), pp. 66–80. London, Sage.

McNamara-Goodger, K. (2017) Transitional care for children and young people with life threatening or life limiting conditions. In: *Children and Young People's Nursing Principles for Practice (second edition)* (eds R. Davies & A. Davies), pp. 247–262. London, Hodder Arnold.

Moore, A., Anderson, C., Carter, B., *et al.* (2010) Appropriated landscapes: the intrusion of technology and equipment into the homes and lives of families with a child with complex needs. *Journal of Child Health Care*, **14** (1), 3–5.

Munro, E. (2011) Munro Review of Child Protection: A Child Centred System. London, Department of Education.

National Collaborating Centre for Cancer (2005) Improving Outcomes in Children and Young People with Cancer: The Manual. London, National Institute for Health and Clinical Excellence.

National Health Service Digital (2015) Health and Wellbeing of 15 Year Olds in England: Findings from the What About Youth? Survey 2014. https://files.digital.nhs.uk/publicationimport/pub19xxx/pub19244/what-about- youth-eng-2014-rep.pdf Accessed 31/01/20.

National Health Service Digital (2018) Mental Health of Children and Young People in England, 2017 [PAS]. https://digital.nhs.uk/data-and-information/publications/statistical/mental-health-of-children-and-young-people-in-england/2017/2017 Accessed 31/01/20.

National Health Service England (2010) Safe and Sustainable: The Need for Change. London, NHS England.

National Health Service England (2018) NHS Youth Forum Activity and Impact Report 2013–17. London, NHS England.

National Health Service England (2019) The NHS Long Term plan. www.longtermplan.nhs.uk Accessed 31/01/20.

National Health Service Scotland (2010) Advanced Nursing Practice Roles: Guidance for NHS Boards. Edinburgh, Scottish Government.

National Leadership and Innovation Agency for Healthcare (2010) Framework for Advanced Nursing, Midwifery, and Allied Health Professional Practice in Wales. Cardiff, NLIAH.

National Specialised Commissioning Group (2010) Children's Heart Surgery: The Need for Change. London, NSCG.

Noyes, J. (2002) Barriers that delay children and young people who are dependent on mechanical ventilators from being discharged from hospital. *Journal of Clinical Nursing*, **11** (1), 2–11.

Noyes, J., Pritchard, A., Rees, S., *et al.* (2014) *Bridging the Gap: Transition from Children's to Adult Palliative Care*. Bangor, Bangor University.

Nursing and Midwifery Council (2007) Advanced Nursing Practice Update. London, NMC.

Nursing and Midwifery Council (2018) The Code: Professional Standards of Practice and Behaviour for Nurses, Midwives and Nursing Associates. London, Nursing and Midwifery Council.

Nursing and Midwifery Council (2019) Evaluation of Post-registration Standards of Proficiency for Specialist Community Public Health Nurses and the Standards for Specialist Education and Practice Standards. Nursing and Midwifery Council. London, NMC.

Pillas, D., Marmot, M., Naicker, K., *et al.* (2014) Social inequalities in early childhood health and development: a European-wide systematic review. *Pediatric Research*, **76**, 418–424.

Pollard, K., Thomas, J. & Miers, M. (2010) *Understanding Interprofessional Working in Health and Social Care: Theory and Practice*. Basingstoke, Palgrave Macmillan.

Price, S. (2018) Community care and care in non-hospital settings for children and young people. In: *Essentials of Nursing Children and Young People*. (eds J. Price & O. Mc Alinden). pp. 101–119. London, Sage.

Redfern, M., Keeling, J.W. & Powell, E. (2001) The Royal Liverpool Children's Inquiry. London, House of Commons.

Robinson, C. & Jackson, P. (1999) Children's Hospices: A Lifeline for Families? London, National Children's Bureau.

Rolfe, G. (2014) A New Vision for Advanced Nursing Practice. *Nursing Times*, **110** (28), 18–21.

Royal College of Nursing (2014) The Future for Community Children's Nursing: Challenges and Opportunities. London, RCN.

Royal College of Nursing (2017) RCN Credentialing for Advanced Level Nursing Practice. London, RCN Professional Services.

Royal College of Nursing (2020) Futureproofing Children's Community Nursing. London, RCN.

Royal College of Paediatrics and Child Health (2012) Bringing Networks to Life – An RCPCH Guide to Implementing Clinical Networks. London, RCPCH.

Royal College of Paediatrics and Child Health (2018a) Child Health in England in 2030: Comparisons with Other Wealthy Countries. https://www.rcpch.ac.uk/resources/child-health-england-2030- comparisons-other-wealthy-countries Accessed 31/1/20.

Royal College of Paediatrics and Child Health (2018b) The Case for Investing in Children and Young People's Diabetes Services | RCPCH. https://www.rcpch.ac.uk/resources/case-investing-children-young-peoples-diabetes-services Accessed 31/1/20.

Royal College of Paediatrics and Child Health (2019). State of Child Health England -Two Years On. London, RCPCH.

Royal College of Paediatrics and Child Health, Royal College of General Practitioners and Royal College of Nursing (2015) Facing the Future: Together for Child Health. London, RCPCH.

SCIE (2009) An introduction to Interprofessional and Interagency Collaboration. London, SCIE.

Scottish Executive (2005) Building a Health Service Fit for the Future. Edinburgh, Scottish Executive.

Scottish Government (2016) Getting it Right for Every Child (GIRFEC). Edinburgh, Scottish Government.

Shaw, J. & Barker, M. (2004) 'Expert patient' dream or nightmare. *British Medical Journal*, **32** (7442), 723–724.

Smith-Stoner, M. (2011) Webcasting in home and hospice care services. *Home Healthcare Nurse*, **29**, 337–341.

TEIS UK (2004) Telemedicine and E-Health Information Service. www.teis.nhs.uk Accessed 31/01/20.

Valentine, F. & McNee, P. (2007) Context of care and service delivery. *In: Nursing Children and Young People with Chronic Illness* (eds. F. Valentine & L. Lowes), pp. 29–54. Oxford, Blackwell.

Vickers, J., Thompson, A., Collins, G.S., *et al.* (2007) Place and provision of palliative care for children with progressive cancer: a study by the paediatric oncology nurses forum/United Kingdom children's cancer study group palliative care working group. *Journal of Clinical Oncology*, **25**, 4472–4476.

Walker, S. (2012) Effective Social Work with Children and Families: Putting Systems Theory into Practice. London, Sage.

Wang, K. & Barnard, A. (2004) Technology-dependent children and their families: a review. *Journal of Advanced Nursing*, **45** (1), 36–46.

Wanless, D. (2002) Securing our Future Health: Taking a Long Term View. Final Report. London, HM Treasury.

Welsh Assembly Government (2004) Nurturing the Future: A Framework for Realising the Potential of Children's Nurses in Wales. Cardiff, Welsh Assembly Government.

Welsh Assembly Government (2005a) National Service Framework for Children, Young People and Maternity Service in Wales. Cardiff, Welsh Assembly Government.

Welsh Assembly Government (2005b) Designed for Life: Creating World Class Health and Social Care for Wales in the 21st Century. Cardiff, Welsh Assembly Government.

Welsh Government (2012) Children and Young People's Continuing Care Guidance. Cardiff, Welsh Government.

Welsh Government (2019) A Healthier Wales: Our Plan for Health and Social Care. Cardiff, Welsh Government.

Wickham, S., Anwar, E., Carr, B., *et al.* (2016) Poverty and child health in the UK: Using evidence for action. *Archives of Disease in Childhood*, **101**,759–766.

Whiting, M. (2004) The future of community children's nursing. *Archives of Disease in Childhood*, **89**, 987–988.

Whiting, L., Roberts, S., Petty, J., *et al.* (2018) Work of the NHS England Youth Forum and its effect on health services. *Nursing Children and Young People* http.//doi: 10.7748/ncyp.2018.e1074.

CHAPTER 3

Impact upon the Child and Parents

Dawn Daniel and Mandy Brimble

Introduction

When a child is diagnosed with a long-term condition, this is often a life-changing event for the whole family. The consequences of such a diagnosis are multiple and ongoing losses. From a parental perspective, these losses can include loss of control, loss of identity and relinquishing the vision of a future with a healthy child (Smith *et al.*, 2015). As changes are made to accommodate the needs of the child, the whole family is presented with challenges that may upset the equilibrium of their daily lives. However, a diagnosis of long-term childhood illness does not only impact upon the family during the peri-diagnostic period, it can have a significant impact upon their life and lifestyle over many years (Lowes, 2007).

Aim of the chapter

The purpose of this chapter is to critically examine the impact of a long-term condition diagnosis on the child and parents, and to identify factors that may contribute to family stress and disruption during the peri-diagnostic period. Issues will be explored from the perspectives of the affected child and parents both immediately and up to 12 months post diagnosis. The impact on siblings will be discussed separately in Chapter 4. This chapter does not intend to be all inclusive concerning the possible impact of childhood long-term illness on the child and family, but to raise an awareness of the topic and the associated theories to stimulate further learning. Issues will be explored within a theoretical framework of grief, loss, change, adjustment and adaptation, which will allow the impact of long-term illness to be considered from various standpoints, including cultural influences. The impact of long-term illness on finances, employment, socialising and relationships within the family will also be examined. Type 1 diabetes in childhood is used as a case study to introduce, examine

Nursing Care of Children and Young People with Long-Term Conditions, Second Edition.
Edited by Mandy Brimble and Peter McNee.
© 2021 John Wiley & Sons Ltd. Published 2021 by John Wiley & Sons Ltd.

and apply some of the theories and social and practical issues that may confront families of children with long-term conditions.

Intended learning outcomes

- To analyse models and theories of grief, loss, change, adjustment and adaptation, and how they apply to children with long-term conditions and their families
- To examine how childhood long-term conditions can impact emotionally, socially and practically on the child and family, taking cultural influences into account
- To explore the effect of childhood long-term illness on the child and family, the factors that may contribute to family stress and conflict, and consider these issues in the context of family-centred care
- To explore the role of the children's nurse in helping children and parents cope with, and adapt to, a diagnosis of long-term illness

Theories of grief, loss and change

The period immediately following a diagnosis of childhood long-term illness is often an anxious and distressing time for the whole family. Parents may find it difficult to come to terms with the diagnosis, which they may view as the end of 'normal' health and a familiar lifestyle. Parents often talk about the loss of the normal healthy child they thought they had (Lowes & Lyne, 2000; Ward, 2011). The profound impact of the diagnosis on family life often triggers feelings of grief arising from the losses imposed by the long-term condition (Smith *et al.*, 2015). Some parents experience a more enduring grief known as 'chronic sorrow' (Bowes *et al.*, 2009; Coughlin & Sethares, 2017; Rifshana *et al.*, 2017). Grief experienced in the context of childhood long-term illness may not have an endpoint and needs to be considered well beyond the time of diagnosis. Some theories of grief, loss and change are introduced here to provide a framework for the discussion throughout this chapter.

Reflection

Before reading the next section, take a few minutes to reflect on your own knowledge and experiences, and identify key points that arise from your understanding of loss and grief.

Much of the work that has been undertaken on grief, as a response to loss, has focused on the bereaved or care of the dying. However, it is well recognised that a diagnosis of long-term illness can trigger a similar grief response in affected individuals and their families (Smith *et al.*, 2015; Pate, 2016; Koch & Jones, 2018) and this is discussed later in the chapter. As you read the following section, you may find it helpful to try to relate the theories of grief, loss and change to the grief response that may arise from losses incurred by a diagnosis of childhood long-term illness. A classic *stage theory* developed by Kubler-Ross (1970) has played a major role in increasing understanding about the grieving process. Kubler-Ross describes five stages of emotional reaction to death and dying: denial, anger, bargaining, depression and acceptance.

The belief that the experience of loss can be divided into stages is common to many grief theories, some of which suggest there is a sequential progression through these stages, which vary in definition depending on the theoretical perspective (Kamm, 1985; Clubb, 1991; Worden, 1995). Traditional *stage* or *time-bound theories* about grief are often developed through work undertaken with the bereaved. They describe similar end stages such as acceptance (Kubler-Ross, 1970) and resolution (Engel, 1962). However, the experience of grief is unique to each individual and influenced by numerous factors, such as the type of loss, circumstances leading up to the loss, and personal, cultural and social values and beliefs (Worden, 1995). Parents can experience negative emotions in addition to sorrow. Some of the emotions can be anger, fear, frustration, and a sense of helplessness (Pate, 2016; Koch & Jones, 2018). Thus, different stages of grieving vary in their intensity for individuals and may not be experienced in their entirety by all, with no predetermined order or pattern to the grieving process (Kubler-Ross & Kessler, 2014).

The idea of grief being experienced in stages or phases, while appropriate to the concept of grieving as a process, implies a kind of passivity – something mourners must pass through (Worden, 1995). Worden discusses *adaptation to loss* in the context of four basic grief tasks: to accept the reality of the loss, to work through the pain of grief, to adjust to the environment of the loss, and to emotionally relocate the deceased (the loss) and move on with life. Worden (1995) believes that tasks offer mourners hope through purposeful activity, which can help overcome feelings of helplessness, but suggests that incomplete mourning can result if all these tasks are not accomplished. The reaction of parents following diagnosis of a long-term illness can include disbelief, confusion, fear, inability to cope, anger and tension (Al-Gamal & Long, 2010). The grief from a long-term condition is related to an ongoing situation of loss. This situation has been referred to in the literature as *anticipatory loss* (Green, 2006; Al-Gamal & Long, 2010), *chronic grief* (Olshansky, 1962; George *et al.*, 2006) and at times *chronic sorrow* (Roos, 2002; Lichtenstein, *et al.*, 2002; Gordon, 2009).

Traditional theories propose that the grieving process normally results in acceptance or resolution, with failure to reach this stage seen as an abnormal response (Moayedoddin & Markowitz, 2015). However, some authors who have studied long-term illness believe it may be very difficult to reach this stage and suggest that failure to achieve acceptance or resolution is not 'abnormal' (Lowes *et al.*, 2005; Kepreotes *et al.*, 2010). Grief may be perpetual, with periods of remission and periods of intensification (Batchelor & Duke, 2019). The perception of grief as a recurring state may have implications for parental adaptation to the diagnosis of childhood long-term illness because, as Clubb (1991) suggests, parents of children with long-term illness may never reach the acceptance or closure stages of time-bound theories. This is because the affected child serves as a constant reminder of the loss, which consequently inhibits resolution of the grief response (Compas *et al.*, 2011; Christie & Khatun, 2019). For example, parents of a child with type 1 diabetes are constantly reminded about the loss of their 'healthy child' when insulin must be administered at least twice a day. Even if the treatment becomes 'part of their daily lives' (Lowes *et al.*, 2004; Compas *et al.*, 2011), their grief may resurface under certain circumstances, such as their child moving to a new school or restrictions on employment choices. Thus, when exploring grief in long-term illness, theories that analyse grief in the context of bereavement may not be wholly applicable (George *et al.*, 2006; Michalopoulos, 2006).

Chronic sorrow is an approach that views the parental reaction to childhood long-term illness as one of functional adaptation to, but not acceptance of, the child's condition (Coughlin & Sethares, 2017; Hockenberry *et al.*, 2019). Chronic sorrow does not resolve over time, and is defined as a frequent sadness, intermingled with phases of neutrality, satisfaction and happiness (Lowes & Lyne, 2000; George *et al.*, 2006). Olshansky (1962) introduced the theory of chronic sorrow to explain the response of lifelong intermittent sadness in parents of children with impaired cognitive abilities. He proposed that parents never fully recover from the impact stage and, although they adjust and adapt to the situation, this does not represent acceptance. So Olshansky (1962) argued that parents of children with long-term illness never reach the closure stage of time-bound grief models and defines chronic sorrow as a normal response to continuing loss. Alternatively, other seminal work by Solnit and Stark (1961) described chronic sorrow as a disturbance to traditional time-bound grief theories. Later, the work of Copley and Bodensteiner (1987) further developed the theory of chronic sorrow. They identified two phases of reaction to loss in parents of children with disability. The first phase being impact, denial and grief, experienced as a cycle of emotional peaks and troughs. This leads to the second phase, within which parents develop coping strategies to resolve crises, and start to adapt to their new situation. Emotional turbulence remains, but reduces in the second phase. While sorrow diminishes with time, it never ends (Lowes & Lyne, 2000).

Coughlin and Sethares (2017) suggest that chronic sorrow occurs when there is no hope of a cure, progress or normality. This can be as true for parents who have a child with a long-term condition without cognitive impairment or severe disability as it is for those who do. This is because the former also experience situations which, from time to time, highlight their child's condition. This leads to a resurgence of sadness and guilt or underlines disparities. Examples of this are being unable to wean their child onto solid food and the subsequent effect this has on the nature of family meals and social occasions or the absence of menstruation due to infertility in certain genetic conditions. Disparity is defined as the difference between a parents' current situation and the way they had envisaged their life with the child (Lowes & Lyne, 2000). When working with parents of children with long-term illness, children's nurses need to accept that chronic sorrow exists and use strategies to reduce its impact (Bolch *et al.*, 2012; Glenn, 2015; Rifshana *et al.*, 2017).

⟨□⟩ Key points

- A diagnosis of long-term illness in childhood can trigger a grief response in the child and family.
- Traditional stage or time-bound theories of grief suggest there is a sequential progression through stages of grief culminating in an endpoint such as acceptance.
- In chronic sorrow, grief is believed to be perpetual with no endpoint, such as resolution, and is characterised by phases of remission and episodes of intense grief.
- Children's nurses can use their understanding of the grief experienced by children with long-term illness and their parents to help them adapt and adjust to the demands of the condition.

🕐 **Time out**

- What key physical and social developmental events may trigger a reminder in parents of children/young people with long-term illness?

A diagnosis of childhood long-term illness represents many losses or consequences for families and these will reflect the different stages of their child's physical and social development. Key milestones that may be adversely affected include those associated with communication, social skills, toilet training, play patterns, motor skills and maturation. For example, in younger children, developmental events such as walking and talking may be delayed, or never realised. In older children, maturation may be problematic – for example, some conditions such as Turner syndrome, delay maturation and development – while others – such as spina bifida, cerebral palsy and some endocrine conditions – may cause premature development (Hockenberry *et al.*, 2019). Young people may also experience problems with events related to increasing independence, such as maintaining steady employment or leaving home.

The grief experienced by parents of a child with newly diagnosed diabetes arises from an awareness of the difference between the future that they were expecting and the situation in which they now find themselves (Smith *et al.*, 2015; Rifshana *et al.*, 2017; Batchelor & Duke, 2019). The new situation in which they find themselves after diagnosis is one into which they need to incorporate the demands and challenges of having a child with diabetes (Compas *et al.*, 2011; Smith, 2018).

Reflection

Reflect on how the above theories might apply to children and young people with long-term conditions.

Much of the work on grief and loss in relation to childhood long-term illness has focused on parents, predominantly mothers, as the main carers, and very little work has been undertaken with children with long-term conditions. Contemporary research ethics and governance frameworks make research with children and young people a complex undertaking, but quite rightly so, because children's rights and well-being must take paramount importance over the need for research (Graham *et al.*, 2015). Research that aims to elicit an understanding of people's experiences of loss and grief is usually qualitative in design, with in-depth interviewing being the main data collection method. Some adult respondents have found being interviewed about emotive topics a helpful, even 'therapeutic', activity (Lowes & Gill, 2006; Hopper & Crane, 2019) but in-depth interviewing can bring feelings and emotions hitherto unacknowledged to the fore and it is not known how this may affect children and young people. Selecting a research sample from this population may also be problematic due to different stages of cognitive, emotional and physical development potentially affecting how children and young people experience loss and grief.

It is difficult to estimate the impact of a diagnosis of long-term illness on a child's life because this will be determined by a number of influencing factors, including age at diagnosis, stage of development, gender, personality, temperament and coping styles (Compas *et al.*, 2011). The impact will also be influenced by the characteristics of the long-term condition, including nature of onset, disease trajectory, effects on appearance, effects on daily functioning, effects on behaviour and ability to relate to others and the care required (World Health Organisation (WHO), 2011). It is also likely that the impact on the child will be influenced by parental response and coping (Compas *et al.*, 2011). For example, children whose social activities are severely restricted due to parental over-concern about safety might experience a greater loss of freedom (Lowes, 2007).

Initial impact

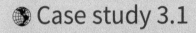

Case study 3.1

Background information

Josie is an 11-year-old girl who developed type 1 diabetes two weeks ago. Her father (42 years of age) is Caribbean, has lived in England for 20 years and is employed as a store manager for a large national computer company. Her mother (39 years of age) is white British and a part-time hairdresser at a local salon. Josie was born in England and has a 13-year-old brother and a 4-year-old sister. The family are social class 2 (based on the National Statistics Socio-Economic Classification (NS-SEC)) and live in a cul-de-sac of four-bedroomed modern detached houses in a semi-rural village. Josie has been attending the local primary school for the past five years but will be transferring to the local comprehensive school in four months' time. Her widowed paternal grandmother lives in Antigua, and her maternal grandparents live a hundred miles away in Leeds and work full time in a family run hardware store. No other family members are known to have diabetes.

Test your knowledge

- What are the classic sequential symptoms that indicate a diagnosis of type 1 diabetes?
- What are the essential elements of type 1 diabetes management?
- Why is it important to obtain and sustain optimal glycaemic control?

Type 1 diabetes

Type 1 diabetes is one of the most common lifelong childhood disorders. In 2013, the incidence in the UK was 24.5 per 100,000 of 0–14-year-olds, the 5th highest in the world, with Finland being the highest at 57.6. The cause is not fully understood (Diabetes

UK, 2019a). A lack or relative insufficiency of insulin results in hyperglycaemia, poly-uria, polydipsia, lethargy and weight loss (Holt *et al.*, 2016). If untreated, severe fluid, electrolyte and acid–base disturbances will lead to vomiting, dehydration, coma and death (National Institute for Clinical Excellence (NICE), 2015). The management of childhood diabetes is relentless and invasive, involving two or more insulin injec-tions a day, blood glucose monitoring up to four times a day, a healthy diet and regular exercise. In addition to the short-term complications of diabetic ketoacidosis and hypo-glycaemia, poor glycaemic control increases the risk of life-threatening microvascular and neurological complications in later life (Diabetes UK, 2019b).

For more information on type 1 diabetes and its management, readers are referred to the suggested reading list and websites at the end of this chapter.

Impact on parents

Taking the case study as an example, parents of a child with newly diagnosed diabetes have been found to experience a grief response similar to that normally associated with bereavement (Rifshana *et al.*, 2017) and a diagnosis of childhood diabetes may repre-sent multiple losses to Josie's parents.

🕐 Time out

- Consider what losses you think may be experienced by parents of a child with newly diagnosed childhood diabetes.

Feelings of loss will vary from family to family depending upon, for example, their view of the world, their past experience, the extent to which their life needs to change and their expectations of the future. Losses that Josie's parents may experience include the loss of the healthy child they thought they had, loss of a certain lifestyle, loss of free-dom, loss of former support systems, loss of social acceptance, potential loss of their child's life, and a loss of confidence in their ability to protect their child from danger (Lowes *et al.*, 2004; 2005; Rankin *et al.*, 2016; Couglin & Sethares, 2017; Hockenberry *et al.*, 2019).

Following the diagnosis, Josie's parents are likely to experience a range of emo-tions such as disbelief, anger, sadness, guilt, anxiety, fear and confusion (Flynn, 2013; Rankin *et al.*, 2016). For some time after diagnosis, diabetes will be at the forefront of Josie's parents' thoughts. They will have received a lot of information about diabetes and its management in addition to having to learn the practical skills of insulin administration and blood glucose monitoring (Rankin *et al.*, 2016). Josie's father works long hours as a store manager and it will fall to Josie's mother to take responsibility for the day-to-day management of her daughter's condition. This includes thinking about the timing and content of meals, and how her new responsibilities will fit in with her part-time job as a hairdresser. Helgeson *et al.* (2012) state that parents of chil-dren with diabetes may experience post-traumatic stress disorder and both Whittemore *et al.* (2012) and Pinquart (2019) identified depressive symptoms in parents of children with long-term health conditions. These effects may interfere with parents' ability to manage their child's condition.

Indeed, parents may find that having a child with a long-term illness impinges on almost all aspects of their life, including finances, employment, childcare, parenting, marital relationships and roles, sibling relationships and socialising (Smith *et al.*, 2015; Nabors *et al.*, 2019). One or both parents must devote extra time and attention to help their child cope with the demands of the condition. This can create problems; for example, with conflict about disciplining the affected child, sibling rivalry, attention seeking behaviour and disagreement about approaches to parenting or management of the long-term condition. Childcare becomes difficult, either because parents are worried about handing over the care of their child to untrained or inexperienced carers, or because carers are concerned about taking responsibility for routine medication or managing potential emergency situations (Coughlin & Sethares, 2017). This can affect the parents' ability to work outside the family home, which in turn may reduce the family income. Childcare difficulties may also severely curtail the social activities of children with a long-term illness and their parents (Kish *et al.*, 2018).

⟨🔑⟩ **Key points**

- A diagnosis of long-term illness can represent a number of losses for affected children/young people and their families.
- The presence of long-term illness in childhood can impinge on almost all aspects of family life.

It is important to remember, however, that some parents of young people with a long-term illness may identify positive aspects of the parenting experience, including recognising family strengths and adopting a healthier lifestyle (Compas *et al.*, 2011).

🕐 **Time out**

- Consider how a diagnosis of long-term illness might impact on children and young people at different developmental stages; for example, preschool, school-age and adolescent.

Impact on the child/young person with a long-term illness

A diagnosis of a long-term illness will have a significant effect on the child. Children with long-term conditions are confronted with a complex interpersonal situation – they have to cope with the fact that their condition is not only affecting their own lives but also those of their parents and siblings (Compas *et al.*, 2011; Hockenberry *et al.*, 2019;

Christie & Khatun, 2019). In addition, while coping with the unique demands of their condition, they also have to navigate the developmental tasks associated with their particular age group (Compas *et al.*, 2011).

A child's stage of development will affect their response to the diagnosis. Although infants (0–2 years of age) will clearly not realise the implications of having a long-term condition, the process of bonding between the parents and infant may be affected. Management of the condition and extended periods of illness or hospitalisation can interfere with 'normal' interaction between the infant and parents (Nabors *et al.*, 2019) and create difficulties with attachment (Tallon *et al.*, 2015). Having a long-term condition is stressful for toddlers and preschool children. Their drive for autonomy and self-control may be hindered due to the restrictions and effects of a long-term illness, and if parents are overprotective, they may lose independence and the opportunity to meet developmental tasks. They will be unable to understand the rationale for, sometimes painful, treatment and their developing self-concept may be strongly influenced by the condition and discomfort experienced (Hockenberry *et al.*, 2019). Preschool children with a long-term illness are at an emotionally vulnerable age and their condition and treatment may adversely affect their feelings of security, their self-esteem and perception of their body image (Kopel & Eiser, 2013). Preschool children often have a 'literal' grasp of language, which has implications both for them and for health care providers. For example, a 4-year-old child who is told that he/she has diabetes might well understand this as meaning he/she is going to 'die of the betes', a frightening misinterpretation, particularly if they feel unable to voice their fears. It is important, therefore, that a child's understanding is assessed and any misinterpretations corrected. Primary school-age children enter the stage of concrete operational thought (Piaget, 1962) at about 7 years of age, when they have an increased ability to understand their condition but only in the present (Kopel & Eiser, 2013). School-age children (6–11 years of age) develop their sense of identity, belonging and self-esteem through involvement and acceptance by their peers (Kopel & Eiser, 2013), and this process can be affected by the presence of a long-term illness. In adolescence, peer relationships take on even greater importance, often to the detriment of family relationships, as young people face the major developmental task of establishing independence from parents. Limitations imposed by a long-term condition can complicate this struggle for autonomy as young people try to integrate management of the condition into their lives (Malik & Koot, 2009; Hockenberry *et al.*, 2019). (Long term illness in adolescence is discussed in detail in Chapters 10 and 11.)

At 11 years of age, Josie is coming to a stage in her life when she is beginning to strive for a degree of independence from her parents, maybe going to friends' houses for sleepovers or to the local shops with friends at weekends. These activities are made more difficult in the presence of diabetes because she now has to consider issues such as insulin injections, blood glucose monitoring and regular consumption of carbohydrates. She has to try to avoid and, when necessary, recognise and treat hypoglycaemic episodes. Her increasing shift towards independence may be hindered due to parental concerns about safety issues and she may start to feel different to her friends who are not subject to these restrictions. Feeling 'different' is often a major problem for school-age children with a long-term condition.

Children with a long-term illness are presented with unique problems in school, where they may encounter a range of academic, social and emotional challenges (Gannoni & Shute, 2010). Depending upon the age of the child and the demands of the long-term condition, they and their parents may rely heavily upon support from school staff to help the child cope with their disease management away from home. Children with long-term conditions such as diabetes, epilepsy, asthma and cystic fibrosis may require some form of intervention during the school day. It is essential that social integration and education are a primary focus within schools and early year provision for children or young people with diabetes (Royal College of Nursing (RCN), 2013). The Equality Act (2010) states that education providers have a duty to ensure reasonable adjustments are made to enable children and young people with diabetes have their needs met. In order for this to occur, it is crucial that staff in schools and early years settings receive appropriate training, advice and support from health services and children's diabetes specialist services (RCN, 2013). To help children cope with a long-term illness in school, a multidisciplinary and interagency approach (see Chapter 2) is essential.

Key points

- It is important that children who are chronically ill are enabled to integrate the management of their condition into school life, participating in sports/activities and achieving their full academic potential.
- To achieve this, there needs to be effective communication between the child and family, school staff and health professionals, including the school nurse and the primary and secondary health care teams.

Before Josie returned to school following her diagnosis, it was important that the children's diabetes specialist nurse educated school staff about diabetes and the extra care and support that Josie would need (RCN, 2013), particularly in relation to hypoglycaemic episodes. This was relatively straightforward in Josie's primary school setting, where her class teacher assumed primary responsibility for her care. However, this will be more difficult when Josie moves to high school where she will move between a range of classrooms and teachers. Although the ideal solution is to regularly educate all school staff about diabetes at an inset day, this is sometimes not possible due to increasingly full agendas at these sessions. Therefore, responsibility for the care of children with long-term conditions often falls to the designated first aider and/or the head of year.

Time out

- Think of four factors that may influence how successfully Josie copes with diabetes management in school.

You may have thought about:

- The level of teachers' knowledge and understanding of diabetes.
- The understanding and support of her peer group and immediate circle of friends.
- The provision of somewhere private to go to undertake blood glucose monitoring.

- Josie's confidence to deal with situations such as hypoglycaemic episodes.
- Whether she is subjected to teasing or bullying for being 'different'.
- Is she included unconditionally on school trips or do the school insist that a family member accompanies her?
- Whether she received support from the school nurse.

School nurses are fundamental to helping children and young people with a long-term illnesses integrate the management of their condition into school life. They have a pivotal role in ensuring effective communication between children with a long-term illness and their parents, teachers and other health care professionals. They also have a remit, alongside specialist health care professionals, to educate school staff about specific long-term conditions and their implications for school life.

Continuing care

Gender differences

Historically, research has shown that girls and boys manage long-term conditions in different ways (Williams, 2000; Arrington-Sanders *et al.*, 2006; Vlassoff, 2007). In both Williams' (2000) study and Vlassoff's (2007) review, the majority of girls showed greater adaptation than boys, incorporating their condition and associated treatment regimens into their social and personal identities. Further, Arrington-Sanders *et al.* (2006) found that adolescent females used more emotion-orientated and problem-orientated strategies than males in relation to coping with cystic fibrosis. Josie's positive transition to high school suggests that she has successfully integrated diabetes into her life outside the home environment.

Parental control

Nevertheless, at a clinic visit, it transpired that there was conflict between Josie and her mother concerning her mother's reluctance to allow Josie the freedom she enjoyed pre-diagnosis. Research has shown that parents, especially mothers, are often afraid to 'let go' following a diagnosis of childhood diabetes (Lowes *et al.*, 2004). Problems with 'letting go' arise mainly from a parental fear that their child might have a severe hypoglycaemic episode when out alone or with friends and no one will know how to treat it. Parents need to feel in control of the diabetes management. This is a difficult problem to resolve because it is important that Josie socialises with her peer group, but equally important that her mother's concerns are addressed. Josie's father suggested that he buy her a mobile phone, thus allowing easy contact between Josie and her mother, a solution that pleased Josie and offered some reassurance to her mother.

Metabolic control

Khanolkar *et al.* (2017) found that children and young people with type 1 diabetes from ethnic minorities living in England and Wales had significantly poorer metabolic control. This related to educational background and insufficient language skills. Josie's mixed-race parentage does not seem to have been problematic in relation to her family's adaptation to the diagnosis. The family are highly respected in the community. Her father has lived in the UK for many years, speaks very good English and holds a well-paid and influential position in a large national company. The family diet is healthy and varied. Although Josie's mother sometimes cooks African-Caribbean meals, she now avoids typical sweet dishes and concentrates on starchy foods (e.g. yam, sweet potato, rice, hard dough bread), fruit and vegetables (e.g. banana, mango, melon, okra, pepper), meat, fish and other protein alternatives (e.g. kidney beans, black-eye beans, lentils).

🕐 Time out

- Can you identify characteristics of specific cultures and religions that may impact on a family's ability to adapt and adjust to a diagnosis of long-term illness in childhood?

Religion and culture

Religion and culturally different beliefs about health and illness can influence coping, adaptation and adjustment to a diagnosis of a long-term illness. For example, in Vietnamese culture, it is disrespectful to ask a doctor a question. The Vietnamese value and appreciate services and believe it is disloyal to question (Donovan & Williams, 2015), which has implications for successful, patient-centred long-term illness management. In some cultures (e.g. India, China and Japan), parents of a child with a long-term illness such as type 1 diabetes or epilepsy will fear social stigmatisation, which may result in families being burdened with a sense of shame and lead to secrecy about the condition (Hockenberry *et al.*, 2019). Dietary management of certain conditions, such as diabetes, may be affected by religious beliefs. Muslim families, for example, may wish to observe Ramadan, which requires fasting from sunrise to sunset, although diabetes is one condition that exempts affected individuals from keeping this rule. Some religious beliefs can result in more serious outcomes. For example, Jehovah's Witnesses believe that blood represents life itself and may consequently refuse blood transfusions even in life-threatening situations, and members of the Church of the First Born believe in prayer rather than medicines to treat the sick. The consequences of this are discussed by Bulman (2017) who reported the case of a 15-year-old boy who died of complications from untreated diabetes. Chapter 5 also discusses psychosocial issues in relation to culture and spirituality in the context of long-term illness in childhood.

Coping, adaptation and change

A diagnosis of childhood diabetes represents a major stressor for parents (Whittemore *et al.*, 2012; Rankin *et al.*, 2016). Parents may approach the process of coping in a variety of ways and these will be influenced by a number of interpersonal and environmental factors. Over the four months since diagnosis, Josie's parents will have used various strategies to help them cope with the changes to their lifestyle necessitated by the diagnosis. Some theories of coping, adaptation and change are introduced below.

Coping strategies that may be used by parents of children with long-term illnesses are also discussed.

Reflection

Think about the last time you experienced stress. Reflect on how you coped with this and the strategies you use to resolve or minimise the stress.

Theories of stress and coping

Coping, or how a person responds to a stressful event, is important in managing stress (Compas *et al.*, 2011). Traditionally, stress has been deemed to be either the physiological and/or psychological response to a threatening or demanding situation (response-based model) or a reaction to an event/set of circumstances which threatens a person's well-being (stimulus-based model). However, neither of these models consider the meaning of events to those who experience them (Blount *et al.*, 2008). Families cope with change in a variety of ways and consequently many theories about coping have been developed.

In this chapter, two theories relating to stress, coping, adaptation and change are introduced: the *family adaptation model* (Roy, 2009) and the classic *cognitive appraisal and coping* model (Lazarus & Folkman, 1984), both of which recognise the numerous factors that may influence individual responses to the same stress experience.

The family adaptation model

Roy's adaptation model (2009) is based on family care-givers' experiences of caring for patients with long-term conditions. It describes the individual as responding to a stressor event through the four phases of adaptive modes. These are the physiological function mode, self-concept mode, role function mode and interdependence mode. Diaz and Cruz (2018) discuss that according to the stimuli (focal, contextual or residual) this will determine the regulatory and cognitive coping that will define the adaptation of the care-giver.

The family's vulnerability to a crisis is believed to be dependent upon the actual stressor event and prior strains, the family's existing resources and the family's subjective perceptions of the seriousness of the stressor event. Adjustment to the stressor event, therefore, varies with individual families. Some families absorb the change into routine family functioning, whereas for other families more adjustment is necessary and can develop into a crisis. The family's adaptation to caring for a child with a long-term illness is a complex process which involves internal and external factors that influence the responses and how they are able to adapt. For example, if other stressful events happen at the same time as the diagnosis, less energy may be available for coping with the long-term illness.

Cognitive appraisal and coping

According to Lazarus and Folkman (1984) and Folkman *et al.* (1986), coping involves the individual continually altering their behavioural and cognitive responses to external and/or internal demands which they perceive to be beyond their personal resources. The stress experience is moderated by two basic cognitive appraisals, through which people assess the level of threat and their own resources for dealing with it. These appraisals will be influenced by the personal characteristics of individuals, such as patterns of motivation (values, commitments or personal goals), beliefs about themselves and the world and personal recognition of resources for coping (social skills, problem-solving skills or finances). Cognitive appraisals are also influenced by environmental variables, such as the nature of the danger, whether it is imminent, whether it is ongoing or short term and whether it is an ambiguous type of threat or not, as well as the existence and quality of social support (Compas *et al.*, 2011). Other influences on individuals' ability to cope include their previous experiences, existing coping strategies, health status and cognitive ability.

Thus, stress is the product of the interaction between a person and their environment. An event is only stressful if it is perceived as such by the individual. Stress is believed to arise when there is an imbalance between the perceived demand and the perceived capability to cope with that demand (Compas *et al.*, 2011). In a long-term illness such as diabetes, the process of coping entails different challenges, tasks and responses at various points in time (Hockenberry *et al.*, 2019).

Coping strategies

It is important for families to develop coping strategies to help them deal with the overwhelming stress of a long-term condition. Jaser and White (2011) used the Responses to Stresses Questionnaire (RSQ) to explore coping and resilience in young people with type 1 diabetes. Ten commonly encountered stressful situations were examined, including caring for diabetes and dealing with peer groups. They identified that coping strategies could be flexible and could be problem-focused or emotionally-focused. Coping strategies are sometimes described as 'adaptive' or 'maladaptive' (Thompson *et al.*, 2010). *Adaptive strategies* are believed to alleviate stress and re-establish equilibrium, enabling the individual to adjust appropriately while gaining from the experience. Adaptive coping might include understanding what is occurring, recognising demands versus resources and taking action to reduce demands. *Maladaptive strategies* are defined as those that exacerbate existing demands, fail to stabilise the situation and do not allow the individual to adjust, resulting in misery and unhappiness. Maladaptive coping might include failing to recognise and understand what is happening, denial, avoiding situations which produce anxiety and withdrawal from social support (Thompson *et al.*, 2010).

A positive outlook can be a helpful coping strategy, for instance Johnson (2000) found that parents who focused on their child's achievements controlled stress more effectively. Furthermore, some authors, such as Ray (2002) and Whiting (2012), have highlighted positive aspects of caring for a child with a long-term condition, in that the relationship between parent and child and indeed the whole family was strengthened by mutual engagement in caring routines.

 Time out

- Can you think of some coping strategies that Josie's parents might use?

A variety of coping strategies are used by parents of children with a long-term illness. Ganjiwale *et al.* (2016) found in their cross-sectional study of children with special health needs that their parents main coping style was active emotional coping. Seminal work by Carver (1997) outlined a 28-item measure of coping style which was developed from the COPE inventory. There are three coping strategies identified within this: *problem-focused coping* which includes active coping, planning, accessing support and religious support; *active emotional coping* includes venting problems, reframing positive thoughts, use of humour, acceptance and accessing emotional support; last is *avoidant emotional coping* which includes self-distraction, denial, disengagement, self-blame and use of substances. It is clear in Ganjiwale *et al.*'s (2016) study that the type of disability will alter the parents coping style. It is also identified that when the parents were able to accept the diagnosis and condition, this helped them to cope. Furthermore, input from schools and other agencies assisted with acceptance and allowed a positive outlook for the future. In addition, accessing support from support groups, friends and family is helpful. Christie and Khatun (2019) discuss that if parents and children are not involved in information sharing and education about the condition, there is a higher risk of low mood and depression. They discuss that it is important to involve the parents and the child in a collaborative partnership as this can provide an emotional buffer for any negative thoughts and feelings. Consequently, children, young people and their parents can feel more optimistic about their future.

Normalisation

A major coping strategy used by parents of children with a long-term illness is normalisation. The aims of normalisation are to reduce feelings of being different and enable children and their parents to have a sense of control over their lives (Knafl *et al.*, 2010). Children with long-term conditions and their families are faced with several challenges in achieving normalisation. Knafl *et al.* (2010) state that families can define normal according to their needs, experiences and circumstances. The role of the children's nurse is key in encouraging and empowering the family to consider delegating care and family tasks, considering ways to deliver care alongside current routines, ensuring adequate support services are in place, and advocating the child has access to age appropriate activities at home (Knafl & Santacroce, 2010).

🗝 **Key point**

- Parents of children with a long-term illness face difficulties not experienced by other parents (Pinquart, 2019).

The experience of having a child with a long-term illness in the family is extremely demanding, with adjustment and adaptation by the family requiring recurrent modification in response to environmental, social and cognitive pressures (Knafl *et al.*, 2010). Parents use normalising tactics to minimise the effects of, and thereby reduce the impact of, long-term illness (Knafl *et al.*, 2010). Parents define normalisation as a continual process of actively accommodating the shifting physical and emotional needs of the child or young person, with the objective of integrating the child into family life (Kuo *et al.*, 2011).

The children's nurse can assist the family in achieving normalisation through assessment of the family's day to day routines, signposting to social support networks, identifying coping strategies and techniques, and assisting with family and community support. The nurse can assist with empowering the family to gradually take charge of their needs (Hockenberry *et al.*, 2019). The role of the children's diabetes clinical nurse specialist (CNS) is particularly important in leading these activities and/or supporting colleagues to achieve these outcomes.

🕐 **Time out**

- Can you think of some coping strategies that Josie might use?

Coping strategies used by children and young people with long-term conditions will depend upon their personal characteristics, which include level of confidence, self-esteem, usual coping style, view of the world, past experiences, developmental stage, cognitive ability, family structure and dynamics, and how parents, family and friends perceive, and cope with, the condition. Josie has reached a developmental stage where friends are important. She is beginning to want to socialise independently of her parents and siblings. Therefore, Josie might:

- Seek information to become expert about her condition.
- Develop a supportive relationship with her health care team.
- Actively participate in decisions about her care.
- Learn self-care skills to minimise the daily effects of her condition and enhance her self-esteem and autonomy.
- Pursue interests and hobbies.
- Explain the condition, its treatment and the restrictions it imposes to supportive friends.
- Normalise diabetes in the context of her life and lifestyle.

🌐 Case study 3.2

A year after diagnosis

Josie's glycaemic control is deteriorating. She is attending clinic with very few blood glucose readings and her HbA1c (12.3%) indicates that she is probably not administering all of her insulin, the dosage of which has been gradually increased as her body is now producing little or no endogenous insulin. The school nurse has contacted the diabetes team due to a concern about Josie's attendance at school. Josie's mother broke down at their last attendance at clinic and appears to be depressed, partly because coping with Josie's diabetes management is causing conflict within the family unit. A multidisciplinary, inter-agency meeting is to be convened at the school to include Josie and her parents.

Psychosocial problems are not unusual in children and young people with a long-term condition, or their parents (Geist *et al.*, 2003; Guthrie, 2003; Theofanidis, 2007), and may occur for any number of reasons. NICE (2016) *Quality Standards: Diabetes in Children and Young People* recognises that diabetes is often more difficult to control during puberty and adolescence. Children and young people with type 1 diabetes may experience psychological disturbances such as anxiety, behavioural and conduct disorders and family conflict, so it is recommended that they and their families should receive timely and ongoing access to mental health professionals (NICE, 2015; Diabetes UK, 2019b). It is recommended that targeted and specialist services should be available to ensure that parents receive appropriate support, when required, at any time during their child's journey to adulthood. Psychosocial distress in young people with long-term conditions often results in poor adherence to treatment, poor behaviour, acting out, and non-adaptive and risk-taking behaviours (NICE, 2015). The target HbA1c (glycosylated haemoglobin) for children and young people with type 1 diabetes is 7.5% or below (NICE, 2015). Thus, Josie's high HbA1c result is cause for concern, and it is clear that, for whatever reason, she is not receiving sufficient quantities of insulin.

🕐 Time out

- Can you identify why Josie may not be receiving enough insulin?

It may be that Josie is omitting or inappropriately reducing some of her insulin doses, or that she has come out of the honeymoon period (i.e. her pancreatic beta cells are no longer producing insulin) and, because she is doing little or no blood glucose monitoring, she is unaware of her resulting high blood glucose levels. She could be omitting some of her insulin doses to lose weight, which is a common reason, particularly for girls, not to adhere to or comply with the insulin regimen. Although Josie is not overweight, she may have an altered perception of her body image (Falcão & Francisco, 2017). She may be testing the boundaries or simply be 'fed up' with the inconvenience of insulin injections and blood glucose monitoring. She may not want to feel 'different' from her non-diabetic peers and be ignoring her diabetes management to fit in with their relatively unrestricted lifestyle, particularly if she is trying to avoid hypoglycaemic episodes. It is possible that she is rebelling against her parents' strict adherence to diabetes care. She might be experiencing bullying at school, feel that no one appreciates what she has to 'suffer' on a daily basis, or resent her invasive diabetes care becoming an accepted part of her life, whereas immediately after diagnosis she was treated as 'special'. Due to her stage of development, Josie may have a growing awareness of the perpetuity of her condition, be frightened about the future or have an increased sense of her own mortality.

These are just a few scenarios that may have been the catalyst for the deterioration in Josie's glycaemic control. What is clear is that psychosocial issues often impact on glycaemic control and, due to an increased risk of diabetes-related complications in later life (Diabetes UK, 2019b), there is a need to try and resolve the underlying problem. It is sometimes difficult for health professionals to understand why children and young people endure high blood glucose levels for extended periods of time because they will undoubtedly experience polyuria, nocturnal enuresis, polydipsia and lethargy, have mood swings and feel generally below par. Children and young people with poor glycaemic control may have frequent readmissions to hospital with diabetic ketoacidosis (DKA), a life-threatening acute complication of type 1 diabetes. Furthermore, it is not unheard of for children and young people with type 1 diabetes to engineer admissions to hospital to escape a threatening situation.

🔑 Key point

- Children's nurses in the ward environment are in a unique position to develop a trusting relationship with children and young people with long-term illness who suffer repeated readmissions, and work with them and other health professionals to uncover the underlying cause.

Josie's mother is concerned and upset about the HbA1c result, which is an average blood glucose measurement over 6–8 weeks. Parents often view the HbA1c as an 'exam' they have to pass at their child's clinic visit (Lowes *et al.*, 2004) and feel guilty or inadequate if it deteriorates, even if they believe they have done all they can to try and achieve good glycaemic control. This is, perhaps, when the concept of chronic sorrow could be applied. Other parents do not have to worry about these sorts of issues. Repeatedly over time, parents are forced to realise that their child or young person with long-term illness is 'different' under certain circumstances (Pinquart, 2019).

NICE (2015) recommends that children with long-term illness and their parents should be offered structural behavioural intervention strategies for reducing diabetes-related family conflict. Morrison et al. (2003) discussed the benefits a therapeutic model to support parents of children with long-term illness. The therapeutic model assumes that childhood long-term illness and disability can represent a trauma that impacts on day-to-day activities for the whole family, as discussed in the first section of this chapter. The study by Morrison *et al.* (2003) identified that families needed ongoing supportive interventions and counselling, referred to as 'psychological first aid', from diagnosis and at subsequent times of crisis. More recently a Cochrane Systematic review (Law *et al.*, 2019) explored the benefit of therapies such as Cognitive Behavioural Therapy (CBT) or Problem Solving Therapy (PST) as a mechanism to improve parenting skills in those who have a child with a long-term condition.

The multidisciplinary paediatric diabetes team worked with Josie and her parents to try to resolve the problem. The approach included ongoing diabetes education, which was age appropriate and in keeping with Josie's stage of growth and cognitive development (NICE, 2015; Diabetes UK, 2019a). The paediatric diabetes specialist nurse consulted with Josie privately because it was felt that she might be experiencing issues she wished to discuss without her parents present. However, considering Josie's age, if there were problems that were detrimental to her well-being, it may not be possible to maintain confidentiality (legal and ethical issues are discussed in Chapter 7). Josie's parents also found it beneficial to discuss their problems and emotional responses to the diagnosis with an experienced member of the paediatric diabetes team. Although not necessarily applicable to Josie and her parents, some children with a long-term illness and their parents will require referral to a mental health professional with expertise in this area.

The multidisciplinary, interagency meeting at the school, which was attended by Josie and her parents, was convened to address her poor school attendance rate of 42%. It transpired that Josie was finding it difficult to incorporate her diabetes management into school life and felt alienated from her peer group because she perceived herself as 'different', a belief compounded by her mixed race parentage in a school attended by predominantly white Caucasian children. Another problem concerned her friends' parents' reluctance to invite her to sleepovers or birthday outings because they were anxious about taking responsibility for Josie's diabetes management. It was agreed that a 'buddy' system would be put in place, where a close friend would be educated about diabetes, allowed to accompany her to do her pre-lunch blood glucose monitoring and attend the outpatient clinic with her during the school holidays. During the meeting, it was also identified that Josie's parents had been allowing her to stay at home if her blood glucose level was more than 15 mmol/l, because they worried about her becoming unwell at school. They were reassured regarding the unlikelihood of this happening and were offered further education about managing hyperglycaemia. Arrangements were also made for school staff to receive further diabetes education at the next inset day to reassure Josie and her parents about her safety while at school.

These interventions resolved the family conflict, and Josie subsequently improved her diabetes control and school attendance. However, life in the presence of childhood and adolescent diabetes is rarely that simple. Children and young people who present with problems relatively soon after diagnosis often continue to experience difficulty with diabetes management (Diabetes UK, 2019b). Problems change in nature as the young person moves through different developmental stages, presenting children, young people, parents and the paediatric diabetes team with different challenges.

🕐 Time out

- Considering the content of this chapter, what is the role of children's nurses caring for families with a new diagnosis of childhood long-term illness?

Children's nurses should not underestimate the impact that a diagnosis of a long-term illness may have on the lives of children, young people and their parents. Parents will need to make multiple adjustments in order to accommodate the needs of the child, both at the time of diagnosis and long after. Lowes *et al.* (2004) identified that parents will often recall the life that they used to lead compared to the reality of their present situation.

Thus, children's nurses need an in-depth knowledge of the theories of grief, loss, adaptation and change, and need to be able to understand and apply the underlying theoretical principles in the context of the care they provide to children with a long-term illness and their families. They need to maintain an acute awareness of the intense grief that may be experienced by children and their parents, and how this may affect their ability to adapt and adjust to the diagnosis. Insensitivity by children's nurses to the grieving process has the potential to inhibit expression of feelings, make affected children and their parents feel that they should be coping better and result in lowered self-esteem. Children's nurses also need knowledge of child development to be able to recognise maladaption or regression and put preventative or remedial strategies into place.

Children's nurses should be non-judgemental (Nursing and Midwifery Council (NMC), 2018). It is important that they accept that different parents cope in different ways and adapt the care they provide in response to individual need. For example, although some parents of a child with newly diagnosed diabetes may be prepared to inject their child with insulin on the day of diagnosis, others may find this extremely distressing. It is essential that children's nurses also take cultural and religious influences into account when addressing the care of a child with a long-term condition. Is there a need to adapt the dietary management? What are the implications of a diagnosis of a long-term illness in relation to stigma or perceived suitability for marriage, particularly if infertility is a characteristic of the condition?

Children's nurses need to tailor education about a long-term condition to the needs of individual parents. Complex regimens may be difficult to understand, depending upon cognitive ability, and the shock experienced at diagnosis may affect the capability to retain information (Rankin *et al.*, 2016). Language barriers may need to be crossed through the use of trained interpreters or pictorial information. Children's nurses should be able to direct parents to voluntary organisations specific to particular conditions that have information in a variety of languages, or be able to download such information via the internet for families; being mindful to use credible sources.

Children's nurses are often best placed to work with children with a long-term illness admitted to hospital. By developing close relationships with these children and their parents during periods of hospitalisation, children's nurses may be privy to information that could ultimately affect the care they receive (Nabors *et al.*, 2019). They need to liaise closely with specialist teams and share information to ensure that children and their parents receive optimal care during hospitalisation and after discharge home.

Conclusion

Children and young people with a long-term illness, their parents and families are faced with coping with the demands of long-term conditions on a daily basis. They live with a lifestyle that changes, and different problems that arise, as the child passes through developmental stages to adulthood. Grief experienced at diagnosis will subside, but may resurface at particular times in the lives of children and young people with a long-term illness and their parents. Different coping strategies will be used by children and parents to minimise the impact of the diagnosis and normalise the illness within the context of their lives, but their lives will always be different and more complicated than those of families who do not have to contend with the demands of a long-term condition.

Despite the challenges, however, many children and young people with long-term illnesses, and their families, cope extremely well. The case study provided in this chapter was designed to illustrate how a diagnosis of a long-term illness may impact upon the child and their parents and give readers an opportunity to reflect upon and examine their understanding and knowledge of the topic.

Acknowledgement

We acknowledge the contribution of Lesley Lowes who authored the previous version of this chapter (Lowes, 2007). NB: the previous chapter included impact on siblings which, in this updated edition, is covered in a separate chapter (Chapter 4).

Useful websites

Diabetes UK
www.diabetes.org.uk

International Society for Pediatric and Adolescent Diabetes
www.ispad.org

Juvenile Diabetes Research Foundation
www.jdrf.org.uk

National Institute for Clinical Excellence
www.nice.org.uk

References

Al-Gamal, E. & Long, T. (2010) Anticipatory grieving among parents living with a child with cancer. *Journal of Advanced Nursing*, **66** (9), 1980–1990.

Arrington-Sanders, R., Yi, M.S., Tsevat, J. *et al.* (2006) Gender differences in health-related quality of life of adolescents with cystic fibrosis. *Health and Quality of Life Outcomes.* http://doi:10.1186/1477-7525-4-5

Batchelor, L.L., & Duke, G. (2019) Chronic sorrow in parents with chronically ill children. *Pediatric Nursing*, **45** (4), 163–173, 183.

Blount, R.L., Simons, L.E., Devine, K.A. *et al.* (2008) Evidence–based assessment of coping and stress in pediatirc psychology. *Journal of Pediatric Psychology*, **33** (9), 1021–1045.

Bolch, C.E., Davies, P.G., Umstad, M.P., *et al.* (2012) Multiple birth families with children with special needs: A qualitative investigation of mothers' experiences. *Twin Research and Human Genetics*, **15** (4), 503–515.

Bowes, S., Lowes, L., Warner, J. *et al.* (2009) Chronic sorrow in parents of children with type 1 diabetes. *Journal of Advanced Nursing*, **65** (5), 992–1000.

Bulman, M. (2017) Parents who let diabetic son starve to death found guilty of first-degree murder. Independent Newspaper Online, Sunday 26 February 2017 14:48 https://www.independent.co.uk/news/world/americas/murder-diabetic-son-diabetes-starve-death-guilty-parents-alexandru-emil-rodica-radita-calagry-canada-a7600021.html Accessed 28/01/20.

Carver, C. (1997) You want to measure coping but your protocol is too long: Consider the brief COPE. *International Journal of Behavioral Medicine*, **4** (1), 92–100.

Christie, D. & Khatun, H. (2019) Adjusting life to chronic illness. *The Psychologist*, **25** (3), 194–197. https://thepsychologist.bps.org.uk/volume-25/edition-3/adjusting-life-chronic-illness Accessed 23/06/20.

Clubb, R.L. (1991) Chronic sorrow: adaptation patterns of parents with chronically ill children. *Pediatric Nursing*, **17** (5), 461–465.

Compas, B.E., Jaser, S.S., Dunn, M.J. *et al.* (2011) Coping with Chronic Illness in Childhood and Adolescence. *Annual Review of Clinical Psychology*, **8**, 455–480.

Copley, M.F. & Bodensteiner, J.B. (1987) Chronic sorrow in families of disabled children. *Journal of Child Neurology*, **2**, 67–70.

Coughlin, M.B. & Sethares, K.A. (2017) Chronic sorrow in parents of children with a chronic illness or disability: an integrative literature review. *Journal of Pediatric Nursing*, **37**, 108–116.

Diabetes UK (2019a) What is Type 1 Diabetes? https://www.diabetes.org.uk/diabetes-the-basics/what-is-type-1-diabetes Accessed 28/01/20.

Diabetes UK (2019b) Complications of Diabetes. https://www.diabetes.org.uk/guide-to-diabetes/complications Accessed 28/01/20.

Diaz. L.J.R. & Cruz. D.A.L.M. (2018) Adaptation Model in a controlled clinical trial involving family caregivers of chronic patients. SciELO Analytics http://www.scielo.br/pdf/tce/v26n4/en_0104-0707-tce-26-04-e0970017.pdf Accessed 28/01/20.

Donovan, R. & Williams, A.M. (2015) Care-giving as a Canadian-Vietnamese tradition: It's like eating, you just do it. *Health and Social Care in the Community*, **23** (1), 79–87.

Engel, G. (1962) *Psychological Development in Health and Disease*. Philadelphia, W.B. Saunders.

Equality Act (2010) http://www.legislation.gov.uk/ukpga/2010/15/contents Accessed 28/01/20.

Falcão, M.A. & Francisco, R. (2017) Diabetes, eating disorders and body image in young adults: an exploratory study about "diabulimia". *Eating and Weight Disorders - Studies on Anorexia, Bulimia and Obesity*, **22** (4), 675–682.

Flynn, R. (2013) Coping with children with diabetes: Is this burden too great for parents to bear? *Journal of Endocrinology, Metabolism and Diabetes of South Africa*, **18** (2), 82–86.

Folkman, S., Lazarus, R.S., Dunkel-Schetter, C. *et al.* (1986) Dynamics of a stressful encounter: cognitive appraisal, coping and encounter outcomes. *Journal of Personality and Social Psychology*, **50** (5), 992–1003.

Ganjiwale, D., Ganjiwale, J., Sharma, B., *et al.* (2016) Quality of life and coping strategies of caregivers of children with physical and mental disabilities. *Journal of Family Medicine and Primary Care*, **5** (2), 343–348.

Geist, R., Grdisa, V. & Otley, A. (2003) Psychosocial issues in the child with chronic conditions. *Best Practice and Research: Clinical Gastroenterology*, **17** (2), 141–52.

George, A., Vickers, M.H., Wilkes, L. *et al* (2006) Chronic grief: experiences of working parents of children with chronic illness. *Contemporary Nurse*, **23** (2), 228–242.

Gannoni, A.F. & Shute, R.H. (2010) Parental and child perspectives on adaptation to childhood chronic illness. *Clinical Child Psychology and Child Psychiatry*, **15** (1), 39–53.

Glenn, A.D. (2015) Using online health communication to manage chronic sorrow: Mothers of children with rare diseases speak. *Journal of Pediatric Nursing*, **30** (1), 17–24.

Gordon, J. (2009) An evidence-based approach for supporting parents experiencing chronic sorrow. *Pediatric Nursing*, **35** (2), 115–119.

Graham, A., Powell, M.A. & Taylor, N. (2015) Ethical research involving children: Putting the evidence into practice. *Family Matters*, **96**, 23–28.

Green, S.E. (2006) Enough already! Caregiving and disaster preparedness-two faces of anticipatory loss. *Journal of Loss and Trauma*, **11** (2), 201–214.

Guthrie, D.W., Bartsocas, C., Jarosz-Chabot, P. *et al.* (2003) Psychosocial issues for children and adolescents with diabetes: overview and recommendations. *Diabetes Spectrum*, **16** (1), 7–12.

Hockenberry, M.J., Wilson, D. & Rodgers, C.C. (2019) *Wong's Nursing Care of Infants and Children* (eleventh edition). St. Louis, Elsevier.

Holt, R.I.G., Cockram, C.S., Flyvbjerg, A., *et al.* (2016) *Textbook of Diabetes* (fifth edition). Chichester, John Wiley and Sons.

Hopper, A. & Crane, S. (2019) Evaluation of the burdens and benefits of participation in research by parents of children with life-limiting illnesses. *Nurse Researcher*, **27** (3), 8–13. http://doi: 10.7748/nr.2019.e1617.

Helgeson, V.S, Becker, D., Escobar, O. *et al.* (2012) Families with children with diabetes: implications of parent stress for parent and child health. *Journal of Pediatric Psychology*, **37** (4), 467–478.

Jaser, S.S. & White, L.E. (2011) Coping and resilience in adolescents with type 1 diabetes. *Child: Care, Health and Development*, **37** (3), 335–342.

Johnson, B.S. (2000) Mothers' perceptions of parenting children with disabilities. *The American Journal of Maternal/Child Nursing*, **25** (3), 127–132.

Kamm, J.A. (1985) Grief and therapy: two processes in interaction. In: *Psychotherapy and the Grieving Patient* (ed. M. Stern), pp. 59–64. New York, Harrington Park Press.

Khanolkar, A.R., Amin, R., Taylor-Robinson, D., *et al.* (2017) Ethnic differences in early glycemic control in childhood-onset type 1 diabetes. *BMJ Open Diabetes Research and Care*, **5** (1). http://dx.doi.org/10.1136/bmjdrc-2017-000423.

Kish, A.M, Newcombe, P.A. & Haslam, D.M. (2018) Working and caring for a child with chronic illness: A review of current literature. *Child Care Health and Development*, **44** (3), 343–354. http://doi: 10.1111/cch.12546.

Knafl. K.A. & Santacroce. S.J. (2010) Chronic conditions and the family. In: *Primary care of the child with a chronic condition* (fifth edition). (eds P.J. Allen *et al.*), pp. 74–89. St Louis, Mosby/Elsevier.

Knafl, K.A., Darney, B.G., Gallo, A.M., *et al.* (2010) Parental perceptions of the outcome and meaning of normalization. *Research in Nursing and Health*, **33** (2), 87–98.

Kuo, D.Z., Cohen, E., Agrawal, R., *et al.* (2011) A national profile of caregiver challenges among more medically complex children with special health care needs. *Archives of Pediatrics and Adolescent Medicine*, **65** (11), 1020–1026.

Koch, K.D. & Jones, B.L. (2018) Supporting Parent Caregivers of Children with Life-Limiting Illness. *Children*, **5** (7), 85. http://doi: 10.3390/children5070085.

Kopel, S. & Eiser, C. (2013) Children's perceptions of health. In: *Perceptions of Health and Illness* (eds K. Petrie and J.A. Weinman), pp. 47–76. London, Routledge.

Kepreotes, E., Keatinge, D. & Stone, T. (2010) The experience of parenting children with chronic health conditions: a new reality. *Journal of Nursing and Healthcare of Chronic Illness*, **2**, 51–62.

Kubler-Ross, E. (1970) *On Death and Dying*. London, Tavistock.

Kubler-Ross, E. & Kessler, D. (2014) *On Grief and Grieving: Finding the Meaning of Grief Through the Five Stages of Loss*. London, Simon and Schuster.

Law, E., Fisher, E., Eccleston, C. *et al.* (2019) Psychological interventions for parents of children and adolescents with chronic illness. *Cochrane Database of Systematic Reviews*, **4** (4), CD009660. http://doi: 10.1002/14651858.CD009660.pub4.

Lazarus, R.S. & Folkman, S. (1984) *Stress, Appraisal and Coping*. New York, Springer.

Lichtenstein B., Laska, M.K. & Clair, J.M. (2002) Chronic sorrow in the HIV-positive patient: issues of race, gender, and social support. *AIDS Patient Care and STDs*, **16** (1): 27–38.

Lowes, L. (2007) Impact on the child and family. In: *Nursing Care of Children and Young People with Chronic Illness* (eds F. Valentine & L. Lowes), pp. 55–83. Oxford, Blackwell Publishing.

Lowes, L. & Lyne, P. (2000) Chronic sorrow in parents of children with newly diagnosed diabetes: a review of the literature and discussion of the implications for nursing practice. *Journal of Advanced Nursing*, **32** (1), 41–48.

Lowes, L. & Gill, P. (2006) Participants' experiences of being interviewed about an emotive topic. *Journal of Advanced Nursing*, **55** (5), 587–595.

Lowes, L., Lyne, P. & Gregory, J.W. (2004) Childhood diabetes: parents' experience of home management and the first year following diagnosis. *Diabetic Medicine*, **21** (6), 531–538.

Lowes, L., Gregory, J.W. & Lyne, P. (2005) Newly diagnosed childhood diabetes: a psychosocial transition for parents? *Journal of Advanced Nursing*, **50** (3), 253–261.

Malik, J.A. & Koot, H.M. (2009) Explaining the adjustment of adolescents with type 1 diabetes. *Diabetes Care*, **32** (5), 774–779.

Michalopoulos, H. (2006) The Greek hospital and community nurse's role of offering support, counselling skills and nursing rehabilitation to parents of children with chronic medical, surgical or genetic conditions or disabilities. PhD Thesis, Cardiff University. http://orca.cf.ac.uk/54252/.

Moayedoddin B. & Markowitz J.C. (2015) Abnormal grief: should we consider a more patient-centered approach? *American Journal of Psychotherapy*, **69** (4), 361–378.

Morrison, J.E., Bromfield, L.M. & Cameron, H.J. (2003) A therapeutic model for supporting families of children with a chronic illness or disability. *Child and Adolescent Mental Health*, **8** (3), 125–130.

Nabors, L., Liddle, M., Graves, M.L., *et al.* (2019) A family affair: Supporting children with chronic illnesses. *Child Care, Health and Development*, **45** (2), 227–233.

National Institute for Clinical Excellence (2015) *Diabetes (Type 1 and Type 2) in Children and Young People: Diagnosis and Management*. London, NICE.

National Institute for Clinical Excellence (2016) *Quality Standards for Diagnosing and Managing Type 1 and Type 2 Diabetes in Children and Young People (Under 18)*. London, NICE.

Nursing and Midwifery Council (2018) *The Code: Professional Standards of Practice and Behaviour for Nurses, Midwives and Nursing Associates*. London, Nursing Midwifery Council.

Olshansky, S. (1962) Chronic sorrow: a response to having a mentally defective child. *Social Casework*, **43** (4), 190–193.

Pate, T. (2016) Families of children with chronic illness and the relational family model. *The Person and the Challenges*, **6** (2), 57–65.

Piaget, J. (1962) *Play, Dreams and Imitation in Childhood*. New York, Norton.

Pinquart, M. (2019) Depressive symptoms in parents of children with chronic health conditions: a meta-analysis. *Journal of Pediatric Psychology*, **44** (2), 139–149.

Rankin, D., Harden, J., Waugh, N., *et al.* (2016) Parents' information and support needs when their child is diagnosed with type 1 diabetes: a qualitative study. *Health Expectations*, **19** (3), 580–591.

Ray, L.D. (2002) Parenting and childhood chronicity: making visible the invisible work. *Journal of Pediatric Nursing*, **17** (6), 424–437.

Rifshana, F., Breheny, M., Taylor, J.E., *et al.* (2017) The parental experience of caring for a child with type 1 diabetes. *Journal of Child and Family Studies*, **26**, 3226–3236.

Roos, S. (2002) *Chronic Sorrow: A Living Loss* (second edition). New York, Routledge.

Roy, C. (2009) *The Roy Adaptation Model* (third edition). Upper Saddle River, Pearson Prentice Hall.

Royal College of Nursing (2013) *Supporting Children and Young People with Diabetes: RCN Guidance for Nurses in Schools and Early Years Settings*. London, RCN.

Solnit, A.J. & Stark, M.H. (1961) Mourning and the birth of a defective child. *The Psychoanalytic Study of the Child*, **16** (1), 523–537.

Smith, J., Cheater, F. & Bekker, H. (2015) Parents experiences of living with a child with a long-term condition: a rapid structured review of the literature. *Health Expectations*, **18** (4), 452–474.

Smith, L.B., Liu, X., Johnson, S.B., *et al.* (2018) Family adjustment to diabetes diagnosis in children: Can participation in a study on type 1 diabetes genetic risk be helpful? *Pediatric Diabetes*, **19** (5), 1025–1033.

Tallon, M.M., Kendall, G.E. & Snider, P.D. (2015) Rethinking family-centred care for the child and family in hospital. *Journal of Clinical Nursing*, **24** (9–10), 1426–1435.

Theofanidis, D. (2007) Chronic illness in childhood: psychosocial adaptation and nursing support for the child and family. *Health Science Journal*, **1** (2), 1–9.

Thompson, R.J., Mata, J., Jaeggi, S.M. *et al.* (2010) Maladaptive coping, adaptive coping, and depressive symptoms: variations across age and depressive state. *Behaviour Research and Therapy*, **48** (6), 459–466.

Vlassoff, C. (2007) Gender differences in determinants and consequences of health and illness. *Journal of Health and Population and Nutrition*, **25** (1), 47–61.

Williams, C. (2000) Doing health, doing gender: teenagers, diabetes and asthma. *Social Science and Medicine*, **50** (3), 387–396.

Ward, A. (2011) The grief experience of caregivers when the child has a life threatening illness. PhD Thesis. Loma Linda University.

Whiting, M. (2012) Impact, meaning and need for help and support: The experience of parents caring for children with disabilities, life-limiting/life-threatening illness or technology dependence. *Journal of Child Health Care*, **17** (1), 92–108.

Whittemore, R., Jaser, S., Chao, A. *et al.* (2012) Psychological experience of parents of children with type 1 diabetes: a systematic mixed-studies review. *Diabetes Education*, **38** (4), 562–579.

Worden, J.W. (1995) *Grief Counselling and Grief Therapy. A Handbook for the Mental Health Practitioner* (second edition). London, Routledge.

World Health Organisation (2011) Evidence for Gender Responsive Actions to Prevent and Manage Chronic Conditions: Young People's Health as a Whole-of-Society Response. Geneva, WHO.

CHAPTER 4

Impact On Siblings

Amie Hodges, Daniel Kelly, and Julia Tod

Introduction

The sibling relationship within a family can be a complex entity in terms of daily interactions and influences. Further complexity can be added when a child is living in the context of a long-term condition. Siblings can experience significant changes in family life when they are journeying alongside their brother or sister in the chronic illness trajectory, as this can impact on their psychosocial and physical well-being. Often, care of the chronically ill child is the key focus within the family and requires greater parental attention as the chronically ill child's needs are considered a priority. However, as a consequence, siblings can feel left out or isolated and their needs can go unnoticed or are unmet. Siblings can be perceived as being 'well' in the absence of having a long-term condition themselves (Hodges, 2016). However, this is not necessarily the case and they may have worries or concerns of their own. Therefore, it is important that children's nurses have a greater insight into the needs of siblings living in the context of a long-term condition, as well as having an understanding of the importance of the sibling relationship within their family.

Aim of the chapter

This chapter will firstly draw on the work of some seminal authors to explore theoretical perspectives surrounding the sibling, the sibling relationship and factors that impact on sibling social development, as this will provide a foundation before exploring and giving an insight into the wider issues and influences that can impact upon them as a consequence of the chronic illness trajectory. Siblings as care-givers will also be explored. The lack of research in recent years pertaining to the theoretical perspectives relating to siblings necessitates the need to draw upon the seminal works which are referred to in this chapter as they still hold relevance in contemporary society. The chapter will also discuss supportive interventions that can be used to help understand the needs and care of siblings within their family. Case studies will be used to explore different aspects of sibling experiences, using cystic fibrosis (CF) as the long-term illness example. Before reading this chapter, readers will need to have an understanding

Nursing Care of Children and Young People with Long-Term Conditions, Second Edition.
Edited by Mandy Brimble and Peter McNee.
© 2021 John Wiley & Sons Ltd. Published 2021 by John Wiley & Sons Ltd.

of CF and its management in children and young people. Chapter 11 provides some insight into the condition of CF.

Intended learning outcomes

- To explore theoretical perspectives pertaining to siblings and their relationship within the family
- To examine how a childhood long-term condition can impact psychologically, socially and physically on the sibling
- To explore the needs of siblings when living in the context of a long-term condition
- To discuss how children's nurses can support siblings within the trajectory of a long-term condition

---

Reflection

Before reading the following passage, consider your own experience of childhood sibling relationships. This could be your own or one that you have observed. Write down your key thoughts.

The sibling relationship

The sibling can be an important and influential person in one's life from the moment that they meet, and throughout their lifespan. The relationship is considered a life-long journey as siblings can share memories and experiences which can be good or bad, pleasurable or painful, conflicting or comforting (Bank & Kahn, 1982; Rowe, 2007; McHale *et al.*, 2012). Siblings within their relational journey can be referred to as co-voyagers that are co-constructed through their family interactions, influences, encouragements and conflicts (Bank & Kahn, 1982; Edwards *et al.*, 2006; McHale *et al.*, 2012). Being a sibling is ascribed rather than a chosen status; however, it can change when child siblings reach adulthood when they can choose whether or not to spend time together. Regardless of a sibling's relationship being good, bad, indifferent or ambivalent, the sibling bond remains because siblings formulate and influence each other's past, present and future (Hodges, 2016).

🔑 **Key points**

- The sibling is an important and influential person in the family.
- Siblings can influence each other's past, present and future.

Sibling identity

It is important for siblings to feel a sense of belonging in being part of a family, but also in having a connection with their sibling. It is through these early connections that siblings formulate their real, innermost private selves (James, 1890 cited in James, 2017; McHale *et al.*, 2006; 2012). However, contradictory to this want for togetherness, the sibling can engage in an inner struggle as they wish to acquire independence and their individuality to be recognised (Edwards *et al.*, 2006). By maintaining togetherness as well as striving for their individuality, siblings identify themselves through the comparative realms of being the same or being different (Edwards *et al.*, 2006).

The intertwined notion of same and different is where siblings are able to express their unique self in terms of physical differences, preferences and personalities. This can frame their sense of identity, which is interconnected with the emotional composite of dependence versus independence (Edwards *et al.*, 2006). The comparisons of these notions are not solely the observations of the sibling, because they also arise from other family members as well as being influenced by an external social world to which they belong. Other influences on sibling identity are gender, race, class, culture and history (Edwards *et al.*, 2006; McHale *et al.*, 2012).

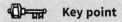 **Key point**

- It is important for siblings to maintain togetherness, as well as to be recognised for their own individuality.

Sibling boundaries

The contradiction of siblings wanting to feel connected but also seeking independence can lead them to begin to set boundaries in their relationships with each other. They can make boundary distinctions of their possessions in terms of what they own themselves and what belongs to another, as they differentiate between what is mine and what is yours (Bak & Ross 1996; Ruble *et al.*, 1980; McGuire *et al.*, 2000; McHale *et al.*, 2012).

Boundary setting is not exclusive to the protection of possessions, but also to that of protecting one's own space within the family home (Hodges, 2016). It is here where siblings may display notices, such as the example provided by Stark (2007, p.11) that states 'No Trespassing'. Such a sign is exhibited to make it clear what space is theirs, giving a definitive message to the brothers and sisters.

Boundary setting is part of sibling's social development in their journey toward independence and it links into the notion of difference that was stipulated by Edwards *et al.* (2006). This aspect of social development and formation of one's temperament can influence the harmonious equilibrium of family life (Brody, 1998).

> **Key point**
>
> • Setting boundaries is part of the sibling's social development in their journey toward independence.

Sibling interaction

The harmonious synchronisation of family life can be influenced by the interactions that siblings have with each other and whether positive or negative feelings are exhibited within their engagements (Edwards *et al.*, 2006; Brody, 1998; Updegraff *et al.*, 2010; McHale *et al.*, 2012; Hodges, 2016). Child siblings can spend much of their time in each other's company, more so than with their parent, and as a consequence they can become aware of each other's idiosyncrasies which provide them with knowledge of what will and will not please their sibling (Klett-Davies, 2008). This privileged knowledge of other can be used when the sibling chooses to be a source of comfort or conflict to their brother or sister.

Such comfort can be provided in times of distress, if a sibling can see that their brother or sister is upset and requires a supportive companion to ease their woes and listen to their concerns (Dunn, 2008; Hodges, 2016). Edwards *et al.* (2006) presented sibling narratives that demonstrated the protectiveness, empathic warmth and caring traits that can occur when siblings are looking out for one another. There is a suggestion that siblings can become dependent on each other for companionship and play, so as to avoid being alone and isolated.

Siblings can also project conflict through arguments, bickering and in moments of antagonism and indifference (Edwards *et al.*, 2006; Hodges, 2016). Conflicts can result from siblings knowing each other so well, which leads them to know what would annoy one another as well as knowing what sibling reaction would prevail (Dunn, 2008). Different temperaments of siblings may also be influential in their conflict where temperaments are seen to be dissimilar (Munn & Dunn, 1989). However, Stoneman and Brody (1993) suggest that if a sibling has more positive temperament attributes, this can help them to counteract the potential unfavourable impact of living with a sibling with a negative personality attribute.

Sibling conflict can result in positive outcomes for siblings as it can help them to develop social competence in terms of dealing with different situations, as well as help in the formation of identity and development of self (Bedford *et al.*, 2000; Hodges, 2016). Sibling experiences of positive, negative and ambivalent feelings towards each other influence their emotional development as well as the quality of their relationship (Edwards *et al.*, 2006; Hodges, 2016).

> **Key point**
>
> • The positive, negative and ambivalent interactions of the sibling can influence their emotional development as well as the quality of the sibling relationship.

Parental influence on the sibling relationship

(Please see Chapter 3 for the impact of long-term illness on parents.)

It is not solely sibling interactions themselves that are seen as responsible for the quality of sibling relationships, but those of family dynamics and differential treatment and quality of attention provided by their parents (Coles, 2003; Mitchell, 2003; Brody, 1998; Brody *et al.*, 1992; Dunbar, 1999; Howe *et al.*, 2001; Sanders, 2004; McHale *et al.*, 2012). Parents are often the role models for the social interactive processes within the family (Sanders, 2004). Children are recipients of their parenting styles and for some siblings an absence or limited amount of emotional and physical attention can lead to a co-dependence of siblings on one another and a stronger sibling bond, as they compensate for this lack in quality of parenting by relying on each other more (Bank & Kahn, 1982; McHale *et al.*, 2012).

When parental attention is available, siblings are quick to notice differential treatment in terms of one being treated more positively than the other. This may include where one sibling is given more time and attention or given a specific role that may be considered a greater accolade than another given role. It may also include differing levels of discipline or exhibition of praise and appearance of favouring one over the other (Sanders, 2004; McHale *et al.*, 1995; Volling & Elins, 1998; Shanahan *et al.*, 2008; McHale *et al.*, 2012; Hodges, 2016). Transitions in approach to parenting at given times can also be an influence in the sibling relationship because parenting patterns are not always consistent and their skills may change over time due to their prior experience. Siblings may be quick to notice their differing decisions and skills and view this as unfair treatment (Sanders, 2004; Shanahan *et al.*, 2008; Hodges, 2016).

Where both siblings are treated fairly and with positive regard, this can lead to positive relationships between siblings. However, if this is not the case and one sibling feels that they are being neglected of attention and treated less favourably, then there can be an upsurge of negative feelings which can include: jealousy, anger, fear and rivalry (Brody, 1998; Hodges, 2016). This can impact on a child's self-esteem as well as the quality of the sibling relationship. It can generate competitiveness as well as the aforementioned sibling conflict, as siblings compete for parental attention.

🔑 Key point

- It is important for approaches to parenting to be considered because this can have an influence on the how siblings view themselves as well as their brother or sister.

🕐 Time out

- Now that you have read the theoretical background information regarding sibling relationships, interactions and development, make a list of the key points that the children's nurse will need to be aware of.

Siblings are forever changing in their transient worlds in terms of their experiences, interactions, developments and influences. The changes encountered, as referred to above, can be complex as siblings remain connected to their brothers, sisters, parents and carers in their parallel worlds and a sibling faced with living in the context of long-term illness adds further complexity to their worlds (Hodges, 2016). The next section of this chapter will explore the impact of having a brother and or sister with a long-term condition.

Reflection

Before reading the following section, reflect on your own experience in practice where you have encountered, engaged with or cared for a sibling who has a brother or sister with a long-term condition.

The impact of a long-term condition on the sibling

Having a brother or sister with a long-term condition can add a new dimension to a sibling's world due to many amendments and challenges that are encountered alongside the disease trajectory within their family life (O'Brien *et al.*, 2009; Knecht *et al.*, 2015).

A new diagnosis

🌐 Case study 4.1

Molly is a 6-year-old girl who lives with her mother Jade (30 years of age), her father Gary (31 years of age) and her new baby sister Nora (4 months of age). The family are of white Caucasian origin, all born in the UK. They live in a detached house in a quiet village in the countryside. Gary works full time as an accountant and Jade is a primary school teacher, but she is currently on maternity leave. Molly attends the local primary school where her mother normally works. Molly's sister Nora has recently been diagnosed with cystic fibrosis (CF). This has come as a shock to Gary and Jade and they are trying to come to terms with the diagnosis. Molly has been told that Nora is a special baby who requires extra care because she has CF. Molly does not really understand what CF is, but she has noticed that family life has changed since Nora had to go to hospital for tests and she has noticed that she is asked to do a lot more for herself, such as having to get herself ready for school, whereas previously Jade used to help her. Molly has also noticed that she can no longer have her friends to come over to stay and play. Molly had been excited about having a baby sister, but now she wants things to be like they used to be before her sister was born.

Changes in family life for the sibling

Siblings like Molly who are living with a child with a long-term condition can encounter changes in family life due to the demands of their brother or sisters' condition. There can often be a need for attention to be focused on the chronically ill child, particularly at treatment giving times and if additional vigilance is required (Hodges, 2016). Siblings can experience loss of life as they knew it in comparison to how it was prior to their brother or sister being ill (Woodgate, 2006; 2016). For Molly, she was used to having all of her parent's attention before her baby sister arrived, and then this became much less when her sister was diagnosed with CF. As a consequence, siblings living in the context of a long-term condition such as CF can experience uncertainty, as they can have periods of time where they may be separated from their parent and or chronically ill sibling, due to the need for hospitalisation or clinic visits. Siblings can feel different, left out and consequently can feel isolated within their family (Hodges, 2016). Siblings may choose to act out to gain attention or they may vie for attention alongside their brother or sister (Hodges, 2016). Siblings can be socialised to take on certain roles within the family, such as care-giving (siblings as care-givers is discussed in more detail later on in this chapter). An alteration in family life can place additional pressure, responsibility and expectations on the sibling when their brother or sister is ill, as is presented in the scenario where Molly has been asked to do more for herself, such as getting ready for school. If the expectations that are placed on the sibling outweigh the resources and their ability to cope with those expectations, it can place them under duress as it may be beyond their capabilities or what they feel able to manage (French & Caplan, 1973; Hamama *et al.*, 2008; Hodges, 2016). Molly has noticed that she no longer has her friends coming over to play or stay over, which can add to feelings of isolation. An alteration in family life can cause a sibling to feel negatively towards the child with the long-term condition.

🕐 **Time out**

- How do you think that Molly might be affected due to Nora's diagnosis of cystic fibrosis?

The effect of a childhood long-term condition on siblings will vary from family to family, and will depend greatly upon parenting styles, family structure and positioning (e.g. where the siblings sit within the family), previous and present sibling relationships, age differences, past experiences, individual characteristics and the nature/demands of the condition. However, Molly may experience jealousy if she thinks that all the care and attention surrounds Nora. She may feel restricted because she cannot do things that she used to do before her sister's diagnosis, including having friends over. Molly may feel sad because her sister is chronically ill and she is not going to get better. She may worry that her sister may die or that she may catch CF herself. She may also be confused as she does not fully understand what CF is and why her sister has it, but she does not. She may also feel angry because family life has changed from how it was before.

> ◉ Case study 4.2 (three years post-diagnosis)
>
> Nora has developed a respiratory infection and requires intravenous antibiotics, which are being administered at home by the nurse who comes to visit every day. Molly watches from a distance during these treatment giving times and often goes to her bedroom to cry after the nurse has been because Nora does not like having the intravenous antibiotics and she screams and shouts when she has to have the medication. This is upsetting for Molly to watch. Molly also feels ignored because the nurse only asks how Nora is and does not ask how she feels.

Emotional labour

Case study 4.2 demonstrates a situation that siblings can find themselves in when moving along the parallel journey with their brother or sister with a long-term condition. Within the scenario, Molly has watched her sister's treatment being given and she has become distressed herself as a witness of care-giving where Nora has become upset. Molly does not express her upset outwardly, but leaves the room as she contains her emotion until she is able to reach a private space. The scenario is congruent with the work of Hodges (2016), who discussed the emotional labour that siblings can encounter when living within the chronic illness trajectory. In the study by Hodges (2016), siblings demonstrated visible emotional upset in relation to living with a child with cystic fibrosis, particularly in relation to diagnosis and/or deterioration in their brother or sisters' condition, along with missing their mother in moments of separation. Siblings also witnessed the stress and worry of their parents. As a consequence, siblings acted out their anxiety and they expressed their feelings of fear, apprehension, uncertainty and frustration. Siblings may need time to transition and adapt to the changing parenting roles and parental absence because of their brother or sister's long-term illness (Hodges, 2016).

Sibling empathy and maturity

Siblings living in the context of a long-term condition can exhibit positive traits that have been gained as a consequence of their experiences. Siblings have been reported to externalise their empathy towards their brother or sister with a long-term illness and they can also demonstrate a level of maturity and wisdom beyond their years as they develop an understanding of the need for the chronically ill child to receive a greater level of parental attention, as a consequence of the demands of the trajectory of the long-term condition (Hodges, 2016; Knecht et al., 2015; Labay & Walco, 2004). Additionally, siblings can develop a protective bond with their brother or sister and can be very loyal towards their family in their social encounters and often they will put their sibling's needs first instead of their own (Hodges, 2016). Mulroy et al. (2008) reported siblings as being more caring, compassionate and considerate of their brother or sister with a long-term condition. They also suggest that the sibling can have a greater appreciation of the value of health and the preciousness of life, which can add to their development of personal skills and attitudes, which may not be available to their peers who are not living in the context of long-term illness. Siblings living with a chronically ill brother or sister can demonstrate social competence with regards to their ability to communicate effectively, co-operate with others and demonstrate commitment towards others (Knecht *et al.*, 2015). Additionally, specific traits identified were those of compassion, patience and empathy (Knecht *et al.*, 2015).

⌗🔑 **Key point**

- Siblings living with a brother or sister with a long-term condition can exhibit positive traits.

🕐 **Time out**

- Now that you have read the passage above, write a list of the positive traits that have been identified in siblings living in the context of a long-term condition.

Siblings as carers

Reflection

Consider your personal experience in childhood; what did caring in your family mean to you?

The definition of 'young carer' is a contested area; it involves determining when normal interfamilial relationships, which involve mutual care, become an issue of concern to the state. The Department of Health (DoH) defines young carers as 'those under the age of 18 who carry out significant caring tasks and assume a level of responsibility . . . which would usually be undertaken by an adult' (DoH, 1999). This definition does not include emotional support (Cree, 2003) or intention to care (Becker, 2000).

This problem of definition is one of several factors that make identifying numbers of young carers problematic. There are estimated to be at least **376 000** young adult carers in the UK aged 16–25, according to census figures (Office for National Statistics (ONS), 2011) making this a significant group of young people who are potentially vulnerable to harms associated with caring, such as poor health and reduced social outcomes.

In certain circumstances, professionals fail to recognise the caring role. The young carer themselves may also fail to recognise their caring role, considering it simply part of family life. They might, however, remain silent about the extent of their caring due to concern that the family will be separated (Metzing-Blau & Schnepp, 2008) or experience stigma, which can also lead to secrecy and social withdrawal (Bolas *et al.*, 2007).

In recent years, there has been an increase in research on the impact of the caring role on the emotions, education and socialisation of young carers (Joseph *et al.*, 2019); examples of detrimental effect include poor school attendance (Dearden & Becker, 1998) and feeling isolated and undervalued (Children Services Network, 2005). In a survey of 4192 children in Northern Ireland, those stating they had caring responsibility scored lower on measures of health and well-being, reported that they were bullied more frequently and had poorer educational aspirations (Lloyd, 2013). It is important to recognise that there are also reported benefits to caring. Studies have shown that caring is associated with increasing maturity and preparation for life in adulthood (Fives *et al.*, 2013) and the ability to foster qualities of compassion and empathy (Stamatopoulos, 2018).

Reflection

Do you think that siblings could be defined as young carers?

As a 6 year-old, Molly may not be very involved in the care of Nora. When professionals look at the family, they will see that there are two parents who provide physical and emotional care for Nora. As the children grow, however, this situation may alter. The continuum can change from caring *about* an individual family member to caring *for* that family member (Becker, 2007). It is important to recognise that children and young people who undertake inappropriate care for a sibling are young carers and will themselves *need* care. Siblings often take part in care tasks alongside parents, such as supervision, feeding, personal care, assisting with therapies and giving medication. Siblings often also support their parents emotionally, especially if parents themselves have anxiety or depression. Professionals need to be aware that a sibling can become a young carer at any time during their childhood.

Key points

- Under section 17 of the Children Act (1989), young carers may be considered children in need.
- If they are considered to be suffering or likely to suffer significant harm, there may be an inquiry under section 47 of the Children Act (1989).

Young carers and carers' assessment

The Care Act (2014) and the Social Services and Well-being (Wales) Act (2014) emphasise a whole family approach in assessment, planning and review processes. Local Authorities have a duty to assess 'on the appearance of need'. They also have a more general duty to 'take reasonable steps' to identify young carers in their area (Children and Families Act 2014). All young carers under 18 have a right to an assessment of their need and the Local Authority must involve the child with caring responsibilities, their parents and any other person the young carer requests in the assessment process. The assessment itself must look at whether the young carer wishes to continue caring, and whether it is appropriate for them to continue caring. When doing this, any education, training, work or recreational activities the young carer is involved in or wishes to participate in must be considered. Where a young carer's eligible needs are identified as requiring support, local authorities are required to provide support directly to the young carer or demonstrate that the 'cared for person's' assessment has provided adequate care and support to prevent inappropriate care being provided by the young carer.

🕐 **Time out**

- Molly wants things to be as they were before Nora's diagnosis of a long-term condition, but the family's experience does not need to be harmful. Who can help support the family to build positive sibling relationships and prevent some of the negative outcomes of caring?

Young carers often highlight that effective care of the person with care needs will reduce the pressure on them. Effective multidisciplinary and multiagency working and service provision will reduce the load on the carer. Young carers also ask for help to take part in education, friendship and community groups and a break from caring responsibility. Health care workers can also signpost to the young carers support groups provided by organisations such as Action for Children, Barnardos, Carers Trust and The Children's Society, who can offer information and group support.

Recognising the unmet needs of siblings

As you read the first section of the chapter, you may have started to think about siblings and the roles they have to play in the lives of children living with a long-term condition. Sometimes it may seem that they barely need to speak to understand each other, and they may seem to be able to read each other's feelings just by being together. If you have siblings of your own, you may easily be able to recognise when they are worried, upset or angry. Such a close bond takes many years to form and as siblings spend so much time in each other's company, especially if they are close in terms of age, they learn to communicate non-verbally. This may change, of course, as they grow up and enter the period of adolescence and guard their privacy more as they seek to separate themselves from such close bonds.

Understanding the nature of the sibling relationship is crucial to children and young people's nursing, as caring for those who are chronically ill may lead us to assume things about siblings (that all is going well for them, for instance) when the opposite may actually be true. As Murray (2000) reminds us, the family members of a child or young person with a long-term or life-threatening condition, such as cancer, usually focus most on the child who is ill, and whose needs are most obvious. However, parents may have limited time and emotional resources to focus on their other children's needs, meaning that it is the healthy sibling who may easily be forgotten. In this section we encourage you to think about the unmet needs of siblings and to consider how to include them in the package of care that you provide for the whole family (Knecht *et al.*, 2015).

🕐 Time out

- If a child with CF has repeated admissions to hospital with their mother or father, what might be the impact on their siblings at home? What feelings might they be experiencing and how might they express these?

If we look back at case study 4.1, we can see that Molly's life has been changed, first by the arrival of Nora, and then with all the changes brought about by CF. We know that she was excited about having a new baby sister, but now Nora's illness has evoked more negative feelings as she wants her previous life back. This will never happen, of course, regardless of how much as she wishes it, so she will have to adapt and learn to incorporate CF into her own life, just as much as her parents will. The challenge for Molly, however, is that she is healthy and will be facing the same challenges of girls her own age. She previously enjoyed a carefree and close relationship with her mother and father, but their attention is now increasingly being drawn to Nora. This may require Molly to *act* as if she is coping well, while she is really feeling confused and angry about this new situation. Who can she tell about her feelings if she feels guilty? Her home is now filled with equipment and medications that serve as reminders of how much her life has changed.

Research by Kelly and Kelly (2013) observed a group of British Bangladeshi children through their treatment for cancer. This longitudinal study, over a period of one year, demonstrated how all family members engaged in the care of the ill child. This may include shopping, cooking, tidying up at home or even translating medical information for their parents. Siblings played a key role, but their own needs were not recognised, despite the pressures they were under due to the illness in their family.

One of the key risks for siblings experiencing unmet needs is the impact of other people's preconceptions. These may include assuming that all is well when siblings may actually be experiencing a range of issues, such as separation anxiety (from the parents or their ill sibling), sorrow for their brother or sister's situation and anxiety about the amount of stress being placed on their parents. They may also experience feelings that are not always easy to express, such as jealousy and anger about the amount of time not being paid to them and their lives (Knecht *et al.*, 2015).

Assessment of a sibling's unmet needs is an important skill to help prevent such negative outcomes, and nurses can pay attention to siblings when they visit and make a point of asking about how they are coping with the situation. This may not be a formal form of assessment, but paying attention to how siblings are coping may help prevent them from becoming an 'invisible patient' themselves (Franklin *et al.*, 2018). Researchers found that it was often parents (or even patients themselves) who would eventually suggest that siblings were not coping well in a cancer situation. For some, the best strategy might be to explore the impact outside of the clinical environment using family support (such as social work) or charity/voluntary services and to spend dedicated time with siblings to help address their needs and prevent long-term emotional problems. These researchers also found that health professionals did appreciate that siblings had unmet needs, and needed better support, but multiple barriers existed that prevented this support being delivered. These included lack of time, lack of opportunity to engage with siblings alone and a lack of appropriate resources to support them even if their needs were known. This situation has been confirmed in other research on the needs of siblings carried out in the context of cancer in young people (Long *et al.*, 2015).

Given the risk of unmet needs of siblings, nurses should remain aware of the pressures that other family members may be under and help ensure that their needs are not invisible. By doing so, siblings may become better able to support others in their family during tough times, but also obtain the support they need to live as well as they can in what may be a very difficult and challenging situation.

Conclusion

This chapter has highlighted that siblings are important members of the family and that they can be a constant in each other's lives as they progress through their childhood years into adulthood. Discussions have focused on the multitude of ways that siblings can present themselves in their family when living with a child with a long-term condition (Hodges, 2016). Additionally, siblings can feel burdened with extra roles if they take on young carer responsibilities and they themselves may require additional support. The unmet needs of siblings do need to be addressed so that they can feel more fully understood and supported, so that they do not feel invisible in their family world. The children's nurse is in a key role that can help to facilitate and support the sibling within their family when there is a child with a long-term condition, so that their needs can be addressed.

Useful websites

Sibling websites

The Sibling Support Project
www.siblingsupport.org

Rainbow Trust
www.rainbowtrust.org.uk

Sibs- For Brothers and Sisters of disabled children and adults
www.sibs.org.uk

Websites for further information and signposting for young carers

Action for children
https://www.actionforchildren.org.uk/what-we-do/children-young-people/support-for-
  young-carers/

Barnados
https://www.barnardos.org.uk/what-we-do/helping-families/young-carers

Carers Trust
https://carers.org/about-us/about-young-carers

The Children's Society
https://www.childrenssociety.org.uk/what-we-do/helping-children/young-carers

References

Bak, I.M. & Ross, H.S. (1996) I'm telling! The content, context and consequences of children's tattling on their siblings. *Social Development*, **5** (3), 292–309.

Bank, S.P. & Kahn, M.D. (1982) *The Sibling Bond*. New York, Basic Books.

Becker, S. (2000) Young carers. In: *The Blackwell Encyclopedia of Social Work* (ed. M. Davies), p. 378. Oxford, Blackwell

Becker, S. (2007) Global perspectives on children's unpaid caregiving in the family: Research and policy on 'young carers' in the UK, Australia, the USA, and Sub-Saharan Africa. *Global Social Policy*, **7** (1), 23–50.

Bedford, V.H., Volling, B.L. & Avioli, P.S. (2000) Positive consequences of sibling conflict in childhood and adulthood. *The International Journal of Aging and Human Development*, **51** (1), 53–69.

Bolas, H., Wersch, A.V. & Flynn, D. (2007) The well-being of young people who care for a dependent relative: an interpretative phenomenological analysis. *Psychology and Health*, **22** (7), 829–850.

Brody, G.H. (1998) Sibling relationships quality: its causes and consequences. *Annual Review of Psychology*, **49** (1), 1–24.

Brody, G.H., Stoneman, Z. & McCoy, K. (1992) Parental differential treatment of siblings and sibling differences in negative emotionality. *Journal of Marriage and Family*, **54** (3), 643–651.

Care Act (2014) London, The Stationary Office.

Children Act (1989) London, The Stationary Office.

Children and Families Act (2014) http://www.legislation.gov.uk/ukpga/2014/6/contents/enacted Accessed 24/06/20.

Children Services Network (2005) *Young Carers*. London: Local Government Information Unit.

Coles, P. (2003) *The Importance of Sibling Relationships in Psychoanalysis*. London, Karnac Books.

Cree, V.E. (2003) Worries and problems of young carers: issues for mental health. *Child and Family Social Work*, **8**, 301–309.

Dearden, C. & Becker, S. (1998) *Young Carers in the UK: A Profile*. London, Carers National Association.

Department of Health (1999) *Caring about Carers: A National Strategy for Carers*. London, Stationary Office.

Dunbar, S.B. (1999) A child's occupational performance: considerations of sensory processing and family context. *American Journal of Occupational Therapy*, **53**, 231–235.

Dunn, J. (2008) Sibling relationships across the life-span. In: *Putting Sibling Relationships on the Map. A Multidisciplinary Perspective* (ed. M. Klett-Davies). London, Family and Parenting Institute.

Edwards, R., Hadfield, L., Lucey, H., *et al.* (2006) *Sibling Identities and Relationships. Sisters*. London, Routledge.

Fives, A., Kennan, D., Canavan, J., *et al.* (2013) Why we still need the term 'young carer': findings from an exploratory study of young carers in Ireland. *Critical Social Work*, **14** (1), 49–61.

Franklin, M., Patterson, P., Allison, K., *et al.* (2018) An invisible patient: healthcare professionals' perspectives on caring for adolescents and young adults who have a sibling with cancer. *European Journal of Cancer Care*, e12970. https://doi.org/10.1111/ecc.12970.

French, J.R.P. & Caplan, R.D. (1973) Organizational stress and individual strain. In: *The Failure of Success* (ed. A.J. Marrow). New York, AMACOM.

Hamama, L., Ronen, T. & Rahav, G. (2008) Self-control, self-efficacy, role overload and stress responses among siblings of children with cancer. *Health and Social Work*, **33** (2), 121–132.

Hodges, A.S. (2016) The family centred experiences of siblings in the context of cystic fibrosis: A dramaturgical exploration. PhD Thesis, Cardiff University.

Howe, N., Aquan-Assee, J., Bukowski, W.M., et al. (2001) Siblings as confidants: emotional understanding, relationship warmth and sibling self-disclosure. *Social Development*, **10** (4), 439–454.

James, W. (1890) in James, W. (2017) *The Principles of Psychology* vol. **I**. London, Createspace Independent Publishing Platform.

Joseph, S., Sempik, J., Leu, A., *et al.* (2019) Young carers research, practice and policy: an overview and critical perspective on possible future directions. *Adolescent Research Review*. https://link.springer.com/article/10.1007/s40894-019-00119-9 Accessed 24/06/20.

Kelly, P. & Kelly, D. (2013) Childhood cancer; parenting work for Bangladeshi families during treatment. An ethnographic study. *International Journal of Nursing Studies*, **50**, 933–944.

Klett-Davies, M. (2008) *Putting Sibling Relationships on the Map: A Multi-disciplinary Perspective*. London, Family and Parenting Institute.

Knecht, C., Hellmars, C. & Metzing, S. (2015) The perspectives of siblings of children with chronic illness. A literature review. *Journal of Pediatric Nursing*, **30**, 102–116.

Labay, L.E. & Walco, G.A. (2004) Brief report. Empathy and psychological adjustment in siblings of children with cancer. *Journal of Pediatric Psychology*, **29** (4), 309–314.

Lloyd, K. (2013) Happiness and well-being of young carers: extent, nature and correlates of caring among 10 and 11-year-old schoolchildren. *Journal of Happiness Studies*, **14** (1), 67–80.

Long, K.A., Marsland, A.L., Wright, A., *et al.* (2015) Creating a tenuous balance: Sibling's experience of a brother or sister's childhood cancer diagnosis. *Journal of Paediatric Oncology Nursing*, **32**, 21–31.

McGuire, S., Manke, B., Eftekhari, A., *et al.* (2000) Children's perceptions of sibling conflict during middle childhood: issues and sibling (dis)similarity. *Social Development*, **9**, 2.

McHale, S.M., Crouter, A.C. & Mcguire, C. (1995) Congruence between mothers' and fathers' differential treatment of siblings: links with family relations and children's well-being. *Child Development*, **66**, 116–128.

McHale, S.M., Updegraff, K.A. & Whiteman, S.D. (2012) Sibling relationships and influences in childhood and adolescence, *Journal of Marriage and Family*, **74** (5), 913–930.

McHale, S.M., Whiteman, S.D., Kim, J., *et al.* (2006) Sibling relationships in childhood and adolescence. In: *Close Relationships: Functions, Forms and Processes* (eds P. Noller & J.A. Feeney), pp. 127–149. New York, Psychology Press.

Metzing-Blau, S. & Schnepp, W. (2008) Young carers in Germany: to live on as normal as possible - a grounded theory study. *BMC Nursing*, **7** (1), 15.

Mitchell, J. (2003) *Siblings*. Cambridge, Polity.

Mulroy, S., Robertson, L., Aiberti, K., *et al.* (2008) The impact of having a sibling with an intellectual disability: parental perspectives in two disorders. *Journal of Intellectual Disability Research*, **52** (3), 216–229.

Murray, J.S. (2000) Attachment theory and adjustment difficulties in siblings of children with cancer. *Issues in Mental Health Nursing*, **21**, 149–169.

Munn, P. & Dunn, J. (1989) Temperament and the developing relationship between siblings. *International Journal of Behavioural Development*, **12**, 443–451.

O' Brien, I., Duffy, A. & Nicholl, H. (2009) The impact of childhood chronic illnesses on siblings: a literature review. *British Journal of Nursing*, **18** (22), 1358–1365.

Office for National Statistics (2011) *Census 2001 Data*. London, ONS.

Rowe, D. (2007) *My Dearest Enemy, My Dangerous Friend: Making and Breaking Sibling Bonds*. London, Routledge.

Ruble, D.N., Boggiano, A.K., Feldman, N.S., *et al.* (1980) Developmental analysis of the role of social comparison in social evaluation. *Developmental Psychology*, **16**, 105–115.

Sanders, R. (2004) *Sibling Relationships: Theory and Issues for Practice*. Basingstoke, Palgrave Macmillan.

Shanahan, L., McHale, S.M., Crouter, A.C., *et al.* (2008) Linkages between parents' differential treatment, youth depressive symptoms, and sibling relationships. *Journal of Marriage and Family*, **70**, 480–494.

Social Services and Well-being (Wales) Act (2014) http://www.legislation.gov.uk/anaw/2014/4/contents Accessed 26/06/20.

Stamatopoulos, V. (2018) The young carer penalty: Exploring the costs of caregiving among a sample of Canadian youth. *Child & Youth Services*, **39** (2–3), 180–205.

Stark, V. (2007) *My Sister, Myself: Understanding the Sibling Relationship that Shapes our Lives, our Loves, Ourselves*. New York, McGraw-Hill.

Stoneman, Z. & Brody, G.H. (1993) Sibling temperaments, conflict, warmth and role asymmetry. *Child Development*, **64** (6), 1786–800.

Updegraff, K.A., McHale, S.M., Killoren, S.E., *et al.* (2010) Cultural variations in sibling relationships. In: *Sibling Development: Implications for Mental Health Practitioners* (ed. J. Caspi) pp. 83–105. New York, Springer.

Volling, B.L. & Elins, J.L. (1998) Family relationships and children's emotional adjustment as correlates of maternal and paternal differential treatment: A replication with toddler and pre-school siblings. *Child Development*, **69** (6), 1640–1656.

Woodgate, R.L. (2006) Siblings experience with childhood cancer – a different way of being with the family. *Cancer Nursing*, **29** (5), 406–414.

CHAPTER 5

A Holistic Approach to Meeting Physical, Social and Psychological Needs

Amie Hodges and Julia Tod

Introduction

The physical needs of children and young people with a long-term condition can often impact on their psychological well-being and social development. As highlighted in the previous chapters, families can become consumed by the care requirements of their child with a long-term condition, to the detriment of other aspects of their life such as education, socialisation and promotion of independence. Therefore, assessment that encompasses all aspects of life for these children and young people and their families is an essential skill in contemporary nursing.

While nurses should have an ability to negotiate and manage resources within the arena of multiagency and interdisciplinary teamworking, partnership and negotiation with children, young people and their families must be inherent in the relationship. Using a strength-based approach to practice will incorporate patients and family members as true partners in care.

Aim of the chapter

This chapter aims to provide an overview of some elements of physical, psychological and social issues that can affect the well-being of children and young people with a long-term condition and their families. A detailed critique of social

Nursing Care of Children and Young People with Long-Term Conditions, Second Edition.
Edited by Mandy Brimble and Peter McNee.
© 2021 John Wiley & Sons Ltd. Published 2021 by John Wiley & Sons Ltd.

and psychological theory will not be undertaken. Before reading this chapter, therefore, learners will need to understand the physiology and function of the skin, allergic response mechanisms, theory of pain and key children's cognitive development theories.

Using the case study of a child with eczema, learners will be able to explore a number of social and psychological factors that are relevant to families who have a child with a long-term health need and, through reflection, also explore their own responses to some of the psychosocial factors described. The physical needs of the child with eczema will be considered and reference made to the continuing needs of the child, and the implications for nursing practice.

Intended learning outcomes

- To explore the physical, psychological and social implications for the child/young person and family living with long-term illness
- To discuss how physical symptoms can impact on social and psychological factors
- To examine the relationship between development theories and management interventions for children/young people with eczema
- To critically evaluate how children's nurses can support children/young people and their families to enable them to achieve 'a good quality of life'

Prevalence of eczema

The child in the case study below will be referred to as Isabella, one of many suffering from atopic eczema, a common skin problem in childhood. Over the last 40 years, the prevalence of atopic eczema has risen throughout the Western world and affects 15–38% of children (Ballardini *et al.*, 2013) and specifically within the UK, one in five children have eczema (National Eczema Society, 2019). Historically, environmental factors such as being 'too clean', with a reduction in exposure to microorganisms that help develop natural immunity in early life, and being exposed to pollution have been suggested as reasons for the increase in prevalence. However, the 'hygiene hypothesis' is now disputed by Scudellari (2017) and further research is needed in relation to the immune system to identify the connection between our immune system and how it reacts to inflammatory triggers (Jones, 2017). There is, however, a genetic element to the condition that cannot be ignored, with studies demonstrating the link between parental atopic skin problems and childhood atopic eczema. Fathers are as likely as mothers to pass on the eczema predisposition (Wadonda-Kabondo, 2004; Hyde, 2015). There is also a strong association between eczema and other atopic diseases, such as asthma and hay fever, as well as an association between parental socioeconomic position and prevalence of atopic disease (Hammer-Helmich *et al.*, 2014). These are important considerations when establishing a patient's history. Isabella's family background and current presentation of her skin is explored below.

⊕ Case study 5.1

Background information

Isabella is a 5-year-old Eastern European child who lives with her parents in an affluent sub-urban area in the UK. The family migrated to the UK six months ago after Goran, Isabella's father, gained promotion in a steel company. His wife, Merelee, has not worked since the move. She had worked as a personal assistant in the steel company in their home country before Isabella's birth. Both parents are in their early 30s and Isabella is an only child.

Isabella was diagnosed with atopic eczema at the age of six months; both her parents have a history of mild atopy. Due to her diagnosis, emollients are Isabella's current main-stay of treatment, but recently her skin has become difficult to manage as she is suffering from an acute exacerbation of eczema. There has been an escalation of the inflammation, swelling and irritation of her skin, which has led to an uncontrollable 'itch scratch cycle'. Isabella is not sleeping and is upset, irritable and in pain. Merelee is extremely tired, as she is sleeping with Isabella to avoid disturbing Goran, is homesick and is distressed about her daughter's condition. Goran is supportive and plays with Isabella but is not involved with her ongoing care needs. Merelee has rudimentary English and is finding it difficult to 'settle' as she misses her extended family and the community she has left.

Isabella has recently started school and, as a lone child, is finding this challenging because she has not previously attended nursery. The headmistress has contacted the school nurse with several concerns about Isabella's care needs and her relationship with other children. There are currently no 'specialists' involved in her care as there has been a delay in her referral to the local children's hospital. Due to the concerns raised, her health visitor and general practitioner have been informed and a clinical appointment has been arranged to review all aspects of her care.

⏲ Time out

- Having read the case study, what do you consider are the key implications that nurses will need to consider when caring for Isabella and her family?

Nursing considerations

It is hoped that you will have recognised from the case study that Isabella and her family require an assessment of their needs so that the nurse can support both the child and the family.

This next section of the chapter will focus on considerations for children's nurses in the following areas:

- Recognising the signs of eczema and the importance of assessing the skin of children/young people with eczema.
- The treatment of eczema with emollients.

- The impact of the itch scratch cycle.
- Family coping mechanisms.

These issues will be discussed in relation to the role of the children's nurse throughout the text. The presentation of eczema will be discussed in the first instance.

Presentation of eczema

> 🔑 **Key points**
>
> - One of the key roles of the children's nurse is to assess the current status of the skin of the child/young person with eczema, as it is an inflammatory skin condition that can present with the following physiological problems:
>   - patches of dry skin
>   - cracked skin
>   - redness and inflammation of the epidermis
>   - scaly and itchy skin.
> - The skin can deteriorate if not assessed regularly and there is ineffective management, which can potentially lead to:
>   - blistering
>   - weeping
>   - infection
>   - lichenification (thickening and hardening of the skin)
>   - scarring.

The problems associated with eczema are multifactorial, and some of the above symptoms are synonymous with the acute exacerbation of Isabella's condition. In Chapter 1, the term 'multifactorial' and some environmental and dietary influences on eczema were briefly discussed. It is not surprising that Isabella is feeling miserable, as she is caught up in an itch scratch cycle, is in pain and unable to sleep, a situation that is exacerbating her inability to integrate properly into her new school.

> 🔑 **Key point**
>
> - Having established the skin status of the child/young person, the children's nurse can begin to assess the effectiveness of the current treatment regimen. Thorough assessment which includes discussion with the child and family will enable changes to be made concerning the choice of skin preparations to be used.

Isabella's assessment will take place at the clinical appointment referred to in the second part of the case study.

Treatment of eczema with emollients

Isabella's current eczema treatment regimen comprises emollients that are applied to the skin. Emollients are necessary to treat eczema due to an associated reduction in the lipid barrier function of the skin. Daily use of emollients promotes the barrier function of the skin, helping to maintain skin health. Bath additives for eczema, soap substitutes and topical emollients are recommended. It is important that health care professionals review the use of treatment products at least once a year to ensure monitoring and optimisation of treatment (National Institute Health and Care Excellence (NICE), 2019).

Topical emollients

Topical emollients are moisturisers, in the form of lotions, creams and ointments, which are used to recreate the moisture barrier of the skin, as they trap water in or allow water to be drawn from the dermis to the epidermis. They can be applied after bathing. Table 5.1 outlines the use of non-soap products and topical emollients. Daily application of emollients creates an additional burden for the family, due to the time

TABLE 5.1   **The use of non-soap products and topical emollients.**

Non-soap products Aqueous cream	Topical emollients Lotions
Can be used as soap, applied on to the skin via a cloth or using hands. When rinsed off there should be minimal irritation from it. Aqueous cream is less greasy than emulsifying ointment. It should be avoided if there is a known sensitivity to it.	Lotions can be helpful for application during the day as they are not very greasy and are quite light in consistency. They are absorbed quickly and require frequent application. Due to their lack of oil content, lotions are not as effective as other emollients, even though they are often preferred due to the unobtrusive nature of the product.
Emulsifying ointment	**Creams**
A greasy product that can be used by whisking the ointment in very hot water to dissolve it and then adding it to a bath.	Children usually accept creams for use because even though they have an increased oil consistency, they do tend to sink into the skin quite easily. Creams are useful for the daytime.
Bath oils	**Ointments**
These help wash the skin and trap moisture into it as it leaves an oily film over the surface of the skin.	Ointments are very greasy products and are often not favoured by children because they leave skin looking shiny and the product does not absorb quickly. Due to the greasy nature of ointments, staining of clothing can occur. Ointments are the most effective type of emollient for a child with extremely dry, fissured skin. Ointments are often applied before a child goes to bed. Some children will need to avoid the use of ointments if they develop sensitivity.

Source: Gould (2001); Lawton (2004); Burr & Penzer (2005); RCN (2013); NICE 2019.

taken to apply the product, gaining the child's cooperation and additional laundering of bedding and stained clothes. Further pressure can occur due to mothers wanting to keep their house clean and free from dust or anything that might cause greater irritation to their child's skin, because environmental factors such as house dust mite and animal dander can cause flare ups of eczema (Royal College of Nursing (RCN), 2013; NICE, 2019).

Safety

It is important for the children's nurse to advise children and families to be careful during bathing of the child, because emollients are greasy on the child's skin and may cause slippage when handling them or cause bath areas to become slippery. Careful handling of the child, the use of a bath mat and regular bath cleaning can be advised to reduce the risk of accidents in the home.

Also, paraffin-based products can be hazardous as there is an associated fire risk if paraffin-based products are over 50% in quantities of 100 grams or more. It is important to check the hazard warning on the product and the risk of fire hazard needs to be provided (RCN, 2013).

Key points

- The treatment regimen of children with a long-term condition can impact on all aspects of family life.
- Proving advice to children and families regarding safety when using treatment products is essential, so as to prevent the occurrence of accidents.

Time out

- Outline the advantages and disadvantages of the various eczema treatments discussed.

Effects of the itch scratch cycle

As identified in the case study, a child with atopic eczema is often caught in an itch scratch cycle, which can be one of the most distressing experiences for the child, and equally distressing for the onlooking adult, who feels helpless. The distress and discomfort caused by the itch scratch cycle can cause significant disturbance to the night-time routine of the child and family, as it is often difficult for the child to settle, and sleep is often disrupted (Rinaldi, 2019). Children may scratch their skin so much that it becomes red, inflamed and breaks down, causing infection, pain and discomfort as a weakness in the skin barrier occurs. Erythema can appear as a result of neuropeptide induced vasodilation that raises the temperature of the skin (Rinaldi, 2019).

Sleep deprivation leads to children and their families being tired, irritable and unable to concentrate in school/work. It can have a huge impact on children/young people in relation to their ability to make friends, schooling and educational achievement, and physically in relation to their height and pubertal development, as sleep is necessary for growth and repair to take place. Children and young people who are not developing at the same rate as their peers can often feel embarrassed and may become withdrawn as they try and cope with their emotions (Rubin *et al.*, 2009). In the longer term, this can lead to more acute mental health problems such as self-harm (Morgan *et al.*, 2017; NICE, 2011; NICE, 2019). The external appearance of the skin can have a huge influence on how a person feels and how others react and treat a person. It can influence socialisation as it affects society's perceptions of accepting or rejecting a person (Rubin *et al.*, 2009). Merelee is very aware of this in relation to her daughter, which adds to her maternal anxiety and is affecting her ability to cope. It can also impact on parents' ability to work effectively, which can influence their economic contribution to their family and society. Parents, fearful of leaving their sick children to go to work, may choose to stay at home, thus limiting their own social contact with others. Working parents, kept awake all night by their sick children, may find their ability to be productive in work during the day affected, which can potentially impact on their ability to maintain employment. As a consequence, the confidence and self-esteem of children with a long-term condition, such as eczema, and their families is often diminished, which, as discussed in Chapter 3, can lead to chronic sorrow (Batchelor & Duke, 2019).

Key point

- The itch scratch cycle can be extremely distressing for the child and equally disruptive to family life as a whole. Children's nurses must incorporate this consideration into their assessment to ensure appropriate strategies are put in place for the child and family.

Family stress and coping

The stress of caring for a child with a long-term condition extends beyond the initial diagnosis. This is demonstrated in the care burden highlighted in the case study. This, together with the move from a supportive community to a new country, has altered Merelee's response to Isabella's condition. Following the diagnosis of a long-term condition, families often seek to define family life as essentially normal (Hodges, 2016), acknowledging the existence of impairment while engaging in behaviour that demonstrates their normality. The effort of managing their child's illness, while presenting family life as 'typical', results in a constant struggle. Periods of transition – such as initial diagnosis, moving to a new setting and an increase of symptoms – can have an impact on the family's equilibrium, affecting emotions and increasing stress, and the family's need to use effective coping strategies to adapt to the changed situation. (See Chapter 3 for further discussion.)

Parent's well-being can also be affected by the nature of the child's condition, causing physical and financial stress and time demands. In parents of children with eczema, the daily care routine, sleep disturbance, concerns about the severity of the skin condition affecting the child's appearance and family functioning all contribute to maternal stress (Yamaguchi *et al.*, 2019). A lack of spousal support and perception of the child's behaviour can add to the stress experience (Faught *et al.*, 2007; Cousino & Hazen, 2013). It is important that nurses recognise that stress is an inevitable part of the lives of families with a child with a long-term condition and assess how stress impacts on the child and parents well-being.

⏱ Time out

- Think of a family that you have cared for. What strategies were used to help alleviate stress?
- Were these strategies effective?

Strategies have been identified that help individuals cope with stress and avoid stress-related illness. How many did you identify?

- A sensible pattern of diet, sleep and physical activity is a simple coping strategy. The cycle of sleep deprivation may lead to a lack of enthusiasm for exercise. Encouraging Merelee to attend group exercise would allow her to be active and establish friendships.

- Social support has a significant effect on coping skills (Nabors *et al.*, 2018). It cannot always be presumed that family will provide support; they may in fact be an additional source of stress. Children's nurses should be able to assess the family member's ability to express their needs, evaluate existing support systems (neighbours, religious groups, work colleagues) and act as a liaison between support services. Support groups such as the Eczema Society can provide local group meetings and meeting other parents in similar situations may provide an extended support network.

- An adaptive response to stress is to create positive feelings. Positive events such as celebrations or improving environmental factors (pleasant music, fragrances) can enhance mood. Encouraging Merelee to avoid dwelling on negative feelings and encouraging her to engage in things that she finds enjoyable will enable her to reassess her response to Isabella's condition.

- Effective coping strategies vary for individuals and some techniques may need to be taught. Some families may benefit from both eczema care education and community-based stress and coping courses.

The transition to school for a child with a long-term condition is often stressful and may represent one of the times that force parents to recognise their child's physical cognitive or social differences (Newton & Lamarche, 2012). Relinquishing the daily care management to teachers and other professionals can also be a source of concern. Children may face teasing and difficulties with friendship, and Isabella's skin condition may result in rejection by her peers. Loss of school-time due to hospitalisation can also affect performance in class, cognitive development and long-term success. Clearly, the educational and socialising experience of school is important, and good liaison between the care and education teams can ameliorate some of these difficulties.

🔑 Key point

- Children's nurses can encourage families to use various strategies to help them cope with caring for a child or young person with a long-term condition and signpost them to local facilities.

🌐 Case study 5.2

A thorough assessment at the clinic appointment by the consultant paediatrician and paediatric dermatology nurse established that Isabella's treatment was ineffective and needed to be reviewed and adjusted. The health visitor, who attended the appointment, explained that Merelee had no support network, was isolated and, as a result, was unable to manage Isabella's condition. The sleepless nights were unacceptable for all the family. Alleviation of Isabella's pain and the itch scratch cycle was seen as a priority. At this clinic appointment, Isabella told the nurse specialist, 'No one will play with me! I get called names in school, please make my skin better.' Isabella was asked where it hurt, and she was able to point to the inflamed areas of her skin. Merelee is worried that Isabella is being bullied and is losing confidence. The health care team discussed the treatments currently being used on Isabella's skin and the frequency of application. Merelee explained that she was applying the lotion to Isabella's skin every day, in the morning and before bedtime. However, she did not think the treatment was helping, so she had been using alternative therapies including homeopathy. A short admission to hospital for immediate intervention was arranged and a multidisciplinary team meeting was organised in order to develop an action plan.

🕐 Time out

- From the case study, what do you think you would need to consider in your assessment and care plan?

Assessment and immediate intervention

Part two of the case study has highlighted the need for assessment and intervention to help improve Isabella's skin condition and meet the needs of the family in relation to her skin status. Priorities for care and immediate management will focus on the following key areas:

- The effectiveness of Isabella's treatment regimen, adherence and application technique.

- Isabella's level of pain as a result of the itch scratch cycle.
- The effects of the exacerbation of eczema on Isabella's psychological and social well-being, particularly as she may be a target for bullying and finding it hard to integrate into her new school.
- The physical, psychological and social effects of Isabella's condition on Merelee and Goran.
- Current family support mechanisms.

NB: Isabella needs to be admitted to hospital to assess her pain and stabilise her condition. Treating her physiological symptoms and promoting comfort will help ease the psychological and social burden that has been highlighted in this chapter

---

🔑 Key points

- Children and their family's psychological well-being and quality of life should be discussed and recorded at each eczema consultation (NICE, 2019).
- Treatment that is offered to children with eczema should be based on recorded eczema severity, using a stepped care plan supported by education, as outlined in NICE (2019).

Current care management plan

Due to the inflammation, swelling and irritation of Isabella's skin, it is evident that her overall treatment regimen is ineffective. This is potentially due to a number of reasons:

- Unsuitable skin care products being used to manage Isabella's eczema.
- Not applying the skin care treatments correctly.
- Changes in the home circumstances/environment.
- Non-adherence with treatment; for example, infrequent application of treatments.

Wet wraps

Children with eczema who are caught up in an itch scratch cycle can often be helped by using wet wraps to treat the skin (NICE, 2007; British Association of Dermatologists, 2017). NICE (2019) describes the process of wet wrapping, which involves the application of warm semi-occlusive bandages over an emollient and, if necessary, a topical steroid. Wet wraps can be applied to any area of skin that is affected by eczema. They have the advantage of cooling and rehydrating the skin, which alleviates the itching, reduces pain due to the soothing effect of the treatment and promotes skin healing. Wet wraps are usually used when other forms of treatment such as bath oils, emollients, lotions, creams and mild steroids have become ineffective.

Wet wrapping is not recommended when eczema has become infected, as highlighted by NICE (2007), which recommends that skin should be clean and the eczema dry. Increased moisture introduced by wet wraps can cause an increase in formation of bacteria if an area of skin is already infected. Potent steroids are not recommended with wet wraps due to the increased permeability of the skin.

Although Isabella's skin was red and inflamed, it was not infected or oozing any exudates, so this form of treatment was an appropriate part of her management for the first 24 hours. Subsequent wet wrap treatments were carried out at night-time only for the next few days. Wet wrapping should not be used on a continuous basis as it is meant for short-term use in acute exacerbations. Prolonged use can increase the chances of skin infection and would be a very time-consuming process for parents to manage (NICE, 2007).

Topical steroids

Children with eczema sometimes require treatment with topical steroids if emollients are ineffective. Topical steroids help to reduce inflammation of the skin, and are available in different strengths, with the level of potency chosen dependent upon the severity of the skin condition. Topical corticosteroids are recommended for application to the affected areas of the skin no more than twice a day over the age of 12, and no more than once in the under 12s (NICE, 2007). An additional burden can be placed on the child and family if treatment is not properly explained.

> ⌸══ **Key point**
>
> • A key role of the nurse is to inform children, young people and parents about the side effects of topical steroids and their rate of absorbency (National Eczema Society, 2020).

Pain assessment

Due to inflammation and swelling of her skin, Isabella is experiencing pain. When skin becomes inflamed, a chemical reaction occurs, which stimulates the nerve endings. The perception of pain occurs as a result of a message being transmitted to the brain via the dorsal horn of the spinal cord (Carr & Mann, 2008; Cheng & Rosenquist, 2018).

Pain is a complex experience that can vary between each child and young person. According to Twycross *et al.* (2013), pain can be influenced by a variety of factors, including cultural background, previous experience and cognitive and emotional responses. Children with a long-term illness such as atopic eczema are in a vulnerable position, and assessment of pain status should always be a priority to ensure appropriate control and management of the condition.

Untreated pain can be overwhelming and traumatic for children and young people (Twycross *et al.*, 2013; Twycross & Saul, 2017). Table 5.2 outlines principles of practice relating to pain management put forward by the Royal College of Nursing (2009). These principles of care need to be considered when assessing any child/young person in pain. A widely recognised model of care that is synonymous with these principles is

TABLE 5.2 Pain management principles of practice.
Pain management philosophy of care
1. Children are listened to and believed
2. Children and their families are viewed as partners in care
3. Children and families are involved in shared decision-making
4. Children and families that require extra support should be identified
5. Children and families are informed of potential risks/complications associated with pain assessment
6. Training is provided in the use of tools for parents/carers
7. A collaborative, multiprofessional approach is provided by knowledgeable professionals
8. Attention is paid to the organisational issues and systems that enable effective management to take place

Source: Based on Royal College of Nursing (2009) *Clinical Practice Guidelines. The Recognition and Assessment of Acute Pain in Children*. Update of full guideline. London, Royal College of Nursing.

QUESTT, which involves **Q**uestioning the child, **U**sing a pain rating scale, **E**valuating behaviour and physiological changes, **S**ecuring parental involvement, **T**aking the cause of pain into account and **T**aking action in evaluating results (Baker & Wong, 1987; Wong-Baker Faces Foundation, 2016; Hockenberry & Wilson, 2018). The RCN (2009) also provides clear recommendations and guidance for the recognition and assessment of pain in children.

After questioning Isabella about her pain, she was able to point to the inflamed areas of her skin and where she was hurting. It is an important role of the children's nurse to obtain a pain history from the child and parent and learn the words that a child uses to describe their pain (e.g. baddie, hurt), as this can help reduce a child's anxiety (RCN, 2009; Hockenberry & Wilson, 2018). Cultural factors, which may influence pain and its management, also need to be identified and therefore nurses require key knowledge and skills in this area. When in pain, some children are very stoic and prefer to be left alone, while others prefer to have company. Response to pain may be dependent on family and societal influences, personality, religion, values and beliefs (Twycross *et al.*, 2013; Twycross & Saul, 2017).

On assessment, Isabella's behavioural and physiological response to her atopic eczema is one of distress, irritability and inability to sleep. Through assessment of this response, questioning and using an age-appropriate pain rating scale, Isabella's level of pain was recognised, enabling the appropriate intervention to promote her comfort.

Key point

- Pain management of the child with eczema is multidimensional and needs to focus on several aspects of care.

To provide holistic care, pain relief such as the use of wet wraps, antihistamines, play and distraction should be used. These methods of pain relief act on the sensation fibres of the skin, known as the 'A beta fibres', preventing the transmission of pain. This closes the 'gate' to pain. (See Recommended reading to learn more about 'gate control theory'.)

Time out

- Considering cultural factors, what signs may indicate that Isabella is in pain?

Antihistamines

Due to Isabella's physiological and behavioural responses of being irritable, not sleeping and continuously scratching, which is increasing her level of pain, the introduction of an antihistamine was found to help. Although an antihistamine is not a usual method of pain relief, it can be useful in an acute episode of eczema due to its sedative effects, which can help re-establish a sleeping pattern and control itching and discomfort. As this treatment is meant for short-term use only, Isabella had antihistamines for three nights.

Play and distraction

Play is an essential element of care when looking after a child with a long-term condition, particularly when they are in pain (Hirani, 2015; Hockenberry & Wilson, 2018). It is important for optimal physical, social, emotional and cognitive child development (Bateson, 2015). Children like Isabella can be suffering from high levels of anxiety because they do not really understand their illness or the reason for particular health care interventions. Introducing play that is appropriate to children's age and stage of development can allow them to express their feelings, as well as enabling them to communicate with others (Nijhof *et al.*, 2018). It can also help them to re-enact events that have occurred to gain a greater understanding of their situation (Hirani, 2015). Play is a way of helping children to gain emotional stability and control that can help them cope with their illness, as well as enabling them to communicate with others. Hirani (2015) discusses the importance of children's choice of toys, suggesting that the toys and type of play selected can be symbolic in helping the child to express specific fears, anxieties and guilt. Children's nurses, alongside hospital play specialists, can prepare children for interventions, support and help them to recognise their own coping strategies and enhance their partnership in care (Gill, 2013). They can facilitate play with the child and family through awareness of cultural beliefs, attitudes towards health, illness and play, understanding family dynamics and having a good knowledge of the . child's condition and prior experience (Trigg & Mohammed, 2010). This can enhance the child's rate of recovery and return to normality.

 Time out

- Reflect on a clinical situation that you have encountered with a child that required distraction techniques to be used. What distraction techniques were used? Were they beneficial?

TABLE 5.3 Examples of play, distraction and coping strategies.

Coping strategy	Examples
Breathing techniques	Blowing bubbles and balloons
Relaxation techniques	Guided imagery
Books, games and puzzles	Where's Wally? I spy
Imagery and make believe	Puppets, dolls
Music and television	Singing, videos
Sensory experiences	Play-dough, fibre optics
Positive reinforcement	Stickers, certificates

Source: From Shapcott (2018); Weaver and Groves (2010); Glasper et al. (2009).

Distraction techniques provide a focus to divert the child's attention by interacting with the child and family using developmentally appropriate play techniques that can improve coping mechanisms as well as relieve stress (Trigg & Mohammed, 2010; Gill, 2013). Distraction techniques are useful when carrying out procedures, and work best in partnership with preparation. For example, before Isabella has wet wraps applied, she could observe or be involved in wet wrapping a doll. Examples of play, distraction and coping strategies are outlined in Table 5.3.

Bullying

Isabella is being bullied in school; no one will play with her and children are calling her names. Nickerson (2019) suggests that bullying occurs among many children and young people and defines bullying as a person purposely causing harm or distress someone else. Nickerson (2019) examines the power relationship between the victim and the bully and agrees that bullying involves targeting an individual to inflict intentional harm. Bullying can involve repetitive actions that are direct or indirect and can be categorised as physical, verbal or relational and can occur in several contexts, for example online bullying (Gladden *et al.*, 2014; Smith, 2014; Nickerson, 2019). Physical harm may include pushing or hitting, whereas verbal bullying may include being isolated by others, teased and being called names, like Isabella in the case study. Such bullying and victimisation can lead to psychological harm such as depression, withdrawal, lack of confidence and low self-esteem (Espelage & Holt, 2013; Smith, 2014). If bullying is not resolved, it can lead to continued psychological problems as the child grows into adulthood. Bullies themselves may also have a low self-concept and develop a depressive state of mind, as they often have problems occurring in their own lives (Espelage & Holt, 2013; Nickerson, 2019), such as problems at home, or they may be frightened themselves of being 'picked on' by others.

When children are being bullied, they may be too frightened to tell anyone and may make excuses not to go to school; for example, they may develop symptoms of illness such as headaches and abdominal pain. Fortunately, Isabella has informed the nurse that she is being called names, giving her physical appearance as the reason she is being bullied. Often, children do not accept other children that they perceive to be 'different' from themselves and their peer group.

School nurses are in a prime position to help children caught up in a bullying cycle, as it is their role to safeguard children in their care. This includes promoting good emotional health and well-being (Smith, 2014; Pigozi & Bartoli, 2016). According to Pigozi and Bartoli (2016), schoolchildren feel they are able to confide in the school nurse and discuss the issue of bullying, which allows the school nurse to make assessments of general mental health and enables liaison and support between the school and families. The school nurse, the nurse in attendance at the assessment visit and the schoolteachers can all work together with the family to help Isabella to feel confident and happy to return to school. The school may have a policy to deal with the issue of bullying. The school nurse may speak to small groups of children within the school to help the situation. The family should be supported and may be advised to log any further bullying so that it can be dealt with in an appropriate and sensitive manner.

◉ Case Study 5.3

Isabella has been in hospital for five days, her skin has improved and she no longer has inflammation following wet wrap treatment. Play specialist intervention and meeting other children with the same condition has enabled Isabella to make friends and become less self-conscious.

While Isabella was in hospital, Merelee chose not to stay overnight with her, to gain some respite, and is no longer feeling as tired. Isabella's grandmother, who has come to stay for a month to help and support Merelee – as Goran has been unable to take time off work, has said that alternative therapies are part of the family's tradition and spiritual belief and that she wishes this to continue to be part of Isabella's treatment alongside medical intervention.

Isabella has gained some weight and the paediatric dietician has been in contact with the family. The dermatology nurse has discussed the new treatment plan with Isabella and her family and has taught them the application techniques. Liaison with the school nurse and health visitor has been arranged to ensure there is appropriate support on discharge.

The headmistress has contacted Merelee and asked if she would like to help in the school at lunchtime. Merelee has agreed, recognising that this would be a way to meet new people and support Isabella in school. A clinic appointment in a month's time has been made, and contact numbers for the hospital and information regarding support groups for children and young people with eczema have been given to the family.

It is evident within the case study that Isabella's condition has now stabilised. Merelee is feeling more settled as she has received support from her mother. Ongoing spirituality needs have been considered when planning care.

⏲ Time out

- What key elements need to be considered by the children's nurse when discharging Isabella?

Research highlights that the following key elements will need to be considered for discharge:

- Providing information about support groups.
- Health promotion and education of the child/young person and family concerning the current treatment regime.
- Providing education appropriate to age and stage of development.
- Involvement of the child and family in decision-making and planning care.
- Liaison with the multidisciplinary team.
- Appropriate liaison with the child's school.
- Ensure appropriate follow-up appointment is made.
- Consider ongoing spiritual needs when planning care.
- Gaining an understanding of alternative therapies (particularly those used in Isabella's care) (WAG, 2005).

Case study 5.3 identifies the family's need to maintain traditional spiritual beliefs. It is the role of the children's nurse to uphold families' beliefs and values. This section will consider some of these issues in detail.

🕒 Time out

- Reflect upon your own understanding of spirituality.
- How does this influence your nursing practice?

Spirituality

Contemporary nursing subscribes to the concept of holistic care provision for children and families. However, if nurses caring for children and young people are to embody the concept of holism, this must include an equal emphasis on spiritual needs. Clarke (2013) highlights that compassionate care of the whole person, body and soul is at the heart of nursing practice that values the individual and respects their dignity. For both staff and patients, spirituality is synonymous with religion. However, in present times, it is recognised that there are different forms and expressions of spirituality. Bash (2004) suggests that there are three ways to define spirituality:

- Secular approach (material world), which is often related to concepts of belonging, meaning and value.
- The theistic approach (belief in a god or gods), which is related to a force or being.
- The media approach, which uses secular terms but relates them to matters, typically the concern of religion, the search for truth and a reverence for the mysteries of life.

Any plan of care should include the spirituality, religion, culture and developmental stage of the child; there are a number of assessment tools that may be of use. The FICA Spiritual History Tool, (Puchalski & Romer, 2000) provides a way for the clinician to efficiently integrate the open-ended questions into a standard medical history and can be used by health care professionals. It explores the families **F**aith belief and meaning, **I**mportance of faith, relevance of spiritual **C**ommunity and how this needs to be **A**ddressed in care (FICA).

McSherry (2006) warns against mechanistic tick box style spiritual assessment. Nursing assessment and the subsequent provision of spiritual care should arise out of recognition of its importance and impact on the child, young person and family, and should avoid becoming a 'paper exercise'. Spiritual meaning for Isabella's family relates to some specific New Age beliefs relating to responsibility for, and interconnectedness with, the environment. This form of spirituality that emphasises the 'mystical', and in which the individual's feelings and experience are paramount, will affect the family's response to long-term illness and some forms of treatment. It will also influence Isabella's beliefs, as children's spiritual development does not occur in isolation from their family's beliefs. Cognitive development will also have direct impact on how she provides meaning to experiences. Fowler's theory of 'stages of faith' (Fowler, 1981) is based on Erikson's (1963) development cycle, which described critical periods of psychosocial development through the life cycle. Fowler's stages offer an explanation of the characteristics of faith development but, as with any stage theory, should not be taken too rigorously. Table 5.4 illustrates his description of the period from infancy to late adolescence. Isabella is at a stage where children are influenced by powerful images and rituals. Her grandmother's visit reaffirms the importance of the ritual of the family's faith and may have as great an influence on Isabella as it does on the rest of the family.

TABLE 5.4   **Fowler's stages of faith.**

Fowlers stages of faith (1981)	Age	
Undifferentiated or primal faith	Infancy	A prelinguistic, preconceptual stage in which the infant is gradually recognising distinction between environment and self. Self-worth is based on unconditional or conditional grounds.
Intuitive – projective faith	2–6	This stage builds on development of language and the imagination. With no cognitive operations that could test perceptions and thus reverse beliefs, children grasp experience in and through powerful images. The child is attentive to ritual and gesture.
Mythic – literal faith	7–12	There is a reliance on stories and narrative that is implied in the family faith experience. Belief is valued in a concrete sense; it can involve testing of meaning.
Synthetic – conventional faith	12–21	Development of life meaning is built on the original faith system and compiled of conventional elements; it is accompanied by a need to keep the faith group together.

Source: Adapted from Robinson et al. (2003). *Spirituality and the Practice of Health Care*. Basingstoke, Palgrave MacMillan.

> ⌨️ **Key points**
>
> ● Spirituality can be vital as a coping mechanism for children, young people and families experiencing a long-term condition.
> ● Where spirituality is an important component of home routine, a lack of assessment may lead to disruption of normal routine and a lack of respect for the family's beliefs.

🕐 **Time out**

- What has been your experience of complementary medicine?
- Has your experience affected your attitudes, behaviour and belief in relation to alternative treatments and therapies? If so, how?

Traditional, complementary and alternative medicine

Traditional, complementary and alternative medicine (TCAM) is an area where conventional biomedical ideas are changing. National Centre for Complementary and Integrative Health (2016, p. 6) defines TCAM as 'a group of diverse medical and health care systems, practices, and products that are not considered to be part of conventional or allopathic medicine'. They can range from home-made remedies, Chinese traditional medicine, aromatherapy and homeopathy to Shamanic healing. Individuals may use TCAM for comfort and symptom management or may consider them to be curative. It has been reported that up to 77% of patients do not disclose TCAM use and practitioners rarely ask parents about TCAM in eczema care (Robinson *et al.*, 2012).

Several factors influence parents' use of TCAM in association with or instead of traditional management. These include cultural determinants, dissatisfaction with treatment and the perception that TCAM is more natural or less toxic. Current research suggests a limited evidence base for a range of TCAM interventions; however, Thandar *et al.* (2014) suggest that further study of Chinese herbal medicine, fish oil and certain probiotics are warranted. NICE (2007) guidelines highlight the importance of caution with herbal medicines that are not labelled with clear information for safe usage; this information should be shared with families. Psychological interventions such as self-hypnosis, habit reversal and cognitive behavioural therapy (CBT) may be valuable in an integrative treatment approach (Chida *et al.*, 2007).

Health care staff should recognise that hostile attitudes do not discourage exploration of alternative therapies and may force parents into covert behaviour, no longer discussing their therapies with health professionals. Nurses can help families discuss their fears and concerns, allowing informed choice. If health care systems set TCAM in opposition to conventional medicine, a barrier to the practice of self-care management may be created.

Encouraging open discussion of TCAM use between the child, the family, the multidisciplinary team and, where possible, the therapists themselves may enable families like Isabella's and the multidisciplinary team to work together to achieve the best care for the child or young person with a long term condition.

Key points

- Families may use TCAM for comfort or symptom management for the child or young person with long-term illness. This should be in conjunction with advice from medical professionals.
- Written records of the families TCAM use will improve patient assessment and promote discussions of treatment plans.

Health promotion

The case study describes the improvement in Isabella's condition. However, it has not been an easy time for Isabella and her family as it is evident that caring for a child with a long-term condition can impact on family functioning as a whole. Before discharge, the continuing care needs of Isabella and her family should be addressed. Health promotion is necessary to ensure the appropriate future management of Isabella's eczema. When children are ill, parents have an overwhelming need to obtain information regarding their child's condition and want to be involved as partners in care (Smith & Coleman, 2010; Smith *et al.*, 2015). Using a partnership approach, the children's nurse can negotiate a programme of care with the family. This can be a diverse role as it involves having prior knowledge of the family situation, their coping mechanisms and their ability and willingness to be involved in particular aspects of care. It also requires the children's nurse to be aware of family support mechanisms.

Hopia *et al.* (2004) and Smith *et al.* (2015) suggest that parental involvement in care can be achieved if the children's nurse:

- Explains the child's illness, diagnosis and prognosis.
- Assesses the confidence and competence of the family to manage their child's condition.
- Offers a plan of care that has been negotiated with the child and family.
- Ensures parental and child understanding of the illness and treatment plan.
- Involves the child and family in the decision-making process.
- Allows the child and family to express their views.
- Supports the parent in their care-giving role.
- Includes parental knowledge and experience of their child in the assessment, planning delivery and evaluation of care.

Having a greater understanding and control of Isabella's physical condition can help improve psychological and social well-being. The condition of atopic eczema was discussed with Isabella and her family and a plan of care was initiated with the support of the health care team. When planning a care regimen, it is important to consider the patient's lifestyle as this helps with adherence with treatment.

Conclusion

Eczema is a common childhood atopic condition that is associated with other atopic diseases such as asthma and hay fever. It is a condition that can lead to deterioration of the physical, psychological and social functioning of a child and family. Physical symptoms can result in altered external appearance of the skin, pain, discomfort and insomnia, as well as the itch scratch cycle. Poor educational achievement, poor socialisation and emotional turmoil can prevail if the condition is not managed effectively. This can impact on family life as a whole, affecting marital relationships, socio-economic function of the family and parents' ability to cope.

During an acute exacerbation of eczema, pain management and diversion therapy are essential elements of care. Family support and guidance with coping strategies is paramount. There are several options available that can help treat and prevent exacerbation of the condition. These include non-soap products, emollients, topical steroids and use of wet wraps. Thorough assessment of the skin is necessary to ensure an appropriate treatment regimen is planned. Ongoing follow-up and support of the child and family is essential to monitor the effectiveness of the treatment regimen. Children's nurses need to promote parental involvement in their child's care to ensure their understanding of the condition, which will allow them to recognise signs and symptoms, encourage adherence to treatment plans and involve them in the decision-making process. Spiritual and cultural requirements need to be considered in relation to all aspects of care. Liaison with schoolteachers and the school nursing team is essential to promote emotional health and well-being. Providing ongoing support and follow-up, and involving the multidisciplinary team in the process, will enable the child and family to adapt to living with long-term illness, helping them on the way to achieve a good 'quality of life'.

Test your knowledge

- Outline the signs and symptoms of eczema.
- List the priorities that need to be considered when assessing the needs of children and young people with eczema.
- Consider the physical symptoms of eczema and write down how these can have an impact on the child, young person and family from a social and psychological perspective.

Useful websites

http://www.bad.org.uk/about/
http://www.bdng.org.uk/
http://www.bma.org.uk/ap.nsf/Content/LIBAlternativeMedicine
http://www.eczema.org/

📖   Recommended reading

Goswami, U. (2011) *The Wiley-Blackwell Handbook of Childhood Cognitive Development*. Oxford, Wiley Blackwell Publishing.

Hockenberry, M.J. & Wilson, D. (2018) *Wong's Nursing Care of Infants and Children* (eleventh edition). London, Elsevier.

McSherry, W. (2006) *Making Sense of Spirituality in Nursing Practice: An Interactive Approach* (second edition). London, Churchill Livingstone.

Smith, P. (2009) *Children and Play: Understanding Children's Worlds*. Oxford, Wiley Blackwell Publishing.

References

Baker, C. & Wong, D. (1987) QUESTT: a process of pain assessment in children. *Orthopaedic Nursing*, **6** (1), 11–21.

Ballardini, N., Kull, I., Soderhall, C., *et al*. (2013) Eczema severity in preadolescent children and its relation to sex, filaggrin mutations: A report from BAMSE birth cohort. *British Journal of Dermatology*, **168**, 588–594

Bash, A. (2004) Spirituality: the emperor's new clothes? *Journal of Clinical Nursing*, **13**, 11–16.

Batchelor, L.L. & Duke, G. (2019) Chronic sorrow in parents with chronically ill children. *Pediatric Nursing*, **45** (4), 163–173. 183.

Bateson, P. (2015) Playfulness and creativity. *Current Biology*, **25**, R12–16.

British Association of Dermatologists (2017) Atopic Eczema. Patient Leaflet, 1–9.

Burr, S. & Penzer, R. (2005) Promoting skin health. *Nursing Standard*, **19** (36), 57–65.

Carr, E.C.J. & Mann, E.M. (2008) *Pain: Creative Approaches to Effective Management* (second edition). Basingstoke, Palgrave.

Cheng, J. & Rosenquist, R.W. (eds) (2018) *Fundamentals of Pain Medicine*. New York, Springer.

Chida, Y., Steptoe, A., Hirakawa, N., *et al*. (2007) The effects of psychological intervention on atopic dermatitis. A systematic review and meta-analysis. *International Archives of Allergy and Immunology*, **144**, 1–9.

Clarke, J. (2013) *Spiritual Care in Everyday Nursing Practice: A New Approach*. Basingstoke, Palgrave Macmillan.

Cousino, M.K. & Hazen, R.A. (2013) Parenting among caregivers of children with chronic illness: a systematic review. *Journal of Pediatric Psychology*, **38** (8), 809–828.

Erikson, E.H. (1963) *Children and Society* (second edition). New York, W.W. Norton and Co.

Espelage, D.L. & Holt, M. (2013) Suicidal ideation and school bullying experiences after controlling for depression and delinquency. *Journal of Adolescent Health*, **53** (1), S27–31.

Faught, J., Bierly, C., Barton, B., *et al*. (2007) Stress in mothers of young children with eczema. *Archives of Disease in Childhood*, **92** (8), 683–686.

Fowler, J.W. (1981) *Stages of Faith*. New York, Harper & Row.

Gill, C. (2013) Helping children cope with renal disease: the role of play specialist. *Journal of Renal Nursing*, **2** (5), 244–247.

Gladden, M.R., Vivolo-Kanter, A.M., Hamburger, M.E., *et al*. (2014) Bullying surveillance among youths. uniform definitions for public health and recommended data elements. Atlanta: Center for Disease Control and Prevention.

Gould, D. (2001). Childhood eczema. *Primary Health Care*, **11** (7), 43–49.

Hammer-Helmich, L., Linneberg, L. & Thomsen, S.F. (2014) Association between parental socioeconomic position and prevalence of asthma, atopic eczema and hay fever in children. *Scandinavian Journal of Public Health*, **42**, 120–127.

Hirani, S.A.A. (2015) The magical role of play therapy. *Reflections on Nursing Leadership*. Sigma Theta Tau International Honour Society of Nursing. https://www. Reflectionsonnursingleadership.org Accessed 29/01/20.

Hockenberry, M.J. & Wilson, D. (2018) *Wong's Nursing Care of Infants and Children* (eleventh edition). London, Elsevier.

Hodges, A.S. (2016) The family centred experiences in the context of cystic fibrosis. A dramaturgical exploration. PhD Thesis, Cardiff School of Healthcare Sciences.

Hopia, H., Paavilainen, E. & Astedt-Kurki, P. (2004) Promoting health for families of children with chronic illness. *Journal of Advanced Nursing*, **48** (6), 575–583.

Hyde, P. (2015) Eczema. Kidshealth.org.uk Accessed 07/03/20.

Jones, K. (2017) Researchers dispel "hygiene hypothesis" linked to eczema study. Research: National Eczema Society. https://nationaleczema.org/hygiene-hypothesis/ Accessed 28/01/20.

Lawton, S. (2004) Effective use of emollients in infants and young people. *Nursing Standard*, **19** (7), 44–50.

McSherry, W. (2006) *Making Sense of Spirituality in Nursing Practice: An Interactive Approach* (second edition). London, Churchill Livingstone.

Morgan, C., Webb, R.T., Carr, M.J., *et al.* (2017). Incidence, clinical management and mortality risk following self-harm among children and adolescents: cohort study in primary care. *British Medical Journal*, **359**, J4351.

Nabors, L. Cunningham, J. Lang, M., *et al.* (2018) Family coping during hospitalization of children with chronic illnesses. *Journal of Child and Family Studies*, **27** (5), 1482–1491.

National Center for Complementary and Integrative Health (2016) Strategic Plan. https://nccih. nih.gov/sites/nccam.nih.gov/files/NCCIH_2016_Strategic_Plan.pdf Accessed 20/01/20.

National Eczema Society (2019) *What is Eczema?* London, National Eczema Society. https:// www.eczema.org Accessed 19/12/19.

National Eczema Society (2020) *Topical Steroids Fact Sheet 1–7.* https://www.eczema.org Accessed 28/01/20.

National Institute for Clinical Excellence (2007) *Atopic Eczema in Under 12s: Diagnosis and Management.* https://www.nice.org.uk/guidance/cg57 9 Accessed 25/01/20.

National Institute for Health and Care Excellence (2011) Self-Harm in over 8s: Short term management and prevention of recurrence. NICE Clinical Guideline CG16.2004. https://www. nice.org.uk/guidance cg16 Accessed 28/01/20.

National Institute for Health and Care Excellence (2019) Atopic eczema in under 12s Quality standard published 2013. Copyright 2020. https://www.nice.org.uk/guidance/qs44 Accessed 28 January 2020.

Newton, K. & Lamarche, K. (2012) Take the challenge: strategies to improve support for parents of chronically ill children. *Home Healthcare Nurse*, **30** (5), E1–E8.

Nickerson, A.B. (2019) Preventing and intervening with bullying in schools: A framework for evidence base practice. *School Mental Health*, **11** (1),15–28.

Nijhof, S.L., Vinkers, C.H., Van Geelen, S.M., *et al.* (2018) Healthy play, better coping: The importance of play for the development of children in health and disease. *Neuroscience and Biobehavioural Reviews*, **95**, 421–429.

Pigozi, P.L. & Bartoli, A.J. (2016) School nurses' experiences in dealing with bullying situations among students. *The Journal of School Nursing*, **32** (3), 177–185.

Puchalski, C. & Romer, A.L. (2000) Taking a spiritual history allows clinicians to understand patients more fully. *Journal of Palliative Medicine*, **3**, 129–137.

Rinaldi, G. (2019) The itch-scratch cycle: A review of the mechanisms. *Dermatology Practical and Conceptual*, **9** (2), 3.

Robinson, N., Lorenc, A., Falinski, A., *et al.* (2012) The challenges of facilitating primary healthcare discussions on traditional, complementary and alternative medicine for childhood eczema: Piloting a computerized template. *Patient Education and Counselling*, **89** (3), 517–524.

Robinson, S., Kendrick, K. & Brown, A. (2003) *Spirituality and the Practice of Health Care.* Basingstoke, Palgrave MacMillan.

Royal College of Nursing (2009) *Clinical Practice Guidelines. The Recognition and Assessment of Acute Pain in Children. Update of full guideline.* London, Royal College of Nursing.

Royal College of Nursing (2013) Caring for children and young people with atopic eczema. Guidance for nurses. https://www.rcn.org/-/media/royal-college-of-nursing/documents/publications/2013/august/pub-00328.pdf Accessed 01/03/19.

Rubin, K.H., Coplan, R.J. & Bowker, J.C. (2009) Social withdrawal in childhood. *Annual Review of Psychology*, **60**, 141–171.

Scudellari, M. (2017) Cleaning up the hygiene hypothesis. New Feature. *PNAS*, **14** (7), 1433–1436. https://www.pnas.org/cgi/doi/10.1073/pnas.1700688114 Accessed 24/06/20.

Smith, L. & Coleman, V. (2010) *Child and Family Centred Care. Concept, Theory and Practice* (second edition). Basingstoke, Palgrave.

Smith, J., Swallow, V., & Coyne, I. (2015) Involving parents in managing their child's long term condition. A concept synthesis of family centred care and Partnership in care. *Journal of Pediatric Nursing*, **30**, 143–159.

Smith, P.K. (2014) *Understanding School Bullying. Its Nature & Prevention.* London, Sage.

Thandar, Y., Botha, J. & Mosam, A. (2014) Complementary therapy in atopic eczema: the latest systematic reviews. *South African Family Practice*, **56** (4), 216–220.

Trigg, E. & Mohammed, T. (2010) *Practices in Children's Nursing. Guidelines for Hospital and Community* (third edition). London, Churchill Livingstone.

Twycross, A., Dowden, S.J. & Bruce, E. (2013) *Managing Pain in Children: A Clinical Guide for Nurses and Healthcare Professionals* (second edition). Oxford, Wiley-Blackwell.

Twycross, A. & Saul B. (2017) Assessment and management of pain in children. In: *Essentials of Nursing Children and Young People* (eds J. Price & O. McAlinden). Thousand Oaks, CA, Sage.

Wadonda-Kabondo, N. (2004) Association of parental eczema, hay fever and asthma with atopic dermatitis in infancy: birth cohort study. *Archives of Disease in Childhood*, **89** (10), 917–921.

Welsh Assembly Government (2005) *National Service Framework for Children, Young People and Maternity Services in Wales.* http://www.wales.nhs.uk/sites3/documents/441/33519%20Main%20Doc%20Complete%20LoRes.pdf Accessed 30/01/20.

Wong-Baker Faces Foundation (2016) QUEST for relief. https://www.wongbakerfaces.org. Accessed 29/01/20.

Yamaguchi, C., Takeshi, E., Hosokawa, R., *et al.* (2019) Factors determining parenting stress in mothers of children with atopic dermatitis. *Allergology International*, **68** (2), 185–190.

CHAPTER 6

Empowering Children, Young People and their Families

Mandy Brimble

Introduction

Advances in care delivery and medical technology have resulted in increased life expectancy for many children with long-term conditions (Wijlaars *et al.*, 2016). The continued and growing redirection of health care service provision from acute to community and primary care settings (National Health Service England *et al.*, 2014) has resulted in many children and young people with long-term conditions being cared for by their parents in partnership with health and social care professionals; locally or in their own homes. This has provided professionals with an opportunity to enhance quality of life for this client group, with the implementation of health promotion advice and strategies. Indeed, *Making Every Contact Count* (Public Health England *et al.*, 2016) is an initiative which encourages health and social care staff to use routine interactions with patients to promote health and well-being.

Aim of the chapter

This chapter considers the challenges and issues surrounding the delivery of health promotion strategies by children's nurses, and the uptake of this advice by those in our care. Exploration of a long-term condition scenario will illustrate how these challenges may be exacerbated in terms of the receptiveness of the child, young person or family and their ability to change behaviour.

It is not the intention of this chapter to provide a detailed critique or in-depth theoretical discussion of health promotion models or the condition of childhood asthma, which is used in the case study. For a broader overview of health promotion,

Nursing Care of Children and Young People with Long-Term Conditions, Second Edition.
Edited by Mandy Brimble and Peter McNee.
© 2021 John Wiley & Sons Ltd. Published 2021 by John Wiley & Sons Ltd.

the reader may wish to access Green *et al.* (2015), Naidoo and Wills (2016) and Scriven (2017), full references for which can be found at the end of this chapter.

The aim of this chapter is to develop the readers' knowledge base to enable them to conceptualise how health education and promotion can be used to inform and empower children/young people with a long-term condition and their families.

Intended learning outcomes

- To define the concepts of health promotion and empowerment
- To apply fundamental theoretical approaches to a case study in order to illustrate aspects of promoting health and well-being in the context of long-term conditions
- To explore strategies used by health care professionals, in particular children's nurses, in the empowerment of children, young people and families
- Through a long-term condition case study, to examine barriers that may affect the uptake of health promotion advice and identify strategies to overcome these

Health promotion

The World Health Organization (WHO) (1946) defined health as 'a state of complete physical, mental and social well-being, and not merely the absence of disease or infirmity'. Although this definition can be criticised for conveying a somewhat unachievable ideal, it does describe health in positive terms, underlining the notion of health as a holistic concept. In today's multicultural and diverse society, it is important for nurses to recognise that there are many factors that can influence our individual ideas and health beliefs, for example culture, social class (Naidoo & Wills, 2016).

The reader should note that although health education and health promotion are terms that are often used interchangeably, they are two different concepts. Generally, health promotion activities contain a component of health education (Naidoo & Wills, 2016). Health education is primarily preventative and aims to increase knowledge, thus enabling informed choice in addressing issues that affect health and well-being. There are currently many health education campaigns aimed at the general population – for example, smoking cessation, healthy eating and immunisation – and although some individuals will act on these campaigns, many do not.

Test your knowledge

Why is it that despite having good quality information about the benefits of healthy eating, many people choose to ignore it? Identify reasons from a child, young person and adult perspective.

> **Key point**
>
> - The reason for inaction by large sections of the population, despite having the necessary information, is that knowledge does not necessarily change attitude or behaviour. The effectiveness of health education activities is likely to be linked to an individual's perception of whether their 'locus of control' is primarily internal or external. In basic terms, this refers to an individual's view of their own strength and ability in influencing their life, versus the influence that external factors have on them. In relation to health choices, young children will ultimately be subject to the decisions their parents make for them and, when they reach an age when they can make their own choices, these will be shaped by views and behaviours learned from their parents.

It is clear, therefore, that health education alone is not widely effective in increasing the health of the population, thus highlighting the importance of other components of health promotion. Just as health is a complex and multifaceted concept, so is health promotion and can, therefore, have a variety of meanings for individuals, communities and nations (Kumar & Preetha, 2012). Health promotion is defined as 'the process of enabling people to increase control over and to improve their health' (WHO, 1984, p. 4). This definition highlights the enabling or empowering facet of health promotion and underlines the role of the health professional in not merely education of clients but facilitation of the conversion of knowledge into health-enhancing actions. This aspect of health promotion is likely, therefore, to involve increasing the individual's concept of their internal locus of control.

> **Key point**
>
> - Within a long-term condition scenario, 'health' in terms of the WHO definition can sometimes be unachievable. Therefore, it is more likely that the aim of health promotion strategies will be to empower the child or young person to perform their social roles and achieve their personal potential.

Reflection

Before reading the following passage, consider your own notion of health promotion and make a note of your key thoughts.

The Ottawa Charter (WHO, 1986) presents health promotion as an 'enabling' concept, which can assist individuals and/or groups to establish a state of well-being. Enabling is an essential aspect of health promotion and WHO identifies several elements that potentially influence lifestyle choice; for example, empowerment, autonomy, egalitarianism, partnership and collaboration. The importance of health promotion in relation to long-term conditions is discussed by Kuper *et al.* (2018), who highlight it as a vehicle for enabling individuals to cope with long-term conditions such as disability, and as a means of improving quality of life for the patient within the confines of the disease or condition.

Reflection

Reflect on why and how you could use health promotion strategies in relation to children and young people with long-term conditions. Make notes of your thoughts.

🔑 Key point

- It is the health professionals' responsibility to ensure that communication with all clients is in a format and at a level that is easy to understand. Children's nurses require knowledge of child development to be able to assess a child or young person's developmental stage and skills to interact appropriately with them, at all levels.

Delivery of health promotion advice and health education strategies to children and young people is likely to pose a challenge to children's nurses as some issues may be complex and will have to be dissected and presented carefully; for example, children who are in the pre-operational stage (Piaget, 1963) will not have an understanding of internal body parts. Therefore, justification for behaviour change that focuses on damage to such organs or body systems will be at best ineffective and at worst frightening for the child. In addition, as children and young people are somewhat reliant on their carers for provision of healthy diet or lifestyle options, it will be necessary to fully engage the family/carer in order to facilitate any behaviour change. Finally, because the factors that influence the uptake of health promotion advice are multifaceted, the practitioner needs to be skilled in assessment of the client's individual situation in order to utilise appropriate strategies.

Within a long-term condition scenario, these challenges increase in complexity, as the disease or condition may greatly influence the child or young person's ability or motivation to adopt healthier behaviours. For example, a 10-year-old who is obese and confined to a wheelchair, due to disability, will be unable to increase their exercise levels significantly. The motivation and ability to change the diet will be affected by a historical relationship with food, which at 10 years of age is likely to be well established, and an overall view of the future will influence motivation to lose weight. Another significant factor that will affect desire to lose weight is the opportunity to interact with peers, such as pride in appearance and/or fitting in with the group. Likely progression of disease and/or prognosis could also impact on children's or young people's overall view of their general health and desire to improve it. Issues for such children, relating to reliance on their family/carers for healthy diet and lifestyle options, are likely to be long-standing, rather than confined to infancy and the young childhood period.

Empowerment

Empowerment is a concept that has been widely discussed in relation to the promotion and achievement of good health. In fact, Green *et al.* (2015) state that it is the most important component of health promotion strategies.

> **Key point**
>
> • WHO (2012) define empowerment as 'a process through which people gain greater control over decisions and actions affecting their health'. It is both an individual and a community process.

Individual and community empowerment are influenced by many political and individual factors, but as nursing care focuses primarily on individuals, this chapter will concentrate on enabling children, young people and families to take control over and make decisions about their lives, rather than how nurses may influence the political agenda in order to empower communities.

Individual empowerment involves a partnership approach, whereby the care provider aims to assist clients to develop the knowledge, skills and attitudes that will enable them to be proactive in gaining control over their life, health and health care (Green *et al.*, 2015). An example of empowering versus non-empowering health promotion behaviour in a ward setting is given below.

A nurse who gives information on and discusses a healthy diet with a child/young person and/or family and then:

- Supports them in making healthy food choices but allows negotiation to take place (empowering).
- Makes menu choices on their behalf, without consultation (non-empowering).

Test your knowledge

What type of knowledge, skills and attitudes do you think may be required by the children's nurse in order to empower:

1. children
2. adolescents
3. parents?

Make a note of your thoughts.

Individual empowerment is associated with psychological characteristics such as self-concept, self-esteem, self-assertiveness and perceived locus of control. It can also be influenced by the possession of life skills which enable young people to take greater responsibility for their own health (Prajapati *et al.*, 2017). For children and young people, the ability to become empowered will be linked to their developmental stage. Naidoo and Wills (2016) state that methods by which care-givers can promote the acquisition of these psychological characteristics and life skills are advocacy, negotiation, networking and facilitation. The empowerment of children, young people and families in coping with long-term conditions, specifically during periods of hospitalisation, has been researched by Coyne (2011) who highlights adaptation to the illness, facilitation of coping strategies and involvement in decision-making in order to promote self-esteem as key factors. Chapter 10 highlights some of the impact of long-term conditions upon young people's self-esteem and coping.

Approaches to health promotion

There are many models of health promotion that can be applied to a wide variety of scenarios, with varying degrees of success depending on numerous internal and external factors. This chapter will use the work of Scriven (2017), who has identified a framework of five approaches to health promotion that are universal to most models. This will assist the reader to gain knowledge and understanding of the principles of health promotion. The approaches to health promotion identified by Scriven (2017), together with a summary of each, are shown in Table 6.1.

The last of these approaches, the societal change approach, will be primarily excluded from this chapter, which aims to focus on individual interactions between the children's nurse and the child/young person or family, rather than community and/or government approaches via legislation, rules and regulations. However, in relation to the issues identified, some brief examples will be given.

Key points

- It is important to note that health promotion advice that involves behaviour change must include a client-centred and educational approach (in certain cases, medical intervention may also be used).

- Other strategies need to be deployed in assisting clients to change behaviour, because merely informing clients that a specific behaviour is undesirable is likely to invoke an emotional response which is unlikely to translate into sustained action (Government Communication Service, 2014).

- It is necessary first to provide information (education) relating to how the undesirable behaviour is likely to affect clients and/or those around them and then work with them to make small changes that will motivate them to sustain and extend these changes.

- Health promotion involving behaviour change is an evolving process that commences with the nurse as an external motivator who provides knowledge and facilitates skills, thus empowering clients by helping them to identify internal motivators that enable them to sustain the change.

TABLE 6.1 Approaches to health promotion.

Approach	Aim	Health Promotion Activity	Important Values	Example - smoking
Medical	Freedom from medically defined disease and disability	Promotion of medical intervention to prevent or ameliorate ill health	Patient compliance with preventative medical procedures	Aim – freedom from lung disease, heart disease and other smoking-related disorders Activity – encourage people to seek early detection and treatment of smoking-related disorders
Behaviour change	Individual behaviour conducive to freedom from disease	Attitude and behaviour change to encourage adoption of 'healthier' lifestyle	Healthy lifestyle as defined by health promoter	Aim – behaviour changes from smoking to not smoking Activity – persuasive education to prevent non-smokers from starting and to persuade smokers to stop
Educational	Individuals with knowledge and understanding, enabling well-informed decisions to be made and acted upon	Information about cause and effects of health-demoting factors Exploration of values and attitudes Development of skills required for healthy living	Individual right of free choice Health promoter's responsibility to identify educational content	Aim – clients will have an understanding of the effects of smoking on health. They will make a decision whether or not to smoke and act on the decision. Activity – giving information to clients about the effects of smoking. Helping them to explore their own values and attitudes and to come to a decision. Helping them to learn how to stop smoking if they want to
Client centred	Working with clients on their own terms	Working with health issues, choices and actions that clients identify Empowering the client	Clients as equals Clients' right to set agenda Self-empowerment of client	Anti-smoking issue is considered only if clients identify as a concern. Clients identify what, if anything, they want to know and do about it
Societal change	Physical and social environment that enables choice of healthier lifestyle	Political/social action to change physical/social environment	Right and need to make environment health enhancing	Aim – make smoking socially unacceptable so it is easier not to smoke than to smoke Activity – no-smoking policy in all public places. Cigarette sales less accessible, especially to children, promotion of non-smoking as social norm. Banning tobacco advertising and sports' sponsorship.

Source: From Scriven, A. (2017). *Ewles and Simnett's Promoting Health: A Practical Guide* (seventh edition). Reproduced with permission of Elseveir.

Of the approaches listed by Scriven (2017), being client centred is a fundamental aspect of children's nursing, as it encompasses the principles of family-focused care. This is a concept that underpins our interactions and care for children, young people and families. However, the true meaning of family-focused care has been and continues to be debated (Smith *et al.*, 2002; Jolley & Shields 2009; Smith & Kendal 2018). The case study that follows, and the interventions discussed, aim to give the reader an understanding of how the concept of family-focused care may be delivered within a long-term condition scenario.

Key points

- Children and young people with long-term conditions, their families and other carers often become experts on their particular condition and have a more comprehensive understanding of the condition itself, how it affects the patient and which treatment or interventions are most effective and appropriate (Smith, *et al.*, 2015; Smith & Kendal 2018).
- In family-focused care, the nurse, child and family truly work in partnership, each taking equal responsibility for care planning, making decisions and care delivery (Arabiat *et al.*, 2018).
- However, it must not be assumed that 'expert parents' wish to undertake the majority of care while the child/young person is in hospital – they may view this situation as a welcome opportunity for respite from the daily burden that this level of care imposes on them.
- An empowered parent should feel confident to negotiate care roles, including refusal to undertake any should they wish to act in a parental role only, rather than as a care-giver (Smith *et al.*, 2015).

Read part 1 of the case study below and answer the questions that follow. This will enable you to start to consider areas of health promotion within a long-term condition scenario and apply the identified approaches to these areas. Throughout the chapter, following each part of the case study, there will be a discussion of the approaches and strategies that could be used to address emergent issues.

Case study 6.1

Megan was a normal delivery, born full term to Sarah, aged 19 years, who smokes 20 cigarettes a day. Sarah is a lone parent with a supportive maternal family network. Currently she does not work. At six months of age, Megan presented in the A&E department with a history of poor feeding and a wheezy chest. On this occasion, she was admitted to the children's medical ward, prescribed bronchodilators and her condition improved. She did not require any further pharmacological intervention on discharge. From this time, she was a healthy child with no respiratory symptoms. At age 6 years, Megan was admitted to hospital with an inspiratory wheeze and diagnosed as asthmatic. She was prescribed bronchodilators and inhaled steroids via an MDI (measured dose inhaler) and spacer, as recommended by the British Thoracic Society (2019), for children 5–12 years. Before discharge, Megan and Sarah were seen by the respiratory nurse specialist who assessed, and deemed competent, their administration of medication.

Over the last two years, Sarah has consulted their GP on many occasions about Megan's condition. Sarah is aware that her smoking impacts upon Megan's condition and has previously discussed this with the GP, health visitor, school nurse and practice nurse. However, to date, Sarah has been unable to stop smoking.

Now aged 8 years, Megan has been admitted to hospital with an acute exacerbation of her asthma. On admission, her measurements and vital signs are undertaken in line with the latest RCN (2017) standard. Her height is 127 cm (50th centile) and she weighs 50 kg (above the 99.6th centile). Her observations are: temperature 36.8 centigrade, pulse 140 beats per minute, respirations 40 breaths per minute, oxygen saturations 91%.

Test your knowledge

- What do you consider are the two main health promotion issues?
- Identify from Scriven (2017) the approaches to health promotion you consider are appropriate for these issues.
- What skills are required to enable the practitioner to effectively promote healthy behaviour for Megan and Sarah?
- What would normal temperature, pulse, respirations and oxygen saturations be for a child who is 8 years of age?

Your answer to question 1 should have been parental smoking and obesity, and you should have identified that all five approaches were appropriate to address these issues. As stated earlier, societal change will not be discussed in this chapter. However, examples of this approach are the ban on smoking in public places to discourage smoking and protect non-smokers from second-hand smoke, the ban on cigarette advertising at sporting events, hiding cigarettes from public view in shops and it being illegal to sell cigarettes to children younger than 16 years of age.

Parental smoking

The remaining four approaches to health promotion will now be examined in relation to assisting Sarah to give up smoking. This will improve Megan's environment and consequently her condition and the future health of her mother. To empower Sarah to help her to stop smoking, we need to take a *client-centred* approach. Sarah has already identified that she wishes to give up smoking but has, so far, been unsuccessful. Some parents do not smoke in the house because they are aware of the risks to their child from second-hand smoke, such as sudden and unexpected death in infancy (SUDI), (Royal College of Pathologists, 2016; Lullaby Trust, 2019), exacerbation of asthma, respiratory and ear infections (Action on Smoking and Health (ASH), 2014); and because parental smoking sets a 'bad example', which may lead to a child taking up smoking later in life through normalisation of smoking and learned behaviour (ASH, 2018). However, although avoidance of smoking in the home reduces a child's exposure to second-hand smoke, it is ineffective in terms of the residual harmful substances that are still present in the environment, often referred to as 'third-hand smoke' (Northrup *et al.*, 2016) so giving up completely is preferable (Orton *et al.*, 2014).

Guidance from a health professional can motivate a client to give up smoking. So it is important that nurses have the health promotion skills and knowledge to deliver this advice effectively and in an empowering manner. However, in Sarah's case, the information/advice given by the GP, health visitor, school nurse and practice nurse had been unsuccessful, a common situation because even those motivated to give up can make numerous attempts before they achieve their aim, due to the difficulty in overcoming an addiction. The WHO (2005) state that all health professionals have a role in helping clients to give up smoking and highlight the effect of second-hand smoke on children. Therefore, children's nurses have a key role and are ideally placed to undertake this.

As Sarah has already demonstrated an insight into the harm she is likely to be causing Megan, it would be easy to assume that she has adequate information relating to the effects of second-hand smoke. However, to be effective and client centred, the practitioner needs to explore Sarah's current level of knowledge and understanding before offering any further advice or intervention. In terms of the nursing process, this is equal to undertaking an assessment before devising a plan of care. Once the assessment process is complete, the practitioner can then begin to formulate a plan in partnership with the individual. It is, therefore, important that the nurse clearly understands the condition or behaviour about which they are advising.

To empower Sarah to undertake the required *behaviour change*, it may be necessary to provide *education* to supplement and extend her current level of knowledge. To help Sarah transfer this knowledge into action, her motivational level will need to be explored to assess her attitude towards the behaviour change. It is possible, for example, that Sarah is using cigarette smoking to help relieve the stress she experiences as sole carer of a child with a long-term condition. Having identified relevant internal and external factors that impact on Sarah's ability to quit smoking, an individualised behaviour change plan can be formulated. An intervention that is sometimes successful in smoking cessation is one-to-one or group support, which involves counselling and/or group therapy. One-to-one counselling could be face to face or via helplines such as those run by the National Health Service (NHS, 2018).

It may also be necessary to help Sarah develop some life skills – such as coping strategies or relaxation techniques – for her to be successful in quitting smoking. It is clear, therefore, that in this particular scenario the *educational* and *behaviour change* approaches are closely linked and interdependent.

A *medical* approach could also be used, for example nicotine replacement therapy (NRT) which has been shown, via systematic review, to increase the success rate of smoking cessation to 60% (Hartmann-Boyce *et al.*, 2018). In addition, certain components of antidepressant medications have been shown to be effective in treating nicotine dependence and are licensed in some countries (Hughes *et al.*, 2014). More recently e-cigarettes have been used as an aid to smoking cessation. As yet there is limited evidence in relation to their effectiveness and the long-term effects are largely unknown. However, a randomised controlled study by Bullen *et al.* (2013) found that nicotine e-cigarettes were modestly effective in helping people stop smoking. They were more effective than patches and placebo e-cigarettes, but the differences were not statistically significant. Despite much publicity regarding alternative therapies, systematic reviews have found that interventions such as acupuncture and hypnotherapy have limited success in aiding smoking cessation (Tahiri *et al.*, 2012; White *et al.*, 2014).

Obesity

Romieu *et al.* (2017) state that being overweight or obese is almost always the result of energy intake exceeding energy expenditure, i.e. a greater number of calories are consumed than expended. Childhood obesity can cause hypertension, is associated with type 2 diabetes, increases the risk of coronary heart disease, increases stress on the weight-bearing joints, lowers self-esteem and affects relationships with peers. There are various methods of determining if an individual is obese, for example waist circumference, skin fold measurements and calculation of Body Mass Index (BMI). Calculation of BMI is achieved by dividing weight (in kilograms) by the square of the height (in metres). In other words, the algebraic expression for BMI is:

$$BMI = Kg/m^2$$

Using the weight and height measurements given for Megan, we can calculate her BMI as follows:

$$50kgs \div 1.27 \ m^2 = 31.00006$$

There are BMI categories for adults and children/young people (up to 20 years of age). Adult bandings are unsuitable for children due to changes in body fat as children grow. In addition, girls and boys differ in their body fatness as they mature. BMI for children, known as BMI for age, is calculated using centile charts published by the Child Growth Foundation, based on the seminal work of Cole *et al.* (1995; 2000).

Whether an adult or gender and age specific means of BMI assessment is used, Megan would be classified as obese. For her to be on the 50th centile of a traditional percentile chart (see Figure 6.1) and, therefore, in proportion, she would need to weigh 26 kg. This correlates with the children's BMI chart (as shown below) in that a weight of 26 kg would give a BMI of 16.12, which is on the 50th centile. If one used adult banding classifications, then a BMI of 16.12 would be in the underweight range, thus illustrating the importance of age and gender appropriate means of assessment.

The National Institute for Clinical Excellence (NICE) (2013) recommend that the goal of treatment for children who are still growing and developing should be weight maintenance rather than weight loss in the short term. However, for Megan's weight and height to align on the 50th centile (assuming her height remains on the 50th centile) she would need to maintain 50 kg until she was 14 years of age; a period of six years, which is too lengthy to remain at risk of the health consequences of obesity. Therefore, weight loss through an evidence-based combination of dietary and physical activity changes, such as the NICE (2017) pathway, would be recommend. Furthermore, some authors recommend focusing attention away from weight loss and toward health gains when implementing an exercise intervention for young people who are obese (Shaibi *et al.*, 2015).

As with smoking cessation, all five approaches to health promotion can be used to address the prevention and/or treatment of obesity. However, the education, behaviour

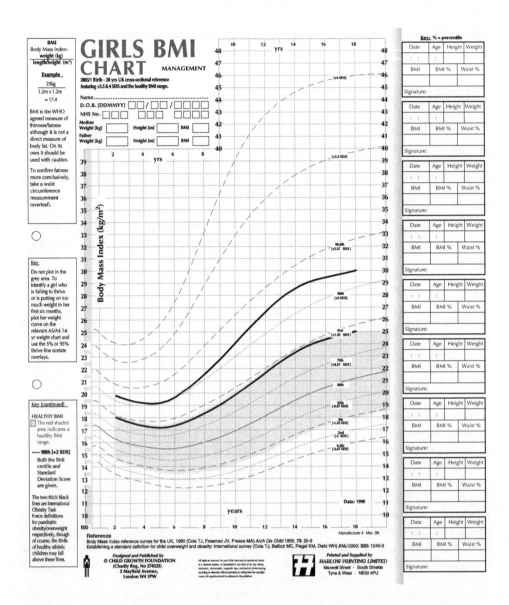

FIGURE 6.1 A BMI chart for girls aged 0–20 years. *Source*: Reproduced with kind permission of the Child Growth Foundation and Harlow Printing.

change and client-centred approaches are most applicable to this case study. Before examining these approaches in detail, the relevance of the societal and medical approaches will be briefly discussed.

Societal approach

Obesity is considered a global epidemic (WHO, 2016) and is therefore a grave cause for concern regarding the effects on the morbidity and mortality of the population and the financial impact on health service resources (Department of Health, 2011). The extent of the problem makes it necessary for a societal approach to be taken, in the first instance by using widespread health education to raise awareness of the problem and related issues. However, as eating habits are personal and likely to have been established in childhood, it is necessary to adopt an individual and client-centred approach to affect behaviour change in treating obesity. If the current, widespread, health education approach continues, and this is targeted at children as they begin to form their eating habits, it is possible that in the long-term a societal educational approach may be effective in actually preventing obesity occurring. This approach may also be successful in perpetuating effective parenting in relation to healthy eating, thereby substantially reducing obesity in future generations.

Medical approach

Pharmacological treatment of adult obesity is long standing (NICE, 2001a, b; Matson & Fallon, 2012). However, a systematic review published by the Cochrane Collaboration found that drugs such as metformin, sibutramine, orlistat and fluoxetine had only a very small effect in reducing the BMI of children and adolescents (Mead *et al.*, 2016)

Gastric banding can be considered for children and adolescents who are severely obese and who have not responded to non-invasive treatments. It has been shown to be successful but is currently available only for severe and complex cases (NHS England, 2017).

Cosmetic surgery, to reduce weight, in the form of liposuction is becoming increasingly popular, particularly in the US. Removal of fat in this way may improve a child or young person's body image and subsequently their self-esteem. However, this may lead to a misconceived perception of a 'quick fix' to weight issues, as opposed to sustained personal effort to address the problem. Furthermore, there is no conclusive evidence that removal of fat by liposuction decreases the risk of developing heart conditions, hypertension or diabetes. This is because liposuction reduces surface fat rather than that which surrounds and infiltrates organs and body systems.

Individual educational, client-centred and behavioural change approaches

From their updated Cochrane review, Brown *et al.* (2019) conclude that strategies for improving nutrition and physical activity levels, or both, are effective in producing modest improvements in BMI for children aged 0–12 years. However, there was less evidence that this would be successful for those aged 13–18 years.

Megan is aged 8, so a *behaviour change* approach to increasing physical activity, diet modification and avoidance of sedentary behaviour would be appropriate to address her weight issues. The intervention is likely to be *educational* in the first instance and, having explored Sarah and Megan's current level of knowledge and motivational level, should be individualised and therefore *client centred*.

A logical approach to making information client centred and more meaningful and relevant to a client is an individualised plan or programme. In addition, the use of graphics or symbols that link information in the plan to specific health education, for example the 'eatwell guide' (NHS, 2016), may help to consolidate this knowledge.

In addition, contemporary tools such as interactive multimedia interventions can enhance effective communication between children and health professionals and subsequently improve knowledge and understanding for children who are overweight (Raff *et al.*, 2014).

Clearly, it is important that children's nurses work very closely with dietitians and paediatricians in delivering this information to Sarah and Megan while maintaining a central role in delivering the personalised intervention. This approach supports effective multidisciplinary team working (Zolotarjova *et al.*, 2018) and promotes continuity of care and effectiveness, since the children's nurses will have already established a relationship with the child and family during the hospital admission. Hospitalisation can affect a child's mental health and cause temporary regression in areas such as speech, educational attainment or behaviour (Li *et al.*, 2016). These potential problems should be discussed with parents so that if they do occur, parents are prepared for them. In addition, the child's school nurse or health visitor should be advised of the admission so that they are similarly prepared.

Many factors can trigger asthma; for example, exercise, colds and viruses, pets, cigarette smoke, cold weather and pollen (Asthma UK, 2019). It is very important therefore, at this stage, to fully explore the factors that appear to trigger Megan's asthma. If exercise is an issue, then behaviour change in relation to increasing physical activity may need to be managed with particular care. By fully exploring this area and designing an individualised activity plan, any concerns that Sarah and Megan may have in relation to exercise induced asthma can be discussed. Any misconceptions should then be dispelled, thereby overcoming such barriers to the uptake of health promotion advice.

Test your knowledge

What specific information could be included in an individualised diet and activity programme for Megan?

◉ Case study 6.2

Megan is now an inpatient on the children's ward. During a conversation with a student nurse, Sarah confides that she has not been administering Megan's preventative inhaled medication. She does not want Megan to take steroids because she is already overweight and does not wish this problem to be exacerbated. Sarah believes that taking steroids will result in Megan gaining even more weight. (See Chapter 7 for a discussion on ethical issues relating to the dilemma of the nursing student.)

Appropriate medications, delivered via a mask and spacer were unsuccessful in alleviating Megan's symptoms. Therefore, these are now being administered via a nebuliser. Unfortunately, Megan has displayed some difficult behaviour when receiving treatment in this way and it has been necessary for the nurses and Sarah to use restrictive physical interventions during the procedure.

Test your knowledge

- What do you consider to be the main health promotion issue?
- Identify approaches to health promotion you would consider to be appropriate regarding this issue.
- Which skills are now required to enable the practitioner to effectively promote healthy behaviour?
- Are there any legal issues relating to the use of restrictive physical interventions with children for medical/nursing procedures?

You will have recognised that non-compliance is the main health promotion issue, in terms of Sarah's resistance to oral steroids and Megan not wishing to comply with nebulised medication. Which approaches to addressing this issue did you identify as being appropriate? These issues can, as in the previous section, be addressed by the medical, behaviour change, educational and client-centred approaches.

Non-compliance

Failure to take medication within a long-term condition scenario is a common problem, particularly in relation to childhood asthma (Burgess *et al.*, 2011). This is due to a number of factors; for example, lack of understanding of the role of 'preventer' medication, fear of side effects and absence of immediate symptom improvement (compared to reliever medication). For Megan to benefit from the correct medical approach, as prescribed, it will be necessary for the practitioner to use an educational, client-centred approach to ensure that Sarah has all the necessary information to make an informed choice regarding compliance with the medical regimen, thereby achieving concordance and the desired behaviour change. Problems experienced during this admission concerning Megan's compliance with the administration of nebulised medication also need to be addressed. (In Chapter 10, compliance is discussed in more detail in relation to adolescent development.)

Steroids

An educational approach is needed to ensure that a full explanation is given to Sarah regarding the safety of low dose steroid therapy, and to reassure Megan and her about the small risk of side effects and exactly what they are. In addition, the practitioner needs to stress that the dangers of uncontrolled asthma far outweigh any risks of treatment (Rottier *et al.*, 2015). It is important that this information is conveyed in a non-judgemental, factual manner to prevent it being misinterpreted as 'scaremongering' to force compliance.

Once this additional information has been internalised and understood by Sarah, and possibly Megan, it may be possible to formulate an individualised self-management plan. This is a client-centred approach that involves keeping an asthma diary, with careful monitoring of peak flow measurements and adjustment of treatment as necessary, together with criteria for seeking further medical advice and/or help. This should enable Megan and Sarah to feel more confident in managing the condition and therefore empowered (Kashaninia *et al.*, 2018).

Restrictive physical interventions and therapeutic holding

Restrictive physical interventions (formerly referred to as restraint) and therapeutic holding, also referred to as clinical or supportive holding, of children for procedures or administration of medication is frequently discussed and occurs in a range of health care situations and settings (Page *et al.*, 2019). The most recent guidance from the Royal College of Nursing (RCN) (2010) highlights the need to distinguish between emergency situations and those where there is no short-term risk of imminent harm. The work of Page *et al.* (2019) uses a case study approach to facilitate ethically sound professional decision-making, inclusive of the views and rights of the child, in situations where some form of clinical holding is required. In addition to the possibility of accidental physical harm to the child, parent or health professional during restrictive physical interventions children's nurses also need to consider the detrimental effects such incidents may have on the mental health of all those involved. Restrictive physical interventions should only be used as a last resort (RCN, 2010). Alternatives such as distraction techniques, for example storytelling and guided imagery (see Chapter 5), are suggested and should be used in negotiation with the child and family to suit their individual needs (i.e. a client-centred approach). In this particular scenario, it may be possible to alter the administration technique slightly to give Megan more control over the situation, thereby empowering her. Many children object strongly to having a mask held over their face, and allowing Megan to hold the mask herself may be all that is required to promote cooperation and compliance.

Test your knowledge

- What developmental stage (according to Piaget) is Megan likely to be at?
- What appropriate educational tools could be used to inform Megan in relation to her asthma and treatment?

As Megan is 8 years of age and has no learning difficulties, it is likely that she is at the concrete operational developmental stage (Piaget, 1963) and able to understand basic information regarding her condition and its management. Staff should aim, therefore, to explain information in an age appropriate way and reinforce this with resources that are specifically designed for children with asthma, for example leaflets available from relevant organisations and suitable websites. These educational interventions should enable Megan to gain a better understanding of her condition and, as she becomes older, increase her level of participation in discussion and decisions about her care.

Being able to interact with other children who suffer from asthma, via forums such as appropriate internet sites and projects such as Asthma Camps (Nabors *et al.*, 2014), should help ensure that Megan does not feel 'different' or isolated from her peers, and potentially improve symptom control.

Colleagues in primary care play a vital role in managing patients' asthma in the community (Lo *et al.*, 2016). It is essential that in relation to this case study, the ward practitioner liaises effectively with the GP, practice nurse and school nurse to support Sarah and Megan. The school nurse is particularly important in supporting pupils with long-term health conditions (National Children's Bureau, 2016) and when this support is effective it can reduce sickness absence (Schuller 2015). Approximately one in ten children in the UK have asthma, i.e. about 1.1 million children (National Education Forum, 2018). This means that about two children in every classroom are affected, illustrating the extent of school nurses' involvement in providing support to children with asthma. It also demonstrates to potential scope for implementing initiatives that are relevant to a large number of their caseload.

Within this scenario, the school nurse should ensure that Megan's teachers are confident and competent in helping with administration of medication, know what usually exacerbates Megan's asthma and are alert to early signs and symptoms of an attack. Education about asthma to Megan's peers (with Sarah and Megan's agreement, so privacy and confidentiality is not compromised) may also be helpful in supporting her, dispelling myths and overcoming prejudice within the school environment.

🌐 Case study 6.3

Eight months later, following a period of good health, the practice nurse sees Megan in asthma clinic. Her peak flow measurements are significantly reduced. Sarah reports that Megan is taking her 'preventer' medication regularly, but it has been necessary for her to take her bronchodilators more frequently over the last two weeks. During the consultation, Megan proudly tells the practice nurse that their kitten, Sooty, will be a year old next week. Sarah also relays a funny story about their experience of pony trekking on a recent holiday in the country.

Test your knowledge

What factors do you think may have contributed to the recent exacerbation of Megan's asthma?

It is likely that Megan and Sarah have been exposed to high levels of pollen, horsehair and cat fur. Assuming that they have not consciously disregarded advice already given on avoidance of such allergens, one assumes that there is a gap in their knowledge. This may have occurred for two reasons. First, the health professionals involved in giving health promotion advice may have focused solely on the main issues, believing that the information provided was substantial and that any additional advice would detract from it. Unfortunately, this viewpoint results in a failure to undertake a truly holistic approach, despite the application of all relevant approaches to health promotion. Second, Sarah and Megan may have received, but forgotten, allergen avoidance advice, perhaps due to information overload or due to a lack of recent reinforcement.

Test your knowledge

- What practical measures could have been taken by the health professionals involved to ensure that Megan and Sarah were fully informed of potential allergens earlier?
- How can children's nurses ensure that families receive all relevant information about a disease or condition, together with health promotion advice, without overloading them?

Allergen testing could have been performed during Megan's hospital admission or followed up at clinic. Although a medical approach was used during that admission to promote compliance and concordance with prescribed medication, an assumption was made that non-compliance was solely responsible for the exacerbation of Megan's condition. As Sooty is now aged 1, it is likely that he would have been with Megan and Sarah eight months ago. One must assume, therefore, that for some reason staff did not ask about pets when admitting Megan or that the information received was disregarded due to oversight or lack of staff knowledge. In this instance, optimum care has not been achieved because only a partially client-centred approach was used, which focused on only one aspect of behaviour change.

Failure to test for allergens earlier and/or discuss potential allergens has now led to a situation where, having become attached to Sooty over a period of months, Megan and Sarah may have to make the difficult decision to find a new home for their family pet.

Educational approaches to ensure that children, young people and their families receive comprehensive information about a disease, symptom control and health promotion will, as already discussed, need to be appropriate to their developmental age and their individual circumstances; that is, client centred. These could include bullet points within an asthma diary so that, when it is used daily by the child and parent, important information is reinforced. Board games that are designed by medication/appliance manufacturers or ward staff could be used during clinics or admissions to convey information, in a fun way, to younger children. Anatomical dolls and mannequins are another resource that can be used, particularly by play specialists, with this age group. Older children and adolescents may prefer to access information via the internet or mobile phone applications (Wiecha *et al.*, 2015). However, care needs to be taken when recommending the access of information via the internet. First, not all sites are suitable or evidence based. Second, some clients may not have access to a computer at home. It is advisable, therefore, to provide details of recommended websites to clients and, if finances permit, provide computers and internet access for clients' use in clinic waiting areas or on children's wards. It is important to note that information needs of parents whose child has a long-term condition are complex (Smith *et al.*, 2013). So nurses should be knowledgeable about the condition and support sources. All verbal information should be reinforced with written materials such as leaflets (Lakhanpaul *et al.*, 2017).

Lakhanpaul *et al.* (2017) examined parental perceptions of childhood asthma and found that knowledge and understanding of the condition was generally poor. Therefore, nurses should deliver opportunistic education in whichever environment the health professional encounters the child, i.e. making every contact count (Public Health England *et al.*, 2016). Parental asthma education programmes, covering topics such as disease process and allergen/trigger avoidance have been shown to impact significantly on understanding, attitude and feelings of empowerment (Agusala *et al.*, 2018; Kashaninia *et al.*, 2018).

Conclusion

This chapter has utilised the work of Scriven (2017) to illustrate how principles of health promotion may be applied in a long-term condition scenario. The individual interpretation of the term 'health' within the general population has been highlighted, together with how this may differ for those with long-standing and non-curable conditions. By addressing specific health promotion issues within a scenario, the aim was to demonstrate the use of relevant strategies by children's nurses to promote healthy behaviours to alleviate symptoms and improve the overall well-being of the child and family.

The effect of external and internal factors on the client's receptiveness to health promotion strategies has also been highlighted alongside suggestions for overcoming barriers to health promotion advice. Potential pitfalls have been outlined in relation to assessment and adaptation to changes in circumstance, thus reinforcing the need for a holistic approach.

The importance of education as a basis for health promotion, and its ineffectiveness if not used in conjunction with other approaches, has been discussed. Empowerment has been identified as the key component of health promotion. The facilitation of empowerment can be summarised as providing client-centred information, retention of this knowledge by the client, facilitation (by the practitioner) of skills development (in the client), which then enable them to effect and sustain health enhancing behaviour change.

Finally, the importance of children's nurses' specialist knowledge of child development and family-focused interpersonal skills has been highlighted. The approaches to health promotion and strategies discussed in relation to the case study have illustrated that children's nurses working in the hospital environment should be as competent and confident in using such knowledge and approaches as their community counterparts. In doing so, opportunities to maximise the health potential of children and young people suffering from long-term conditions will be fully utilised so that they, and their families, feel supported and empowered.

🔑 Key points

- Knowledge does not necessarily change attitude or behaviour.
- Empowerment is 'a process through which people gain greater control over decisions and actions affecting their health' (WHO, 2012) and has been identified as the most important component of health promotion strategies (Green *et al.*, 2015).
- Health promotion advice that involves behaviour change must include a client-centred educational approach (in certain cases, medical intervention may also be used).

- Behaviour change is an evolving process that is primarily concerned with the nurse influencing the client's perception of their locus of control.
- Within a long-term condition scenario, 'health' in terms of the WHO definition can sometimes be unachievable. Therefore, it is more likely that the aim of health promotion strategies will be to empower the child or young person to perform their social roles and achieve their personal potential.

Useful websites

An Introduction to Health Promotion and the Ottawa Charter https://www.youtube.com/watch?v=G2quVLcJVBk

Asthma https://www.asthma.org.uk

Obesity https://www.nationalobesityforum.org.uk

Obesity https://www.aso.org.uk

Staying Healthy http://kidshealth.org/kid/stay_healthy/

Smoking cessation http://www.patient.co.uk/showdoc/40000776/

Smoking cessation http://www.givingupsmoking.co.uk/

Tobacco and smoking policy https://www.gov.uk/government/collections/tobacco-and-smoking-policy-regulation-and-guidance.

NHS BMI Calculator https://www.nhs.uk/live-well/healthy-weight/bmi-calculator/

References

Action on Smoking and Health (2014) The health effects of exposure to secondhand smoke. https://ash.org.uk/information-and-resources/secondhand-smoke/ash-research-report-secondhand-smoke/ Accessed 28/01/20.

Action on Smoking and Health (2018) Fact sheet no. 24: Smoking in cars. https://ash.org.uk/information-and-resources/secondhand-smoke/smoking-in-cars-2/ Accessed 28/01/20.

Agusal, V., Vij, P. & Ag, V. (2018) Can interactive parental education impact health care utilization in pediatric asthma: A study in rural Texas. *Journal of International Medical Research*, **46** (8), 3172–3182.

Arabiat, D., Whitehead, L., Foster, M., *et al.* (2018) Parents' experiences of Family Centred Care practices. *Journal of Pediatric Nursing*, **42**, 39–44.

Asthma UK (2019) Understanding asthma triggers. http://www.asthma.org.uk/advice/triggers/understanding/ Accessed 28/01/20.

British Thoracic Society and Scottish Intercollegiate Guidelines Network (2019) *British Guideline on the Management of Asthma: A National Clinical Guideline*. London: British Thoracic Society and SIGN. Available at: https://www.brit-thoracic.org.uk/quality-improvement/guidelines/asthma/ Accessed 2/7/20.

Brown, T., Moore, T., Hooper, L., *et al.* (2019) Interventions for preventing obesity in children. *Cochrane Database of Systematic Reviews*, **7** (7), CD001871. https://doi.org/10.1002/14651858.CD001871.

Burgess, S., Sly, P. & Devadason, S. (2011) Adherence with preventive medication in childhood asthma. *Pulmonary Medicine*. doi:10.1155/2011/973849.

Bullen, C., Howe, C., Laugesen, M., *et al.* (2013) Electronic cigarettes for smoking cessation: a randomised controlled trial. *Lancet*, **382** (9905), 1629–1637. https://doi.org/10.1016/S0140-6736(13)61842-5.

Cole, T.J., Freeman, J.V. & Preece, M.A. (1995) Body mass index reference curves for the UK, 1990. *Archives of Disease in Childhood*, **73** (1), 25–29.

Cole, T.J., Bellizzi, M.C., Flegal, K.M., *et al.* (2000) Establishing a standard definition for child overweightand obesity worldwide: international survey. *British Medical Journal*, 320. https://doi.org/10.1136/bmj.320.7244.124

Coyne, I. (2011) Children's experiences of hospitalization and their participation in health-care decision making. In: *Ethical and Philosophical Aspects of Nursing Children and Young People* (eds G. Brykczynska and J. Simons), pp. 127–143. Chichester, Wiley.

Department of Health (2011) *Healthy Lives, Healthy People: A Call to Action on Obesity in England*. London, The Stationary Office.

Government Communication Service (2014) *The Government Communication Service Guide to Communications and Behaviour Change*. London, Government Communication Service.

Green, J., Tones, K., Cross, R., *et al.* (2015) *Health Promotion: Planning and Strategies* (third edition). London, Sage.

Hartmann-Boyce, J., Chepkin S.C., Ye W., *et al.* (2018) Nicotine replacement therapy versus control for smoking cessation. *Cochrane Database of Systematic Reviews*. https://doi.org/10.1002/14651858.CD000146.

Hughes, J., Stead, L., Hartmann-Boyce, J., *et al.*, (2014) Antidepressants for smoking cessation. *Cochrane Database of Systematic Reviews*. https://doi.org/10.1002/14651858.CD000031.

Jolley, J. & Shields, L. (2009) The Evolution of Family-Centered Care. *Journal of Pediatric Nursing*, **24** (2), 164–170.

Kashaninia, Z., Payrovee, Z., Soltani, R., *et al.* (2018) Effect of family empowerment on asthma control in school-age children. *Tanaffos: Journal of Respiratory Diseases, Thoracic Surgery, Intensive Care and Tuberculosis*, **17** (1), 47–52.

Kumar, S. & Preetha, G. (2012) Health promotion: an effective tool for global health. *Indian Journal of Community Medicine*, **37** (1), 5–12.

Kuper, H., Smythe, T. & Duttine, A. (2018) Reflections on health promotion and disability in low and middle-income countries: case study of parent-support programmes for children with congenital Zika syndrome. *International Journal of Environment Research and Public Health*, **15** (3), 514–522.

Lakhanpaul, M., Culley, L., Robertson, N., *et al.* (2017) A qualitative study to identify parents' perceptions of and barriers to asthma management in children from South Asian and White British families. *BMC Pulmonary Medicine*, **17**, 126. https://doi.org/10.1186/s12890-017-0464-9.

Li, W., Chung, J., Ho, K., *et al.* (2016) Play interventions to reduce anxiety and negative emotions in hospitalized children. *BMC Pediatrics*, **16**, 36. https://doi.org/10.1186/s12887-016-0570-5.

Lo, D., Gaillard, B., Bullous, L., *et al.* (2016) Diagnosis and management of childhood asthma in primary care. *Practice Nursing*, **27** (10), 488–493.

Lullaby Trust (2019) *SIDS and SUDC Facts and Figures*. London, Lullaby Trust. https://www.lullabytrust.org.uk/wp-content/uploads/Facts-and-Figures-for-2017-released-2019-1.pdf Accessed 28/01/20.

Matson, K. & Fallon, R. (2012) Treatment of obesity in children and adolescents. *Journal of Pediatric Pharmacology and Therapeutics*, **17** (1), 45–57.

Mead, E., Atkinson, G., Richter, B., *et al.* (2016). Drug interventions for the treatment of obesity in children and adolescents. *Cochrane Database of Systematic Reviews*. https://doi.org/10.1002/14651858.CD012436.

Nabors, L., Mason, M. & Bernstein, J. (2014) Asthma camps for children. *Journal of Asthma*, **51** (4), 339–340.

Naidoo, J. & Wills, J. (2016) *Foundations for Health Promotion Practice* (fourth edition). London, Elsevier.

National Children's Bureau (2016) *Nursing in Schools: How School Nurses Support Pupils with Long-term Health Conditions*. London, National Children's Bureau.

National Education Forum (2018) Asthma in Schools. https://neu.org.uk/advice/asthma-schools Accessed 28/01/20.

National Health Service England, Care Quality Commission, Health Education England, Monitor, Public Health England, Trust Development Authority (2014) *NHS Five Year Forward View*. London, NHS England.

National Health Service (2016) *The Eatwell Guide*. London, NHS. www.nhs.uk/live-well/eat-well/the-eatwell-guide/ Accessed 28/01/20.

National Health Service England (2017) *Clinical Commissioning Policy: Obesity Surgery for Children with Severe Complex Obesity*. London. NHS England Specialised Services Clinical Reference Group for Severe and Complex Obesity.

National Health Service (2018) *NHS Stop Smoking Services Help You Quit*. London, NHS. https://www.nhs.uk/live-well/quit-smoking/nhs-stop-smoking-services-help-you-quit/ Accessed 28/01/20.

National Institute for Clinical Excellence (2001a) *Orlistat for the Treatment of Obesity in Adults. Technology Appraisal Guidance No. 22*. London, NICE.

National Institute for Clinical Excellence (2001b) *Guidance on the Use of Sibutromine for the Treatment of Obesity in Adults. Technology Appraisal Guidance No. 31*. London, NICE.

National Institute for Health and Care Excellence (2013) *Weight Management: Lifestyle Services for Overweight or Obese Children and Young People*. London, NICE.

National Institute for Health and Care Excellence (2017) *Lifestyle Weight Management Services for Overweight or Obese Children and Young People Overview*. London, NICE.

Northrup, T., Jacob, P., Benowitz, N., *et al.* (2016) Thirdhand smoke: state of the science and a call for policy expansion. *Public Health Reports*, **131**, 233–238. www.ncbi.nlm.nih.gov/pmc/articles/PMC4765971/pdf/phr131000233.pdf Accessed 28/01/20.

Orton S., Jones L.L., Cooper, S., *et al.* (2014) Predictors of children's secondhand smoke exposure at home: a systematic review and narrative synthesis of the evidence. *PLOS ONE*, **9** (11), e112690. https://doi.org/10.1371/journal.pone.0112690.

Page, A., Elven, B., Seabra, S., *et al.* (2019) Clinical holding: ethical guidance for children's nurses working in the UK. *Nursing Children and Young People*. doi: 10.7748/ncyp.2019.e1021.

Piaget, J. (1963) *The Origins of Intelligence in Children*. New York, W.W. Norton and Company, Inc.

Prajapati, R., Sharma, B. & Sharma, D. (2017) Significance of life skills education. *Contemporary Issues in Education Research*, **10** (1), 1–6.

Public Health England, NHS England and Health Education England (2016) *Making Every Contact Count (MECC): Consensus Statement*. London, Public Health England.

Raff, C., Glazebrook, C. & Wharrad, H. (2014) A systematic review of interactive multimedia interventions to promote children's communication with health professionals: implications for communicating with overweight children. *BMC Medical Informatics and Decision Making*, **14** (8) https://bmcmedinformdecismak.biomedcentral.com/articles/10.1186/1472-6947-14-8 Accessed 28/01/20.

Romieu, L., Dossus, L., Barquera, S., *et al.* (2017) Energy balance and obesity: what are the main drivers? *Cancer Causes Control*, **28** (3), 247–258.

Rottier, B., Ernst, E., Hedlin, G., *et al.* on behalf of the ERS Task Force (2015) Monitoring asthma in childhood: management-related issues. *European Respiratory Review*, **24** (136), 194–203.

Royal College of Nursing (2010) *Restrictive Physical Intervention and Therapeutic Holding for Children and Young People: Guidance for Nursing Staff*. London, Royal College of Nursing.

Royal College of Nursing (2017) *Standards for Assessing, Measuring and Monitoring Vital Signs in Infants, Children and Young People*. London, Royal College of Nursing.

Royal College of Pathologists (2016) *Sudden Unexpected Death in Infancy and Childhood: Multi-agency Guidelines for Care and Investigation* (second edition). London, Royal College of Pathologists.

Schuller, L. (2015) Providing better asthma care for children in school. *Nursing Times*, **111** (40), 12–14.

Scriven, A. (2017) *Ewles and Simnett's Promoting Health: A Practical Guide (seventh edition) London*, Elsevier.

Shaibi, G., Tyder, J., Kim, J., *et al.* (2015) Exercise for obese youth: refocusing attention from weight loss to health gains. *Exercise and Sport Sciences Reviews*, **43** (1), 41–47.

Smith, J., Cheater, F. & Bekker, H. (2013) Parents' experiences of living with a child with a long-term condition: a rapid structured review of the literature. *Health Expectations*, **18** (4), 452–474.

Smith, L., Coleman, V. & Bradshaw, M. (2002) *Family-centred Care: Concept, Theory and Practice.* Basingstoke, Palgrave.

Smith, J., Swallow, V. & Coyne, I. (2015) Involving parents in managing their child's long-term condition—a concept synthesis of family-centered care and partnership-in-care. *Journal of Pediatric Nursing*, **30**, 143–159.

Smith, J. & Kendal, S. (2018) Parents' and health professionals' views of collaboration in the management of childhood long-term conditions. *Journal of Pediatric Nursing*, **43**, 36–44.

Tahiri, M., Mottillo, S., Joseph, L., *et al.* (2012) Alternative smoking cessation aids: a meta-analysis of randomized controlled trials. *American Journal of Medicine*, **125** (6), 576–584.

White, A.R., Rampes, H., Liu, J.P., *et al.* (2014) Acupuncture and related interventions for smoking cessation. *Cochrane Database of Systematic Reviews*. http://doi.org/10.1002/14651858.CD000009.

Wiecha, J., Adams, W., Rybin, D., *et al.* (2015) Evaluation of a web-based asthma self-management system: a randomised controlled pilot trial. *BMC Pulmonary Medicine*, **15** (17). https://doi.org/10.1186/s12890-015-0007-1.

Wijlaars, L., Gilbert, R. & Hardelid, P. (2016) Chronic conditions in children and young people: learning from administrative data. *Archives of Disease in Childhood*, **101** (10), 881–885.

World Health Organization (1946) *Constitution*. Geneva, World Health Organization.

World Health Organization (1984) *Health Promotion. A Discussion Document on the Concept and Principles*. Copenhagen, World Health Organization.

World Health Organization (1986) Ottawa Charter for Health Promotion. *Journal of Health Promotion*, **1**, 1–4.

World Health Organization (2005) *The Role of Health Professionals in Tobacco Control*. Geneva, World Health Organization. www.who.int/tobacco/resources/publications/wntd/2005/bookletfinal_20april.pdf Accessed 28/0120.

World Health Organization (2012) *Regional Office for Europe. Health 2020 Policy Framework and Strategy Document*. Geneva, World Health Organization. http://www.euro.who.int/__data/assets/pdf_file/0020/170093/RC62wd08-Eng.pdf Accessed 28/01/20.

World Health Organization (2016) *Report of the Commission on Ending Childhood Obesity*. Geneva, World Health Organization. www.who.int/end-childhood-obesity/publications/echo-report/en/ Accessed 28/01/20.

Zolotarjoval, J., ten Veldel, G. & Vreugdenhill, A. (2018) Effects of multidisciplinary interventions on weight loss and health outcomes in children and adolescents with morbid obesity. *Obesity Reviews*, **19**, 931–946.

CHAPTER 7

Ethical Issues

Peter McNee

Introduction

This chapter will examine two of the ethical theories commonly used in the teaching of nursing ethics, followed by an exploration of four ethical principles. This is not an exhaustive list of principles and other authors use additional principles, which will not be included here. Similarly, beneficence and non-maleficence will be considered separately and not in this instance together as used by Beauchamp and Childress (2012). It is intended that this chapter will offer the reader a fundamental understanding of nursing ethics that will be useful in the care of children and young people with long-term illness. Both seminal works and contemporary literature will be used to achieve this aim.

This chapter will apply the identified ethical theories and principles to clinical situations through the use of some of the practice case studies examined in other chapters of this book. It will raise and explore ethical dilemmas that can potentially occur in the care of children and young people with long-term illness.

Aim of the chapter

The purpose of this chapter is to explore some of the ethical theories and principles that can be used in practice. The study of these should help provide a possible framework for ethical decision-making. The care of children and young people with long-term illness can present professionals, families and carers with ethical dilemmas. There is no easy answer or clear solution, but knowledge of ethics will empower the reader and support decision-making. Case studies from other chapters in the book will be used to apply these theories and principles to practice. This text does not include a critique of philosophical methods of decision-making that may be found in other published works; for example, Seedhouse (2009). The aim of the chapter is to examine ethical theories and principles and their application to clinical practice through case study and clinical practice examples.

Nursing Care of Children and Young People with Long-Term Conditions, Second Edition.
Edited by Mandy Brimble and Peter McNee.
© 2021 John Wiley & Sons Ltd. Published 2021 by John Wiley & Sons Ltd.

Intended learning outcomes

- To examine the ethical theories of utilitarianism/consequentialism and deontology, rights, duty and obligation, in relation to delivering nursing care to children, young people and families with long-term illness
- To explore the ethical principles of autonomy, beneficence, non-maleficence, justice and veracity and their application to practice
- To analyse a range of ethical dilemmas arising from case studies within this book
- To explore the use of ethical theories and principles as a possible framework to aid ethical decision-making in practice

---

⏱ Time out

- Consider why it is important to study ethics.
- Produce your own definition of ethics and a rationale for its application and relevance to your practice.

Why study ethics?

The study and use of ethics is essential for children and young people's nurses as there is an ethical component to all aspects of care in any setting, whether or not this becomes a dilemma (Brykczynska & Simons, 2011). Care is improved by a comprehensive knowledge of ethics and its application to an individual situation (Wheeler, 2012). The study of ethics provides a challenge and is something that takes time to learn and understand before it can become useful. The application of ethical principles needs to be incorporated into everyday practice to ensure that children, young people and their families receive optimum care.

A definition of ethics

Before examining ethical theories and principles that may be used in decision-making, it is necessary to define ethics or morals. Wheeler (2012) defines ethics or moral philosophy as the examination of how people conduct themselves and their behaviour in a morally acceptable or unacceptable sense. In a literal sense, ethics is a practical study of the actions of human beings as members of social groups.

Children's nurses are one such social group. How then do individuals within such a group achieve moral competence and the ability to make decisions which they can recognise as ethical? Some theorists would suggest that this morality is learnt through observation of society and by conforming to moral rules and codes of behaviour. This does not mean that individuals always behave as they ought to, or even that they know how they should behave. (See Kohlberg's theory of moral development for further reading/study.) Buka (2008) offers a more simplistic definition of ethics to do what is right and how people within society should live their lives.

Introduction to ethical theories

In reading various texts, it can be observed that the relationship between the theories of teleology, consequentialism, utilitarianism and deontology and the principles of ethics can be confusing. This may arise from the fact that the study of ethics is a very old subject and the language used by theorists such as Bentham (1748–1832), Kant (1724–1804) and Mill (1806–1873) has changed over time. These ethical terms will be discussed later and applied to practice situations.

Additionally, the concepts surrounding ethical theories and principles are complex and need careful reading to gain understanding. The realm of ethics is far removed from the normal practice area of children and young people's nurses but is an essential knowledge base to aid ethical decision-making. There is only one solution to the acquisition of this knowledge; these theories and principles have to be learnt, just like, for example, drug calculations or anatomy and physiology, for they are equally important. In the study of ethics, nurses should set out to learn the underlying theories and principles of personal and social morality (Cranmer & Nhemachena, 2013).

There is a division between the theories of normative and non-normative ethics. General normative or prescriptive ethics forms and defends a system of moral principles, which decide what actions are right or wrong. Applied normative ethics are used in making concrete decisions in daily life to resolve particular moral problems in the care of children and young people.

Non-normative descriptive and scientific ethics fall into two categories: namely, descriptive ethics, which is a factual investigation of moral behaviour and beliefs; and meta-ethics, which is an analysis of the meaning of ethical terms, for example 'rights', 'obligations', 'virtue' and 'responsibility'. They are applied to try to ascertain what factually and/or conceptually is the case, not what ought to be the case. In contrast to normative ethics, non-normative ethics has little practical application (Tschudin, 2003).

Consequentialism, utilitarianism, and deontology and non-consequentialism are all normative theories, which tend to look for moral absolutes, so avoiding relativism. In other words: that which is good is simply what the nursing community defines as good. These theories are the most frequently used and have influenced moral thinking. Examples are given later in the chapter.

Theory of consequentialism

The theory of consequentialism is the starting point for learning about the two theories of ethics discussed in this chapter. Consequentialism is also called teleology, from the Greek meaning 'end' or 'purpose'. In this theory, the rightness or wrongness of an action depends upon its consequences. The morally right action is that which produces the best consequence or outcome (Wheeler, 2012). In other words, for children and young people's nurses, the correct or moral thing to do is that which produces the optimum outcome for each child or young person. In the care of children and young people with long-term illness, the relevant outcome may be the control of disease, relief from pain, promotion of health or the prolongation of life. The outcome may also depend upon the teleological theory used. The best-known consequentialist theory is the theory of utilitarianism or utility.

Utilitarianism

The theory of utilitarianism, as espoused by Bentham (1748–1832), Mill (1806– 1873) and Smart and Williams (1989), among others, seeks the promotion of the greatest good for the greatest number. It focuses mainly on the consequences of an action. In modern terminology, it is called consequentialism or teleology: right in terms of the good arising from the consequences of an action.

Early ethical theories, which make the quest for pleasure and the avoidance of pain the basis for making moral choices, have been called hedonistic. Later applications of utilitarianism were also hedonistic and sought to base moral judgements on their usefulness or practical value in adding to our pleasure, diminishing our pain, and so adding to the sum total of human happiness (Avery, 2013). Examples will be discussed in the case studies.

Utilitarianism is particularly associated with Jeremy Bentham (1748–1832) and John Stuart Mill (1806–1873). Bentham defined the greatest happiness principle; put simply, it seeks the greatest good for the greatest number, the least pain, and the greatest happiness, focusing mostly on the consequences of an action. Mill refined this principle by using measuring criteria for happiness and noting the complexity of moral decision-making. Bentham's felicific calculus for measuring happiness was replaced by a cost–benefit analysis of the consequences of actions towards the greatest good–right in terms of the good arising from the consequences of an action (Smart & Williams, 1989). Utilitarians do not regard their actions as inherently good or bad, but as a means to an end with the intent of their actions having more importance (Chobi, 2015). In the context of caring for children and young people with long-term illness, it is the outcome and quality of life that matters and not how it is achieved. Modern philosophers such as Frankenna (1973) have recognised a difference between act and rule utilitarianism.

Act utilitarianism

Act utilitarianism considers the consequences of an act. Using past experience, act utilitarianism tries to predict possible outcomes for various courses of action (Wheeler, 2012). The principle of utility is the ultimate standard of rightness and wrongness for all utilitarians. The act utilitarian justifies actions not by using rules but by appealing directly to the principle of utility (Beauchamp & Childress, 2012). The action of a children and young people's nurse must achieve the optimum balance of good over bad with everyone considered.

Rule utilitarianism

This form of utilitarianism does not judge an action as right or wrong because of the predicted or actual consequences, but judges an action correct if it was based upon a general rule, which if followed should lead to the best consequences – even if short-term consequences could be worse (Avery, 2013).

Obedience to certain rules is fundamental to morality, but there are flaws with rules. Rule utilitarianism considers the consequences of adopting certain rules (Beauchamp & Childress, 2012). A nurse's actions are considered morally right if they are following the rules, for example the Nursing and Midwifery Council (2018). *The Code: Professional Standards of Practice and Behaviour for Nurses, Midwives and Nursing Associates*. These rules, if followed, will usually produce the best possible outcome as *The Code* is based on both moral and ethical principles to guide practice.

Case study from Chapter 6: Respiratory

Megan's case study outlines a range of issues associated with non-compliance with treatment and the need to access a range of services to control the symptoms of asthma. Megan is first seen at six months of age and treated for a wheeze that did not require ongoing medication at discharge. In treating Megan, we see a morally right action producing the best consequences for the child and family, in that Megan's symptoms have been resolved and she has been successfully discharged home. At 6 years of age, Megan is admitted to hospital again, where a diagnosis of asthma is made. She is prescribed appropriate medication and the respiratory nurse specialist deems her inhalation technique competent. In terms of service provision, again we see a morally right action. Services have been configured to produce the best outcomes for children with asthma. Inpatient beds are available for treatment and a nurse specialist is available to provide the appropriate health education and promotion. At 8 years of age, again Megan is admitted to hospital. On this occasion, it is apparent that there are clear ethical issues facing the children's nurse.

Reflection

Reflecting back on Megan's case study, what do you consider to be the ethical issues and challenges arising from it?

Medication

- First, Megan's mother, Sarah, is not administering Megan's preventative medication due to concerns about Megan's weight.
- Second, Megan needs to be restrained to administer her medication.
- Third, non-compliance with treatment raises a number of issues for the student nurse in whom Sarah confides.

Confidentiality

It is the duty of all children's nurses to act in the best interests of the child. There is also a need to ensure confidentiality in the information that we receive from those in our care. What should the student nurse do? If the student nurse was to withhold the information provided by Sarah, she would be acting against the best interests of

Megan, as Megan has been admitted with an exacerbation of her asthma and has had repeated GP visits related to her condition. The student nurse would also be colluding with Sarah in relation to the non-compliance in Megan's treatment. This would be a morally unjustified act, as potentially there could be severe consequences for Megan's health and well-being. Following the theory of consequentialism, the morally right action to take is to disclose the information provided by Sarah to senior nursing staff and the doctors involved in Megan's care. Obviously, there is a role here for negotiating care and discussing with Sarah the anxieties that have led to the non-administration of medication. It is within the parameters of the role of the children's nurse to attempt to achieve the best outcome and consequences for both Megan's family and the professionals involved in Megan's care.

Restrictive physical interventions

Restrictive physical interventions (formerly referred to as restraint) and therapeutic holding, also referred to as clinical or supportive holding, is a difficult and complex issue within children's nursing. It raises a number of legal, professional and ethical issues. In terms of consequentialism, the nurses restraining Megan need to consider the best outcomes for the alleviation of her symptoms. Clearly, the administration of her medication is in her best interest as it will treat and alleviate her symptoms. The consequences of the nurse's actions will produce a morally justifiable outcome. However, the distress caused to Megan by restraining her may exacerbate her symptoms and negate the benefits of the treatment. Therefore, the action of clinical holding becomes morally unjustifiable, as the outcomes will not provide a benefit for Megan. It has often been said of ethics that there are no right or wrong answers. In terms of consequentialism, what is important is the morally justifiable outcome. For the children's nurse, again, the role of negotiation is important. Megan would need to be prepared for the administration of nebulisers by involving other members of the multidisciplinary team, including the play specialist. Clinical holding should always be an action of last resort and only used if other avenues have been exhausted. Clinical holding can be used to achieve the necessary outcome of administering the nebuliser as long as it remains in Megan's best interest and provides the best outcome.

Key points

- It is within the legal, professional and ethical role of the children's nurse to ensure that confidentiality is maintained in all information gained from children, young people and their families.
- This includes both written and verbal information.

Case study from Chapter 10: chronic renal disease

In Chapter 10, Thomas is presented as a 15-year-old boy who was diagnosed with chronic renal failure when he was a 5-year-old. Thomas' condition is now beginning to deteriorate as a consequence of his non-compliance with a conservative management regime. A number of reasons are presented as contributing to this situation, including the influence of his peers. This is a common issue encountered across a range of long-term conditions. In terms of the wider clinical issues, the utilitarian approach considers the cost and benefits of a potential intervention.

Key issue

In Thomas' case, a regional specialist centre has managed his care over a number of years. This ongoing care is expensive, particularly during a time where value for money, clinical effectiveness and cost effectiveness are all issues within the modern NHS. The question is then posed:

> If Thomas is unwilling to comply with conservative treatment, he will require closer monitoring and an increase in the resources of the multidisciplinary team managing his care, and potentially he may require renal transplantation. Should these services be provided to a potentially non-compliant patient?

Utilitarianism looks to provide the greatest good for the greatest number. If Thomas continues on his current conservative management regime, resources could be applied to children and young people who are compliant with treatment or diverted to children and young people with other long-term conditions. This is a pertinent issue, particularly in times of health care rationing. Withholding these interventions from Thomas will ultimately lead to deterioration in his condition. Therefore, this act is against utilitarian principles, as the greatest good would not be achieved for Thomas, his family or the health care professionals involved in his care.

Clearly, no children's nurse or health care professional is going to refuse Thomas further care provision. In terms of rule utilitarianism, children's nurses are bound by their code of conduct which clearly states that at all times we must act in the best interest of our patients (NMC, 2018). In this scenario, it is incumbent upon the children's nurse to negotiate with Thomas to help ensure his compliance and participation to achieve the best health outcomes in his care delivery; this may involve the children's nurse liaising with the wider multidisciplinary team.

Key points

When caring for children and young people the following points should be considered. It is incumbent on the children's nurse to:

- Deliver the greatest good for the greatest number.
- Ensure that children and young people experience the least possible pain and suffering.
- Adhere to Bentham's happiness principle and focus on the legal, professional and ethical consequences of any action taken.

Theory of deontology

Having started with the theory of consequentialism, we now examine the theory of deontology, which has a very different approach.

Deontology, from the Greek *deon* meaning duty, argues that what makes an action right or wrong is clearly defined by rules. Our moral duties and rights are guided by rules. The focus here is on morally right actions, which if the rules are followed will be right in all situations regardless of any consequences (Avery, 2013). Deontology is often described as duty ethics. It may require doing what is right regardless of the consequences. For this reason, it is also sometimes called non-consequentialism (Tschudin, 2003).

The theory of deontology was advanced by Kant (1785) as cited in Avery (2013). It advocates determining what is right by considering the intrinsic features of an action – for example, duty – often independently from its consequences. It is mostly concerned with the determination of duties and obligations using moral principles and rules; for example, respect for the individual and telling the truth. According to Kant, actions are right if they conform to a moral law and are not to be judged by the consequences. Kant propounded the categorical imperative, a principle that should govern all moral behaviour. It may be formulated in various ways. These are:

- So act that the principle of your action can become a universal law for all rational beings.
- So act as if the principle of your action were to become by your will a universal law of nature.
- So act as to treat humanity, whether in your own person or in that of any other, in every case as an end, never as a mere means.

Another aspect of deontological theory is rights theory. Rights may be defined as a justified claim to have or receive something, or to act in a certain way. There is an obvious link between 'rights', in this sense, and obligations and duties. They could be said to be different sides of the same deontological coin. Using rights theory, the morality of an action can be judged by whether or not it falls within the scope of a right. There are different means of categorising rights, for example:

- Positive rights – rights to do something or have someone else do something.
- Negative rights – which are the forbearance or omission to act by others.

However, the most important distinction to be made between rights is that of natural or human rights and legal rights. Natural or human rights are sometimes said to be self-evident – for example, those in the American Declaration of Independence – and are the most important moral rights, overriding all conflicting rights and being shared equally by all humans by virtue of their humanity. They include positive and negative rights, examples being the right to life and the right not to be tortured.

Legal rights are those rights allowed by law, either by express legislation or based on legal principles, and upheld by the courts. They are necessarily narrower in scope than natural or human rights, being confined to the legal jurisdiction in which they are formulated, and being concerned with more parochial matters, such as property rights.

Rights theory is often employed in an effort to promote the interests of minorities, such as a counter to utilitarian arguments. The United Nations (1989) declared that the child has a right to express an opinion and to have that opinion taken into account in decision-making affecting the child. This was an expression of a natural or human right. However, subsequent legislation in the UK Children Act (1989; 2004) and the Human Rights Act (1998) has specifically provided for the wishes and feelings of the child to be taken into account in decisions affecting the child. Accordingly, it is now a legal right when applying deontological theory that children and young people's nurses have a duty to take account of the moral and legal rights of the child, such as the right to family life, and those explicit in their *Code* (NMC, 2018).

Case study from Chapter 5: Eczema

In this case study, Isabella has eczema and so far treatment has been ineffective. The problems encountered by the child and family are compounded by their recent move to the UK, Isabella's reduced diet and nutritional intake and possibly by the use of alternative treatments. In this case study, a number of health care professionals have been involved in Isabella's care including the paediatrician, nurse specialist, health visitor and school nurse. All professionals involved have a duty of care.

In terms of deontology, it is the role of the individual to perform their preordained duty. On a simplistic level, this can be seen in the referral process that has led to Isabella receiving care as an in-patient. Also, we can see that the family is struggling to manage Isabella's condition, with her mother losing sleep and feeling isolated and unsupported. To help to resolve this situation, the multidisciplinary team has liaised in order to provide effective treatment and support, thus fulfilling their duty.

In the UK, Isabella and her family have a number of rights, including free access to health care at the point of delivery. One of the main principles of the Children Act (1989) is that the rights of the child are paramount. Her mother Merelee is entitled to receive appropriate and evidence-based care to ensure the effective treatment of Isabella's condition. Merelee also expresses the need for Isabella to interact and play with other children. Again, the Children Act (1989) highlights the need to take children's views into account in any decisions surrounding care. Here, the children's nurse has fulfilled her duty by ensuring the involvement of the play specialist in an attempt to engage Isabella in activities with other children. The United Nations (1989) *Convention on the Rights of the Child* also identifies the need to actively consult with and facilitate children's participation in their care. By providing a multidisciplinary approach to the care of Isabella and the support of Merelee, the children's nurse is fulfilling the principles of deontology. Health policy has changed in recent years with a move to greater involvement by children and young people in their care and decisions made about them. This is evident in the publication of *You're Welcome: Quality Criteria* for children and young people friendly health services (Department of Health (DoH) UK, 2011) and *Liberating the NHS: No Decision About Me Without Me* (DOH UK, 2012). The rights of children and young people are also enshrined in wider legislation such as the Health and Social Care Act England (2012) and the Social Services and Well-being Act (Wales) 2014.

⊲◻⇱ Key points

In deontology:

- What makes an action right or wrong is defined by rules.
- Our moral duties and rights are guided by rules.
- Deontology is often described as duty ethics.
- In some instances, doing what is right is the correct course of action regardless of the potential consequences.

Ethical principles

Kant (1724–1804) argued that the concept of 'person' is fundamental to ethics and is a formative principle of ethics (Thompson *et al.*, 2006). If there is no idea of a person who has rights and responsibilities, then ethics cannot work. A person must be treated as an end and never as a means to an end. Therefore, 'persons' are to be treated with respect, whatever their age or cognitive ability. If a person has rights and responsibilities, there must be in this person some degree of morality or self-determination which is exercised freely. Kant calls this moral independence or autonomy. He argues that the principle of autonomy is necessary, both theoretically and practically, for a working system of ethics.

Respect for persons, as a principle, informs codes of ethics such as the International Council of Nurses (ICN) (2012) *Code of Ethics for Nurses* and the NMC (2018) *The Code: Professional Standards of Practice and Behaviour for Nurses, Midwives and Nursing Associates.*

Ethical principles are fundamental moral norms that are used to guide actions (Beauchamp & Childress, 2012). A principle, as suggested by Thompson *et al.* (2006), is a starting point for moral reasoning, and refers to the basic questions the nurse must ask. Principles are guides to give direction. They are pointers but do not tell nurses where they will finish, or what will happen along the way. Thiroux (1995) argues that principles can act like a compass, giving direction but not a road map. They are not rigid like theories, but flexible without being too specific. They do not provide answers, but help direct thinking to achieve an agreement about what ought to be done.

Some of the best-known ethical principles are those described by Beauchamp and Childress (2001; 2012). They used the *Belmont Report* (Presidents Commission for the Study of Ethical Problems in Medicine and Biomedical Research, 1981), which was the outcome of the National Commission for the Protection of Human Subjects of Biomedical and Behavioural research. The *Belmont Report* stated that respect for persons, beneficence and justice should be the ethical principles governing research. Beauchamp and Childress (2012) added non-maleficence, making four principles.

1. Respect for autonomy.
2. Beneficence.
3. Non-maleficence.
4. Justice.

These four principles are general guidelines that leave plenty of room for judgement in particular cases.

⏲ Time out

- What do you understand by the term autonomy?
- What is the role of the children's nurse in relation to autonomy?

Principle of autonomy

There are many views of autonomy, a word that comes from the Greek *autos* (self) *nomous* (rule of law) (Dworkin, 1988). It is a term associated with ideas such as self-determination, self-government, self-mastery, voluntariness and choosing one's own moral position (Beauchamp & Childress, 2012). Autonomy can be defined as the capacity to think, decide and act on the basis of such thought and decision freely and independently and without let or hindrance (Gillon, 1985). To be an autonomous person, therefore, means being able to live one's own life according to a set of self-chosen rules and values. A cardinal principle of autonomy means recognising children and young people as persons who are entitled to such basic human rights as:

- The right to know.
- The right to privacy.
- The right to receive care and treatment (Thompson *et al.*, 2006).

In relation to a capable person's autonomy, Hendrick (2004) refers to an individual's ability to come to his/her own decisions and requires nurses to respect the choices patients make concerning their own lives. Respect for autonomy also means the protection of those incapable of autonomy because of illness, injury, mental disorder or developmental age.

Respect for a child or young person's autonomy, and the right to consent to or refuse treatment, are now widely accepted as central values in health care (DoH UK, 2011).

The principle of autonomy according to Seedhouse (2009) can be defined in three ways:

1. Autonomy as a single principle. This view of autonomy suggests that there is a basic principle that asserts that the wishes and needs of children and young people ought to be respected.
2. Autonomy as a right. The child or young person's ability to choose should be acknowledged and the choice made should be respected, as a right.
3. Autonomy as a quality. The basic intrinsic quality of children and young people. Simply to be autonomous is to be able to do something, rather than nothing.

Autonomy, therefore, means some element of choice for the child or young person and their families. The choice may be wide-ranging; for example, to receive care or to refuse care. However, one child's choice may conflict with another's interests; for example, one child may want a night light on, but it may keep the other children awake. A further example would be an adolescent who wishes to watch a '15' rated film but is unable to because there are much younger children within the same clinical area. Freedom of choice may not be possible because of circumstances:

- If a child is unconscious and therefore a choice must be made on his/her behalf. Someone acts in the best interests of the child at this time, such as the parents, doctor or nurse caring for the child.
- The child is vulnerable in another way, or unable to communicate well; for example, deaf, mute, blind, physically or mentally ill. These children must have

their autonomy protected and have a competent person to make choices for them. This could be called preference utilitarianism, indicating what the child may have chosen.

Autonomy may not be possible because somebody in a position of power is withholding choice from the child or young person; for example, children in young offender institutes or oppressive regimes in a global context. Those in power can control the child's choice, and that may mean that there is a limited choice or none at all, which means they have lost their autonomy. Children's nurses must be very careful if a child or young person's autonomy is unprotected or lost, because then that child is at risk of harm.

Nursing has many definitions but may be said to encompass the care of the sick, frail and vulnerable child. It covers the provision of comfort, services and care in any situation, whether in the hospital or community, employing the virtue of selfless caring. There is an onus on the children's nurse, for these reasons, to become the guardian of autonomy for the child or young person and their family.

When examining the professionalism of nursing, some criteria ought to be considered, such as autonomy. It is sometimes difficult for the children's nurse to be autonomous. If nurses are to achieve autonomy, they must also become accountable for their practice. This may arise from personal moral standards or from a code of ethics or professional code, such as NMC (2018).

The idea of autonomy is central to the NMC (2018) code. The thing that distinguishes a 'person' is the fact that he/she is a rational human being. The code includes the obligation that the nurse respects the independence of the child/young person and family and respects their involvement in the planning and delivery of care. This invokes the ethical principle of autonomy and it is implicit in the reference to patient involvement that the child/young person is given sufficient and truthful information to make that involvement meaningful and provide autonomy, while incorporating the ethical principle of keeping trust.

Case study from Chapter 9: Oncology

In this case study, Katie is presented as a 3-year-old girl with a diagnosis of acute lymphoblastic leukaemia. Katie has been treated with chemotherapy and has acquired an infection that necessitates transfer to a children's high dependency unit. Katie's mother, Claire, is 18 years old and is supported by her own parents. This case study is a good example of the provision of care for a non-autonomous patient or client. As Katie is only 3 years of age, she is reliant on Claire to make key decisions for her and consent to treatment on her behalf. It is the role of the children's nurse to protect the autonomy of both Katie and Claire, who could both be considered vulnerable.

The children's nurse should facilitate the decision-making process to enable Claire to make autonomous decisions. Autonomy is a central concept of health care rights. It is the role of the children's nurse to safeguard this position and prevent paternalism, which has been a feature of health care in recent years. Marriott (2004) advocates the requirement to focus on the needs of children rather than professional groups. In the decision-making process, it is important to involve and encourage children with long-term illness to make decisions about their care. In Katie's case, the facilitation of this process is geared towards Claire acting in the best interests of her child. Some authors have identified that autonomy and childhood have often been perceived as mutually exclusive (Glasper & Richardson, 2010). This has been based on society's view of children as incompetent to make effective decisions for themselves. In Katie's case, it is important that Claire is supported in the difficult decisions that she will have to make about Katie's care.

In this case, the children's nurse can ensure Katie's autonomy by supporting Claire as she makes difficult and complex decisions. One of the key aspects of this decision-making process is the consent to ongoing invasive treatment. There is recognition that, wherever possible, children should be involved in the process of gaining consent to treatment. Griffith and Tengnah (2017) highlight the importance of consent being legally and ethically gained. For this to occur, the individual consenting has to be competent to do so. They must be fully informed of the procedure, understand the information that has been presented to them, give consent voluntarily and authorise the intervention or procedure. Clearly, there are limitations to Katie's understanding of her illness, and she cannot give consent due to her age. However, her autonomy and her right to self-determination should still be uppermost in the minds of those professionals involved in her care.

Key points

- An essential attribute of professionalism is autonomy: the ability to make independent decisions.
- Knowledge of ethics equips the nurse, so far as possible, to make such decisions.

Ethical principle of beneficence

Beneficence has been explained in many ways but can be defined as a principle that generates an obligation to act in ways that promote the well-being of others, or a moral injunction to do good (Beauchamp & Childress, 2012; Butts & Rich, 2013). As the point of nursing action is to promote the well-being of others – for example, children and young people – it follows that such actions accord with the principles of beneficence (Edwards, 2009).

Beneficence is a major part of a nurse's professional duty and requires nurses to benefit children and young people. It has been said to be the cornerstone of nursing ethics and is enshrined in the NMC (2018) *Code*; for example, to act in such a manner as to safeguard and promote the well-being of patients. The principle of beneficence generates significant obligations towards all children and young people who may be affected, directly or indirectly, by a nurse's conduct. Beneficence poses several questions for the nurse:

- What may count as a benefit?
- Who decides what is in the children and young people's best interests?
- Whom do nurses have to benefit; that is, to whom do they owe a moral obligation?

Reflection

Consider the three questions above, reflect upon your own clinical experiences and identify some answers based upon clinical care. What do the words benefit, well-being and interests mean? They all mean a 'good' that the children's nurse is expected to promote both physically and psychologically (Edwards, 2009). This may include the prevention of disease, the restoration of health, and a reduction in pain and suffering.

Who must nurses benefit? There is a primary duty towards children and young people on their own wards, neighbouring wards (Edwards, 2009), other nurses, patients, relatives, the public and themselves (NMC, 2018).

Beneficence demands that the children's nurse respects the rights of the children and young people; for example, to informed consent. Strict justice may have to be compromised, as attention to the special needs of children and young people with long-term illness may result in less attention being given to other children and young people in a busy ward setting. Conversely, special regard for the rights of children and young people has to be balanced against consideration of the common good, as in a case where children and young people have to be quarantined to protect others in an epidemic.

Acting beneficently, immunisations for children and young people may inflict some degree of pain or discomfort but have longer term health benefits. A surgical procedure may also be viewed as causing harm in order to promote a positive outcome. Beneficence also requires an assessment and balancing of 'trade-offs' in situations where decisions are often made against a background of uncertainty.

Case study from Chapter 11: Cystic fibrosis

In the case study, it becomes clear that Sophie is at a crossroads in her life as she is about to undergo the transition to adult services. A number of children with long-term conditions will experience this change, which can have a major impact on the confidence of young people in the management of their conditions. Sophie has got a job and a circle of friends in whom she has not confided about her condition. Sophie has been admitted to hospital for the treatment of a chest infection and nutritional input. During this stay in hospital, the nurse specialist discusses and guides Sophie through the transition process. In this way, the children's nurse is acting beneficently as she is allowing Sophie time and space to reach a decision of her own choosing about when to transfer to adult services.

Issues

Health policy over a number of years (DoH UK, 2004; 2011; 2012; NHS, 2019) advocates the need for children/young people to be listened to and their views taken into account when care decisions are made. In this scenario, it is the role of the multidisciplinary team to make effective and ethical decisions. This can often result in a need to make fateful decisions that they may have to justify (Botes, 2000). To act beneficently, there is a responsibility to do good (Butts & Rich, 2013). Not to support Sophie in her decision about transition would be a breach of duty and therefore counter to the beneficent view. Breaches of duty have been seen in a number of high-profile cases across the NHS, including the cases of Beverly Allitt (DoH UK, 1994), the Bristol heart scandal (Kennedy, 2001) and Mid Staffs (Francis, 2013). Above all, the children's nurse within the case study must be guided by the thoughts and actions of Sophie and support her in making autonomous and effective decisions to ensure a good outcome.

> **⚷ Key points**
>
> - To act beneficently, there is an obligation to act in a way that promotes the well-being of children/young people, or a moral injunction to do good.
> - As the role of the nurse is to do good and promote health and well-being, nursing actions correspond to the principles of beneficence.
> - Beneficence is a major part of the duty of care of the children's nurse.

Ethical principle of non-maleficence

Non-maleficence may be defined as the avoidance of harm to the interests of others, or at least the minimisation of the risk of harm befalling individuals. The principle of non-maleficence generates obligations not to harm others. This differs from beneficence in the sense that it imposes few obligations on others (Edwards, 2009).

The principle of non-maleficence requires that nurses have a duty not to harm children and young people, nor to subject them to risk of harm (Hendrick, 2004; Beauchamp & Childress, 2012). As with beneficence, it is enshrined in the NMC (2018) *Code*, which in contrast to earlier versions (NMC, 2004) refers to harm explicitly.

What counts as harm to an individual child and young person with a long-term condition may not be harm at all to another person. Harm may be physical, pain, disability and death. Harm may also be psychological, such as mental stress. Beauchamp and Childress (2012) give a broad definition of harm, which includes the following:

- thwarting or defeating of interests;
- self-harm;
- actions of another party;
- intimidation;
- undue influence or pressure;
- misleading or misinforming children and young people;
- abuse;
- assault;
- exploitation.

Non-maleficence is less morally demanding than beneficence and generates fewer obligations. It does not demand positive action, and only requires that the children and young people's nurse does not harm anybody (Hendrick, 2004).

Beneficence and non-maleficence are closely related. Both promote the moral objectives of medicine and nursing – beneficence to help those who are sick and suffering, and non-maleficence to prevent harm, preventing deterioration of existing illness, damage or disease (Gillon, 1985). Frankenna (1973) puts the two principles together. Beauchamp and Childress (2012) treat them as separate principles, but recognise that they are entwined. Many nursing or medical interventions that aim to benefit a child or young person may at the same time result in some degree of harm. Beneficence and non-maleficence have to be weighed together and the benefits and harms balanced against each other.

Sometimes, the principles of beneficence and non-maleficence conflict and there is a dilemma as to which one should have priority. For Gillon (1985), the claim that non-maleficence should normally override beneficence is untenable. Nevertheless, in some situations, non-maleficence should override beneficence. If the risks of a procedure or treatment are very high and serious, it will be morally indefensible to carry out the procedure if the benefit is small. On the other hand, there is the example of immunisation programmes. If non-maleficence were to be prioritised, it would mean that nobody could be immunised because of the risk to a minority who may suffer side effects. This is illogical, because the benefit to the wider community carries more moral weight when considering the value of herd immunity (Mallory *et al.*, 2018).

The principles of beneficence and non-maleficence provide a moral foundation for the obligations set out in the NMC (2018) *Code*. The *Code* gives some guidance on using ethical principles to underpin practice. Practically, children and young people's nurses could link these with other concepts, such as accountability and responsibility.

Case study from Chapter 3: Diabetes

In this case study, Josie has recently been diagnosed with type 1 diabetes. Initially, this has been managed well, but following Josie's transfer to secondary school it becomes apparent that Josie is not administering all of her insulin. Josie is also upset by the apparently protective nature of her parents limiting her freedom.

Issues

The key issue within this case study is to minimise any harm caused by the non-administration of insulin. The role of the children's nurse here is to facilitate an open dialogue between Josie, her parents and members of the multidisciplinary team to ensure compliance with treatment. Harm can befall a number of people within this scenario. Josie's parents are experiencing some stress over the management of her condition and to ignore this would negate the principle of non-maleficence and would be working outside the NMC (2018) *Code*. If the nurse were to ignore Josie's non-compliance with treatment, she is likely to experience a further deterioration in her condition. To ensure that the principle of non-maleficence is upheld, the children's nurse must provide continued access to services for Josie and her family. Josie must be allowed time to discuss her thoughts and feelings about her condition and treatment regimen. Above all, the children's nurse must negotiate a way forward, empowering Josie to take control of the management of her condition, thus ensuring her autonomy and upholding the identified principle.

Key points

- In any nursing action it is important to avoid harm, whether that is on a physical, spiritual or psychological level.
- Where harm cannot be totally avoided, it should be minimised at all costs.
- Non-maleficence generates a clear obligation not to harm others.

Ethical principle of justice

Justice as defined by Beauchamp and Childress (2012) is divided into four parts:

1. Justice as fairness; that is to say, one acts justly towards a child or young person when one has given them what is due or owed, what he or she deserves or can legitimately claim.

    Justice is concerned with the fair distribution of benefits, risk and costs. The idea is that children and young people in similar positions should be treated in a similar manner.

2. Distributive justice; that is, pertaining to an equal distribution of benefits and harms for children and young people.

    Distributive justice refers widely to the distribution of rights and responsibilities in society, including, for instance, civil and political rights.

3. Justice and equality: the presumption that children and young people should be treated equally, unless there is a difference between them that is relative to the care in question.

    Justice and equality, according to Aristotle, mean treating equals equally and unequal's unequally. In other words, whatever respects are relevant, children equal in those respects should be treated the same.

4. Justice as desert, concerned with equal distribution – which may also be referred to as material or needs principles. Various philosophers have proposed the following principles as a valid material principle of distribution justice:

    a. To each child and family an equal share.

    b. To each child and family according to need.

    c. To each child and family according to effort.

    d. To each child and family according to contribution.

    e. To each child and family according to merit.

    f. To each child and family according to free market changes.

    Adapted from Beauchamp and Childress (2012).

Thompson *et al.* (2006) describe the principle of justice as the duty of universal fairness, equal opportunity for children and young people. Equity is the equality of outcomes for groups such as children. Rawls (1997) describes justice as fairness. The distribution of burdens and benefits should be considered from the point of view of the least advantaged in society; for example, poor children should share the benefits in society equally with all others. Benefit to the least advantaged becomes the 'norm' for decision and policy-making. Brykczynska (1994) states that the principle of justice provides equal opportunities and access to treatment for all children.

Justice incorporates the ideals of fairness, equality and non-discrimination. The application and relevance of this principle for children and young people's nurses may be shown in discussions about the allocation of resources and nursing priorities and time allocation.

🔑 Key point

- Justice is concerned with the fair distribution of benefits, risk and costs. The idea is that children and young people in similar positions should be treated in a similar manner.

A nursing ethic

With respect to nursing, the meaning of the term ethics has been considered and explained in various ways. Rowson (1990) defined ethics as thinking and reasoning about morality, and morality as respect for a person's autonomy or self-rule. This suggests a dutiful view of ethics consistent with deontology. Another definition is provided by Thompson *et al.* (2006), namely that ethics refers to science, or a study of morals, or moral philosophy. They also suggest that 'an ethic' can refer to the morals of a group, such as a 'nursing ethic'.

On a more practical level, ethics is often seen to focus on the study and practice of what is right and good for people. Thompson *et al.* (2006) suggested that ethics teaches humankind the practice of duties in human life and the reasons for what they should do and what they should leave undone. In the nineteenth century, nursing ethics were entirely concerned with duty and there was a demand for unquestioning obedience from nurses. At about that time, Nightingale wrote of the need for those with practical knowledge of nursing's real moral dilemmas to engage in common study with those of other disciplines, including those with some skill in asking pertinent ethical questions and exploring their implications. This remains true for children and young people's nurses today. To achieve this, individual nurses will need to use their professional and personal life experiences, and social and cultural influences, which have shaped their previous moral upbringing and current moral status.

It is suggested by Jameton (1990) that in order to understand the terms 'culture' and 'morality', they must be considered more closely. Culture can be said to cover the basic aspects and ideas of a society. It also covers settings of life, traditions and work, and it gives explanations for conduct. Morality, which forms part of a culture, assists with the formation of societal beliefs and conduct and also provides laws, standards, ideals and statements of value.

In the absence of ethical theories, society determines whether or not an act is moral on the basis of what is acceptable to it (relativism). Thus, within the nursing community, by tradition nurses are not allowed to run in the ward. However, an exception to this general rule is in an emergency, when it is perfectly correct to run. Even then, nurses must not run fast, because they will consequently be out of breath on arriving at the emergency and limited in their ability to help. Tradition dictates they must simply 'walk quickly'.

Increasingly, nurses are spurning traditional practices in favour of new thinking, leading to rational rather than traditional actions. The nursing profession then examines the resulting practices to assess their morality. This illustrates the need for the application of ethical theory and principles to nursing practice.

Morality, whether learned by observation, intuition or the application of theories and principles, may be influenced by society and also by situations. (See also *Situation Ethics*, Fletcher, 1979.) The individual needs a moral sense, and the ability to grasp and make moral judgements. This is sometimes called conscience and may be said to be a prerequisite for social existence. The moral growth of a nurse may depend upon the extent of his/her autonomy; that is, an individual making his/her own decisions rather than having them determined by outside forces. Thus, ethical rules must be freely arrived at and be reasonable rather than enforced.

In the context of children's nursing, nursing ethics may be defined as a moral code that they apply when caring for children and young people with long-term conditions and their families. Nursing ethics may also be construed as a set of moral standards by which nurses live and work. These ethics or moral standards should not be confused with other codes, for example NMC (2018), which may include ethical and behavioural guidance. The grounding for the nursing ethic may be a personal moral code, a professional code (NMC, 2018) or a moral framework such as Cooper's (1988) covenantal relationship, triple contract or covenant theory (Veatch, 1981; 2016). When a comparison is made between models, mutuality and reciprocity are found to be common to all. These suggestions for grounding the nursing ethic echo the two basic principles of Trusted (1987), namely keeping trust and benevolence.

Having reflected upon the nursing ethic, it is now possible to consider how a framework for ethical decision-making may help children and young people's nurses in practice with issues surrounding long-term illness.

Definition of an ethical dilemma

Thompson *et al.* (2006) define an ethical dilemma as a choice, of whatever kind, between two equally unsatisfactory alternatives. This may involve a conflict between moral principles and values where there are no rules or precedents to follow. This has been established within the case studies presented in this chapter.

Ethical dilemmas demand the attention of children and young people's nurses and other members of the multidisciplinary team. They are not confined to the obvious ethical dilemmas, such as decisions about abortion, euthanasia, transplants and research on humans, but also arise every day in nursing and medical decisions; for example:

- What nurses and doctors should tell children and young people and their families regarding their diseases and treatments.
- On a larger scale, decisions about resource allocation, for example how much of society's money should be spent on health care, and how much should be spent on the provision and delivery of children and young people's services.

To decide upon a particular course of action is to decide that it is better than, or preferable to, the available alternatives; this means making value judgements. Such judgements involve ethical choices, but not every ethical decision or value judgement requires conscious thought, and sometimes can be made intuitively using long held beliefs, commitments and habits.

Sometimes intuition fails and gives no clear answer, or it may deceive and give the wrong answer. Furthermore, there is the risk that intuition can vary from person to person. Intuition is therefore unreliable, making it essential to use another method of ethical decision-making using a framework or a model such as the NMC (2018) *Code*.

Ethical decision-making

Ethical decision-making is not some kind of hidden process but is a problem-solving process similar to many others. Demystifying ethics and using common sense will enable the solving of an ethical problem (Burkhardt & Nathaniel, 2020).

All ethical decisions and judgements are made within a cultural tradition. From traditions come the formation of the idea of what is moral, and how and when moral decisions should be made. MacIntyre (1981) suggests that these traditions could arise from a historical background. Perhaps both individuals and societies are actors in a play, in which they act out previous life experiences, which in turn influence their subsequent behaviour.

Within the society of a hospital, ethics is employed as a moral guideline, and may be used to make comparisons between personal and professional moral benefits. The value for nurses of using nursing ethics is that by looking at these areas, they may improve their powers of observation and pursue insights into morality by clarifying cultural traditions. This enables them to make clearer decisions, having established moral beliefs, and also gives them the power and ability to make autonomous decisions, as seen in the case studies presented within this book. In recent years, high-profile cases have come before the courts where judges have been asked to decide whether ongoing treatment is in the best interests of the child (Close *et al.*, 2018). The cases of both Charlie Gard and Alfie Evans captured the public imagination and led to heated debates on both sides of the argument as to whether treatment should be continued or withdrawn. In both emotive cases, courts have decided the direction of care. In the case of Charlie Gard there were multiple cases both in the United Kingdom and European courts in which ethical arguments on the right to life and treatment were presented (Wilkinson & Savulescu, 2018). Ultimately, medical staff and Charlie's parents reached agreement that ongoing treatment was not in Charlie's best interests and he died in 2017. The Access to Palliative Care and Treatment of Children Bill, which is currently making its way through parliament, has the potential to change the relationship between parents and professionals when disagreements of this type occur (Access to Palliative Care and Treatment of Children Bill, 2019).

One of the purposes of an ethical education for nurses is to enable them to justify their decisions. There are a number of different situations in which nurses may be required to justify their decisions. For example, the most obvious is when a nurse must defend their decision to the doctor. This is of great importance, because such defence goes to the root of their professional autonomy and accountability (NMC, 2018).

In addition to doctors, nurses have to justify their decisions to children/young people and their families, nursing colleagues and managers. It is possible that they may also have to justify their decisions to the general public; for example, when deciding to stand up for what they believe at a subsequent public enquiry or in care proceedings.

All the above have a common objective, namely the promotion of improved practice and care of children and young people with long-term conditions. Nurses need the confidence and assurance when making decisions that can only be engendered by ethical knowledge and education.

Nurses ought to be encouraged to think about why and how they deliver care and the possible consequences of their actions. It is in this area that children and young people's nurses need help and guidance but they do not need another set of rules, because they are inappropriately rigid with respect to complex situations and reduce autonomy by providing a ready-made answer. However, nurses do need a framework with which they can determine what is best and most appropriate. An ethical model or framework could be said to be a systematic construction and evaluation of arguments that can be used when making ethical decisions.

Benjamin and Curtis (1992) argue that frameworks are important for two reasons. First, a framework may provide common ground for resolving dilemmas, or at least a starting point for developing a satisfactory resolution. Second, it can provide the individual with personal integrity and continuity when they are making decisions.

There are a wide variety of ethical models and frameworks for use when attempting to make ethical decisions, which can range from a simple set of steps to a complex grid of many layers. Their common feature is that they all require significant thought and analysis before reaching a conclusion, albeit this may be achieved in different ways. Readers are directed to Beauchamp and Childress (2012), Husted and Husted (2005) and Seedhouse (2009) for information on a number of ethical models and frameworks that can be applied to the ethical dilemmas described in this book.

A simple model to follow involves the achievement of an ethical education to facilitate ethical decision-making:

1. *Learning* ethical theories, principles and models to establish a sound theoretical knowledge base for use in practice.
2. *Discussing* ethical theories, principles and models to improve understanding and comprehension for use in practice.
3. *Applying* ethical theories, principles and models to case histories to demonstrate comprehension and for use in practice.
4. *Using* ethical theories, principles and models for practical decision-making in any setting.

A suggested model for ethics in practice/decision-making

The model illustrated in Figure 7.1 is intended to guide practitioners through ethical dilemmas they may encounter in clinical practice. The model aids the decision-making process in attempting to apply ethical theories and principles to clinical scenarios, thus allowing the individual practitioner to consider the potential outcomes of their own professional actions. To illustrate the use of the model, a case study from earlier in the chapter is now discussed and the model applied.

In Chapter 10, Thomas is presented as a 15-year-old boy with chronic renal disease. The identified ethical dilemma is Thomas' non-compliance with treatment. This is clearly a problem as it impacts upon his ongoing health and well-being. On a wider scale, it also has an impact on the resources needed to care for Thomas from the multidisciplinary team, and potentially the deviation of those resources from other children. The ethical theory that has been applied to this situation is utilitarianism, which advocates the greatest good for the greatest number. Here we see that the tenets of this theory may not be achieved as Thomas, his family and the multidisciplinary team may all be affected by his decision not to comply with treatment. A variety of principles may also be applied to this situation, including autonomy, in terms of Thomas' ability to make his own decisions; beneficence, in terms of the role of the children's nurse in being obliged to act in ways to promote the well-being of others; non-maleficence, again relating to the role of the children's nurse in avoiding the risk of harm to Thomas or minimising that risk, while facilitating his own autonomous decision-making processes.

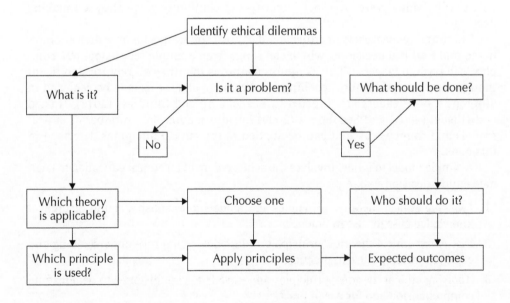

FIGURE 7.1 A model for ethics in practice/decision-making.

Once the practitioner has identified the appropriate ethical theory and principles, it is incumbent on them to find solutions. In Thomas' case, this is around negotiation and partnership, in attempting to find a way forward to ensure that Thomas is compliant with his treatment to assure his ongoing health and well-being. When applying this model in practice, it would be beneficial to identify a range of possible outcomes and the ethical implications of each action and their impact on the individual child or young person, their families and the children's nurse responsible for their care.

Conclusion

The aim of this chapter was to identify and apply a range of ethical theories and principles to clinical practice. For the application of ethics to be pertinent to individual nurses, they must have a clear understanding of the guiding theory and principles. Within the case studies we have used to aid the discussion, we have seen that children and young people with long-term conditions experience a range of difficulties and dilemmas as they pass through the care setting, whether this is within the acute or community setting. Children's nurses are constantly involved in the decision-making process within a range of clinical settings. We have seen that there are no easy solutions to a number of ethical dilemmas; the onus is on individual nurses to be aware of the ethical dimensions of the care that they deliver to ensure that at all times they do no harm and act within the legal, professional and ethical boundaries of their role.

Key points

- There is no such person as a moral expert.
- Children's nurses must make their own ethical decisions and must not blindly follow the dictates of others.
- In particular, they must recognise that the doctor or any other member of the multi-disciplinary team is potentially no more morally competent than themselves.
- Children's nurses must appreciate that not all ethical dilemmas have solutions, but nevertheless be equipped to make the best possible decision.
- The study and application of ethical principles to the often difficult decisions made during the care trajectory of children and young people with long-term conditions will enhance the decision-making capabilities of individual children's nurses and allow them to contribute to the decision-making process and support the child, young person and their family.

Acknowledgement

I acknowledge the contribution of Maggie Furness with whom I jointly authored the previous version of this chapter (McNee & Furness, 2007).

Useful websites

Kohlberg's theory of moral development
http://psychology.about.com/od/developmentalpsychology/a/kohlberg.htm.
UK clinical ethics network http://www.ethics-network.org.uk

📖 Recommended reading

Beauchamp, T. & Childress, J. (2012) *Principles of Bio-Medical Ethics* (seventh edition). Oxford, Oxford University Press.

References

Access to Palliative Care and Treatment of Children Bill (2019) https://services.parliament.uk/bills/2019-19/accesstopalliativecareandtreatmentofchildren.html Accessed 30/01/20.

Avery, G. (2013) *Law and Ethics in Nursing and Healthcare*. London, Sage.

Beauchamp, T.L. & Childress, J.F. (2001) *Principles of Bio-Medical Ethics* (fifth edition). Oxford, Oxford University Press.

Beauchamp, T.L. & Childress, J.F. (2012) *Principles of Bio-Medical Ethics* (seventh edition). Oxford, Oxford University Press.

Benjamin, M. & Curtis, J. (1992) *Ethics in Nursing*. Oxford, Oxford University Press.

Botes, A. (2000) An integrated approach to ethical decision making in the health team. *Journal of Advanced Nursing*, **32** (5), 1076–1082.

Brykczynska, G. (1994) *Ethics in Paediatric Nursing*. London, Chapman and Hall.

Brykczynska, G. & Simons, J. (2011) *Ethical and Philosophical Aspects of Nursing Children and Young People*. Chichester, John Wiley and Sons Ltd.

Buka, P. (2008) *Patients' Rights, Law and Ethics for Nurses*. London, Hodder Arnold.

Burkhardt, M. & Nathaniel, A. (2020) *Ethics and Issues in Contemporary Nursing*. Missouri, Elsevier.

Butts, J. & Rich, K. (2013) *Nursing Ethics: Across the Curriculum and into Practice* (third edition) Jones and Bartlett Learning, Massachusetts.

Children Act (1989) London, The Stationery Office.

Children Act (2004) London, The Stationery Office.

Cholbi, M. (2015) Kant on euthanasia and the duty to die: clearing the air. *Journal of Medical Ethics*, **41** (8), 607–610.

Close, E., Wilmott, L. & White, B. (2018) Charlie Gard: in defence of the law. *Journal of Medical Ethics* **44**, 476–480.

Cooper, M. (1988) Covenantal relationships: grounding for the nursing ethic. *Advances in Nursing Science*, **10** (4), 48–59.

Cranmer, P. & Nhemachena, J. (2013) *Ethics for Nurses: Theory and Practice*. London, Open University Press.

Department of Health, UK (1994) *The Allitt Inquiry*. London, The Stationery Office.

Department of Health UK (2004) *National Service Framework for Children, Young People and Maternity Services*. London, The Stationery Office.

Department of Health, UK (2011) *You're Welcome: Quality Criteria for Children and Young People Friendly Health Services*. London, The Stationery Office.

Department of Health, UK (2012) *Liberating the NHS: No Decision About Me Without Me*. London, The Stationery Office.

Dworkin, G. (1988) *The Theory and Practice of Autonomy*. Cambridge, Cambridge University Press.

Edwards, S.D. (2009) *Nursing Ethics: A Principle-based Approach* (second edition). Basingstoke, Palgrave Macmillan.

Fletcher, J. (1979) *Situation Ethics*. London, S.C.M. Press.

Francis, R. (2013) *Report of the Mid Staffordshire NHS Foundation Trust Public Inquiry*. London, The Stationery Office.

Frankenna, W.K. (1973) *Ethics (second edition)*. Englewood Cliffs, NJ, Prentice Hall.

Gillon, R. (1985) *Philosophical Medical Ethics*. Chester, Wiley Blackwell.

Glasper, E. & Richardson, J. (2010) *A Textbook of Children and Young People's Nursing*. London, Churchill Livingstone.

Griffith, R. & Tengnah, S. (2017) *Law and Professional Issues in Nursing* (fourth edition). London, Sage.

Heath and Social Care Act (2012) London, The Stationery Office.

Hendrick, J. (2004) *Law and Ethics in Nursing and Health Care*. Cheltenham, Nelson Thornes.

Human Rights Act (1998) London, The Stationery Office.

Husted, G.L. & Husted, J.H. (2005) *Ethical Decision Making in Nursing: The Symphonoligical Approach* (third edition). New York, Springer Publishing

International Council of Nurses (2012) *The ICN Code of Ethics for Nurses*. Geneva, ICN.

Jameton, A.I. (1990) Culture morality and ethics: twirling the spindle. *Critical Care Nursing Clinics of North America*, **2** (3), 443–451

Kennedy, I. (2001) *Learning from Bristol: The Report of the Public Inquiry into Children's Heart Surgery at the Bristol Royal Infirmary 1984–1995*. London, The Stationery Office.

Macintyre, A. (1981) *After Virtue* (second edition). London, Duckworth.

Mallory, M., Lindesmith, L. & Baric, R. (2018) Vaccination induced herd immunity: success and challenges. *The Journal of Allergy and Clinical Immunology*, **142** (1), 64–66.

Marriott, S. (2004) Right from the start. *Nursing Management*, **11** (6), 16–18.

McNee, P. & Furness, M. (2007) Ethical issues. In: *Nursing Care of Children and Young People with Chronic Illness* (eds F. Valentine & L. Lowes), pp. 131–155. Oxford, Blackwell Publishing.

National Health Service (2019) NHS Long Term Plan. www.longtermplan.nhs.uk Accessed 30/01/20.

Nursing and Midwifery Council (2004) *Code of Professional Conduct Standards of Performance and Ethics*. London, Nursing and Midwifery Council.

Nursing and Midwifery Council (2018) *The Code: Professional Standards of Practice and Behaviour for Nurses, Midwives and Nursing Associates*. London, Nursing and Midwifery Council.

Presidents Commission for the Study of Ethical Problems in Medicine and Biomedical Research (1981) *Protecting Human Subjects: the Belmont Report*. Washington, DC, US Government Printing Office.

Rawls, J. (1997) *A Theory of Justice*. Cambridge, Harvard University Press.

Rowson, R. (1990) *An Introduction to Ethics*. Harrow, Scutari Press.

Seedhouse, D. (2009) *Ethics: The Heart of Health Care* (third edition). Chichester, Wiley.

Smart, J. & Williams, B. (1989) *Utilitarianism: For and Against*. Cambridge, Cambridge University Press.

The Social Services and Well-Being Act (Wales) (2014) Cardiff, Welsh Government.

Thiroux, J. (1995) *Ethics, Theory and Practice* (fifth edition). New Jersey, Prentice-Hall.

Thompson, I., Melia, K., Boyd, K., *et al.* (2006) *Nursing Ethics* (fifth edition). Edinburgh, Churchill Livingstone.

Trusted, J. (1987) *Moral Principles and Social Values*. London, Routledge and Keegan.

Tschudin, V. (2003) *Ethics in Nursing: The Caring Relationship* (third edition). Edinburgh, Butterworth Heinemann.

United Nations (1989) *Convention on the Rights of the Child*. Geneva, UN.

Veatch, R. (1981) *A Theory of Medical Ethics*. New York, Basic Books.

Veatch, R. (2016) *The Basis of Bioethics*. Oxford, Routledge.

Wheeler, H. (2012) *Law, Ethics and Professional Issues for Nursing: A Reflective and Portfolio Building Approach*. Abingdon, Routledge.

Wilkinson, D. & Savelescu, J. (2018) Hard lessons: learning from the Charlie Gard case. *Journal of Medical Ethics*, **44**, 438–442

CHAPTER 8

Children and Young People's Continuing Care

Melda Price and Sian Thomas

Introduction

Due to developments in medical care and technology, the survival of children with complex needs and long-term illness has become more prevalent (Perrin *et al.*, 2014). A qualitative study undertaken by Whiting (2019) with WellChild suggests that this growing population is cared for at home '24 hours per day, 7 days a week'. The needs of this group of children and young people may be so complex that they cannot be met by the general health care services provided in the hospital and community and additional health support may be needed (WellChild, 2018a); this is known as continuing care.

The first part of this chapter will explore the impact of changing service boundaries and the development of children's nursing roles on children/young people and their families.

An analysis of assessment methods and models of delivery of continuing care and support will follow this. It is important to note that there are differences due to variances in legislation and statutory guidance across UK, this chapter will focus on the overarching principles around meeting the continuing care needs of children and young people (Welsh Government (WG), 2012; Department of Health UK (DoH UK), 2016).

A case study approach will be used to explore the care pathway of a child with a neurological degenerative condition, namely Batten's disease, in a variety of settings. This condition manifests itself in various supportive care issues that can be applied to a number of neurological conditions, and these will be discussed throughout the chapter.

Nursing Care of Children and Young People with Long-Term Conditions, Second Edition.
Edited by Mandy Brimble and Peter McNee.
© 2021 John Wiley & Sons Ltd. Published 2021 by John Wiley & Sons Ltd.

Aim of the chapter

The aim of this chapter is to explore the context of care for children and young people who require continuing care in the community setting.

Intended learning outcomes

- To discuss the importance of multiagency and partnership working across boundaries of care; to explore discharge planning and its application to the child and young person
- To discuss the importance of joint working in planning appropriate services by exploring models of needs assessment
- To examine aspects of assessment and care delivery for children and young people with continuing care needs
- To explore the relationships between the child/young person and their family and the children's nurse involved in the care

Continuing care needs and integrated children services

Within the literature, there is no agreed definition for children with complex health care needs and it has been shown (Whiting, 2019) that the number of these children is difficult to estimate but anecdotally this is an increasing population. Together for Short Lives (2013) state that there are an estimated 49,000 children under 19 in the UK with a life-threatening condition. WellChild (2018b) state that there are 30,000 children with undiagnosed genetic or rare disorders and 6000 children and young people who are dependent on assistive technology. Additionally, the Department of Works and Pensions (2014) estimated that there are 800,000 children in the UK with a disability. These children are quite diverse, with variance in cause, age of onset, duration, severity and frequency of use of services and technology.

The role of a care coordinator is beneficial in supporting and planning service provision for children with complex needs to coordinate the wide range of services involved in meeting the child's care needs (Hillis et al., 2016). This is to recognise that the nature of their complex needs means that their care is provided by a wide range of services which would benefit coordination to ensure the child's care needs are met. The importance of family-centred care and the role of parents being allowed to be parents is vital. The child and family should be central in negotiating packages of care, and these should be agreed between health care providers, local authorities and their partners.

⊕ Case study 8.1

Initial background information

David is 4 years old and lives with his parents and 2-year-old brother on a farm in a rural area of North Wales. His mother is his main carer and feels quite isolated as her husband works long hours managing the farm. The family is Welsh speaking and David attends a mainstream Welsh primary school. Over a period of a few months, his walking became increasingly unsteady and he continually fell over. Also, at this time, David had his first seizure, which was initially thought to be a febrile convulsion. David was admitted to his local hospital where he was investigated for a focus for the infection that might have caused a febrile convulsion. However, it was found to be neurological in nature and he was diagnosed with epilepsy. Due to his deterioration in walking and the continuation of convulsions he required more specialised care and was referred to a consultant paediatric neurologist. As they live in North Wales, the nearest specialist centre for paediatric neurology is at a children's hospital, 60 miles away, in England.

Hospital admissions and travelling long distances for assessment and treatment present many practical difficulties for parents. There are a variety of factors impacting on the family; for example, siblings, distance, travel and financial circumstances. As Welsh is David and his family's first language, staff caring for them need to consider this during the admission and holistic assessment of his needs. David may only have had limited exposure to the English language and consequently may not be able to understand and express himself as well in English as he can in Welsh. This could significantly influence the accuracy of the assessment.

Reflection

- Reflect upon the children and young people you have cared for whose first language is not English.
- Consider the social, emotional and environmental factors that may impact on these children and their families.

David has a right to be able to communicate in his first language and in Wales the Welsh Government Language Measure (2011) and Welsh Language Standards (2016) require the bilingual provision of public services. Commissioned care from an English health care provider delivers David's tertiary care and therefore the Welsh Government Standard does not apply.

🌐 Case study 8.2

When David was 4 years old, he was referred to and assessed by the paediatric neurologist, and following many tests was diagnosed with CLN3 Batten disease. David's newly born sibling was also tested, and his results were negative. Batten's disease is an inherited disorder and has an autosomal recessive characteristic.

Test your knowledge

- In an autosomal recessive disorder, what incidence is there for each pregnancy?
- If one parent is the carrier, what chances are there that the child would be affected?

The term Batten Disease includes several rare life-limiting, life-threatening inherited neurological disorders (National Institute of Neurological Disorders and Stroke, 2019). It is estimated by the Batten Disease Family Association (BDFA, 2014) that 'approximately 11–17 children, young people and adults are diagnosed with a form of the disease each year; this results in between 100–150 affected individuals currently living with Batten disease in the UK'. These disorders are termed neuronal ceroid lipofuscinosis (NCL) and include nine forms. Included in these are CLN1 (gene) infantile onset; CLN2 disease late infantile; CLN3 disease, juvenile (BDFA, 2014). The NCLs involve defective lysosomal processing enzymes or receptors. This then causes cognitive and visual impairments, seizures, deterioration of motor and language skills and premature death (Rosenberg *et al.*, 2019). They differ in symptoms, age of onset and order of progression of the disease (Mink *et al.*, 2013). The different forms of NCL are caused by the mutation of a specific gene resulting in a collection of problems that inhibit normal recycling of molecules at a cellular level (National Institute of Neurological Disorders and Stroke, 2019). The diagnosis has been improved by use of DNA-based tests that screen for a variety of genes. The identification of the actual mutation in 13 genes has enabled the development of targeted therapies (Mole *et al.*, 2018). Recent research undertaken by Mole *et al.* (2018) has shown positive results in treatment with intracerebroventricularly administered enzymes specifically for the neuronal type 2 disease. An example of an innovative research programme is the BATCure, funded by EU Horizon 2020, which supports research to develop new therapeutic options for NCLs (Hartnett, 2019). NHS England has recently announced that all children in England with Batten Disease will be offered Cerliponase alfa to slow the progression of the disease (NHS England, 2019).

Reflection

Reflect upon the children with neurological degenerative disorders that you have cared for in practice. Make a list of their conditions.

Due to the devastating nature of a diagnosis of a life-limiting condition such as Batten's disease, David and his family will need support. The communication of bad news to families requires careful planning and consideration and needs to be delivered by a health professional with good communication skills in a calm, well-prepared environment. Specialist nurses, community children's nurses, social services or voluntary organisations such as Contact and Together for Short Lives, can provide support to families, which is vitally important given that families are known to experience stress and grief arising from their child's condition (Smith *et al.*, 2015), as discussed in Chapter 3.

🌐 Case study 8.3

David is now 5-and-a-half years old, his eating and drinking have gradually deteriorated since diagnosis and he is losing weight. When David swallows fluids, he frequently splutters, and is finding it increasingly problematic to swallow food and drink. He has also suffered from several chest infections and now requires admission to hospital to investigate whether these are being caused by inhalation of fluids and food into his lungs.

Reflection

Consider children you have cared for with feeding difficulties. What are the common symptoms associated with this and why?

Children with Batten's disease or similar neurodegenerative disorders frequently have feeding and swallowing difficulties and may develop gastro-oesophageal reflux (GOR). GOR is associated with chronic vomiting leading to inadequate weight gain, recurrent cough or wheeze following feed aspiration, blood streaked vomit due to oesophagitis, and feed refusal due to the severe pain on feeding (National Institute for Clinical Excellence (NICE), 2016). GOR is often difficult to manage and may be treated medically or surgically. The child's nutritional requirements may not be met despite every effort being made by the child and carers. This in turn results in poor bone and tissue growth, decreased muscle strength (with consequent reduction in the ability to cough), decreased cerebral function with possible exacerbation of neurological impairment, disturbances of the immune system and poor circulation, with delayed healing of pressure sores (Groce *et al.*, 2014).

In addition to a poor ability to chew and swallow, there are various reasons why children with neurodegenerative disorders may not achieve adequate food intake, including:

- Limited communication skills preventing the child from requesting food when hungry.
- A lack of mobility hindering the child from seeking snacks independently.
- Poor hand function hindering self-feeding.
- Weak head and trunk control with extensor posturing limiting self-feeding opportunities.

Test your knowledge

Make a list of care practices you have seen used for children who are disabled and have difficulties with feeding.

Children with neurodegenerative disorders may find fluid difficult to tolerate in the mouth. In a formula-fed infant with frequent regurgitation associated with marked distress, the clinical team which includes the paediatrician/paeditric gastroentero-logist, speech and language therapist and dietitian will review the feeding history. They may recommend to reduce the feed volumes if excessive for the infant's weight. They may also offer a trial of smaller, more frequent feeds, while maintaining an appropriate total daily volume. They may also offer a trial of a feed thickener which can be added to any liquid and allows the fluid to be more easily controlled in the mouth. If the stepped-care approach is unsuccessful, the clinical team may then consider further investigations and pharmalogical treatment (NICE, 2016; Rosen et al., 2018).

The physical and emotional burden on parents and carers of children with severe feeding and swallowing difficulties is constant (Craig, 2013). Eating is not only beneficial for physical growth and development but is also a central part of social activity. Mealtimes for this group of children can be prolonged and stressful due to severe oromotor dysfunction causing feeding difficulties, which often extends the time it takes to complete their meal. Despite the time and care taken, the child may still be malnourished due to the high calorie expenditure usage to complete the feeding process. The nurse should assess the impact of psychological and emotional factors on the child and family (refer to Chapter 5 to reinforce your knowledge about meeting children's psychological needs). Failure to establish a safe, effective feeding method that is satisfying and rewarding to both the child and parents can disrupt the bond between them. Families and schools need expert advice on how to make mealtimes safe, nutritionally adequate and enjoyable. A children's nutrition nurse, community children's nurse, community dietitian, school nurse, health visitor or specialist health visitor can provide this advice.

It is beneficial to the child to establish a routine and ensure that all carers who feed the child use a consistent approach. In some areas, there is a coordinated approach to dealing with feeding problems through the establishment of multidisciplinary feeding teams who hold joint clinics. Where a team approach is not available, the parents, child and dietitian should work with the speech and language therapist, referring to other professionals as necessary, to meet the child's needs.

🌐 Case study 8.4

After a detailed assessment, it was decided that David (aged 5-and-a-half years) would require referral to a paediatric surgeon for insertion of a gastrostomy tube to meet most of his nutritional requirements.

Children with a degenerative condition such as Batten's disease may reach a stage where their poor swallow reflex is classed as unsafe, and the need for enteral feeding methods are explored. Ethical and professional issues regarding the parents' and child/young person's consent to the insertion of the gastrostomy tube should be considered. For consent to be valid and informed, the child and/or parent must be capable of taking that decision, acting voluntarily (not under pressure or duress) and given sufficient information to enable a decision to be made (DoH UK, 2009). This will enable all children and young people and their families to be involved in all decisions regarding their care (WellChild, 2018b).

Guidance from the Department of Health, UK (DoH UK, 2009, p. 33) suggests that:

> In the case of Gillick, the court held that children who have enough understanding and intelligence to enable them to understand fully what is involved in a proposed intervention will also have the capacity to consent to that intervention.

Thus, Gillick competence is a term used in English medical law to describe the ruling made by the House of Lords relating to the rights of children under the age of 16 years to consent to treatment without their parents' knowledge, but the term Frazer competence (after Lord Frazer who made the ruling) is preferred. However, even if children and young people are not able to give legal consent, it is important to involve them in the process. Consideration of their developmental age and understanding is important when explaining procedures or providing information. They should be involved in decision-making, be informed about what is going to happen and given choices about, for example, the timing of procedures. The beneficence of the child and the advocacy role of the nurse in providing information and support for the parents to make an informed decision are key skills required of the children's nurse. (Refer to Chapter 7.)

Test Your Knowledge

- Consider the different types of feeding routes you have observed in practice.
- What were the advantages and disadvantages of each method?
- How did the child and family cope with the feeding method and regime?
- Make a note of your reflections.

Transition to home care

To enable parents and carers to effectively care for a child or young person with complex health care needs at home, a robust and comprehensive education programme needs to be developed and implemented as part of the pre-discharge care. The education programme should provide information about theoretical and practical aspects and should include opportunities for supervised practice before a suitably qualified practitioner undertakes an assessment of the competence of the parent/carer. Discharge

TABLE 8.1 Advantages and disadvantages of enteral feeding methods.

Method	Description	Advantages	Disadvantages
Nasogastric	Feeding tube that enters the gastrointestinal tract via the nose	Easily inserted Method of first choice Short-term feeding	Easily visible Causes discomfort to nasopharynx May block or be easily removed Tube re-insertion is distressing to child and family Risk of aspiration
Gastrostomy	Direct long-term access to stomach via a soft plastic tube or button that is flush to the skin	Easily hidden under clothes Suitable for long-term feeding	Requires general anaesthetic May increase reflux if present before surgery Risk of skin irritation, infection, granulation tissue, leakage, gastric distension Stoma will close within a few hours if accidentally removed
Nasojejunal	Nasal feeding tube enters the jejunum via the gastrointestinal tract	Short-term feeding Less risk of aspiration than nasogastric feeding	Difficult to insert Risk of perforation Abdominal pain and diarrhoea if continuous feeding is not used Discomfort to nasopharynx
Jejunostomy	Delivers feeds via a tube inserted directly into jejunum or via the stomach through gastrostomy tube Suitable for children with persistent GOR	Reduced risk of aspiration Long-term feeding	Risk of perforation Feed needs to be infused constantly Risk of bacterial overgrowth Dumping syndrome can occur

Source: Adapted from Holden, C. and MacDonald, A. (2000). *Nutrition and Child Health*. London, Baillière Tindall.

planning is a process during which the child and family's needs are identified and negotiated in order to prepare them for transition of care from hospital to home. Effective discharge planning takes time to do well and requires good collaboration between hospital and community services (Hewitt-Taylor, 2005; 2012).

The DoH UK (2009) stated that planning for any child to go home should begin on admission, and this remains current practice. However, coordinating a smooth transition from hospital to home for a child or young person with long-term care needs is often challenging and diverse (Council for Disabled Children, 2010). The care of a child or young person should be seamless and the key to this is a multiprofessional team not restricted by organisational boundaries and with clear roles and responsibilities. This is sometimes called the Team around the Child. Effective partnerships are the only way of delivering fully integrated services (WellChild, 2018b).

The WellChild organisation appointed its first WellChild nurse in 2006 and in 2016 they appointed their 32nd nurse. The aim of these children's nurses is to improve the provision of community nursing care for children with complex health needs. This is achieved by improved coordination and planning for discharge of children from hospital and support of children and families at home (Whiting, 2019).

🌐 Case study 8.5

David is now 6 years old and it is a year since his gastrostomy was inserted. On a home visit to David, his mother mentions to you that at their support group a parent had told her about the use of a blended diet. The parent had talked to her about how their child's vomiting was much improved on the diet. David's mother asked if the blended diet could be an option for David? What would you say to the mother?

Blended diets

The use of blended food administered into an enteral feeding tube as an alternative or in addition to commercial feed prescribed by the dietitian has been increasing in practice in the UK. Some professionals have concerns around the mode of feeding and this is due to the perceived increase in risk of nutritional deficiency, feeding tube blockage and infection (British Dietetic Association (BDA), 2013). Initial research in this area has suggested a blended diet can have physiological benefits, such as improvement in the symptoms of vomiting, reflux and abnormal bowel habit (Durnan, 2018; Gallagher *et al.*, 2018). In addition to this, there have been social and emotional benefits reported by the parents and carers of tube-fed children and young people (Phillips, 2018). Considering the growing evidence base in this area, the BDA have issued a policy statement (2019) which aims to support UK dietitians in clinical practice to ensure tube-fed individuals receive effective, evidence-based, equitable and quality care.

Test your knowledge

- What would be the individual roles of the multidisciplinary feeding team?
- In David's case, which professionals would need to be in this team?

The specialist multidisciplinary feeding team should include:

- A paediatric gastroenterologist for clinical management of the gastrointestinal aspect of the condition.
- A paediatric neurologist to manage the neurological aspect of the condition.
- A paediatric dietician to provide advice on dietary requirements.
- A speech and language therapist who would focus on assessment and observation of feeding skills.

- A children's nutrition nurse to provide education, care and advice to children and families on the management of enteral feeding.
- A paediatric psychologist to advise on the behavioural aspects.

⊶ Key point

- No one profession is adequately equipped to single-handedly manage the feeding difficulties of a child with disability.

⊛ Case study 8.6

During David's admission at 5-and-a-half years of age, the nursing staff realised the pressure that his family was under due to his high level of nursing care needs. The nursing staff discussed this with his family and the consultant. A multidisciplinary discharge meeting was organised to discuss David and his family's needs. It was identified from this meeting that David's family required additional financial, social, psychological and health care support at home, and a referral was made for continuing health care.

Reflection

- Reflect on your practice area and consider why a child with complex care needs might have a delayed discharge from hospital.
- Write down the factors the nurse should consider in preparation for David's discharge.

Children and young people's continuing care

Planning of complex care packages via continuing care is challenging for families and professionals. The term continuing care is used to describe the care that a child and young person needs as a result of a disability, accident or illness that cannot be met by existing universal or specialist services alone. In Wales, in 2012, the Children and Young People's Continuing Care guidance was produced. It was developed to provide a framework for planning and provision of continuing care in health boards. This was to ensure fairness and consistency for provision across Wales. This updated guidance is due for publication early 2020 (WG, 2019). This is replicated in England with guidance from DoH UK (2016).

TABLE 8.2   Issues to be considered in discharge planning.

Factors that delay children with complex health needs being discharged from hospital	Factors that need to be considered in preparation for home care
Time taken for planning	Key worker role Communication and liaison between multidisciplinary/multiprofessional teams or services Collaboration between health, social care and education agencies are vital
Priority given by health care staff/ management to discharge planning	Establish funding for respite care package
Recruitment of community staff with relevant experience Issues around who will fund the respite care in the community	Understanding of child's condition – implications for home management, for example medical/ social/ financial needs, home adaptations required Clinical skills training for parents and/or carers
A lack of collaboration between services	Organisation of equipment and/or supplies Health and safety issues Identification of level of nursing and social care support required Development of an action plan for professionals with clear lines of responsibility

Parents may find the responsibilities of caring for their child at home physically and mentally exhausting (Carter & Bray, 2017) and following extended stays in hospital, a period of adjustment is required to empower parents to be the main carers for their child's needs at home (Hewitt-Taylor, 2012). Government policies and guidelines have been developed in order to guide services to meet the supportive needs of families in a cost-effective way (WG, 2012; Children and Families Act, 2014).

Any professional can instigate a referral for continuing care. The process typically comprises of three phases:

- assessment phase
- decision-making phase
- arrangement of provision phase.

Identifying an appropriate care package

Once it is recognised that a child or young person may have needs that require additional health services, a referral may be made through a number of routes and should follow the local process. The assessment is led by a community children's nurse or a children and young people's health assessor. Having gained consent from the parent (or young person, where appropriate) for sharing information, the individual will gather advice from relevant professionals to determine whether a full assessment is necessary.

The lead assessor will draw together all relevant evidence, which will include the preferences of the child/young person and family, a nursing assessment, the key reports and risk assessments from the multidisciplinary team. The information is then collated and will be the focus of the multidisciplinary meeting.

Reflection

- Who should be involved in David's multidisciplinary discharge meeting and what are their key responsibilities?
- Make a list of your thoughts and compare these to Table 8.3.

Everyone who has significant ongoing involvement in the care of the child or young person should be invited to attend the multidisciplinary team (MDT) planning meeting or provide a report, in order to coordinate a seamless discharge plan. The child or young person and their parents should the focus of the MDT meetings; utilising person-centred practice and a 'what matters approach' in line with the Social Services and Well-being (Wales) Act (WG, 2014) can help problem solve issues for families.

The care coordinator/key worker is generally identified at this meeting to take a lead role in future care coordination (WellChild, 2018b). The role of the key worker is important as they have knowledge of local services and can liaise between hospital, community and home, and work closely with the other members of the multidisciplinary team. The WellChild nurse if available can liaise and coordinate this process (WellChild, 2018b).

Key worker role/care coordinator

A systematic review by Hillis *et al.* (2016) found that there isn't a consistent term in the international literature for key worker. Other titles are used family care coordinator, care coordinator counselor, nurse care coordinator and key worker (Hillis *et al.*, 2016). The provision of 'key workers' who work across health, education and social services has been recommended in policy guidance and, most recently by the WellChild (2018b) organisation.

Community children's nursing services

The aim of community children's nursing (CCN) services is to provide nursing and support to children and young people within the family home (Carter *et al.*, 2012). Providing care close to home is an important Welsh government agenda (WG 2018). This is substantiated by the DoH UK (2011) which suggests that nurses can provide expert nursing care for children in their own homes and schools (Dunlop & Maunder, 2019). The *Facing the Future: Together for Child Health* (RCPCH, 2015) document published by the Royal College of Paediatrics and Child Health (RCPCH), Royal College of Nursing (RCN) and Royal College of General Practitioners (RCGP), standard 5 states that 'every acute general children's service should be supported by a CCN

TABLE 8.3   Example of multidisciplinary team members and associated responsibilities.

Multidisciplinary team members	Responsibilities
Parents	24-hour care
Paediatric neurologist (specialist)	Appointments to monitor condition and provide medical support
Community paediatrician (local service)	Health assessments of needs for support in school
General practitioner (local service)	Support to family, ongoing prescriptions for medications and enteral feeding
Named nurse – ward (specialist)	Key worker before discharge (to be discussed later in chapter)
Paediatrician (local acute hospital)	Local medical support and liaison with paediatric neurologist
Community children's nurse (if available – local service)	Local support to family on nursing care issues and key worker role following discharge; referral to continence advisor for continence supplies
Special needs health visitor (if available – local)	Support to family; advice on local services
Dietitian (specialist)	Enteral feeding advice, planning dietary requirements
Nutrition nurse (specialist)	Organising enteral feeding supplies and regular monitoring and problem-solving advice on nursing care of enteral feeding; direct access to paediatric gastroenterologist
Epilepsy nurse specialist (specialist)	Advice and support on management of epilepsy; direct access to paediatric neurologist
Occupational therapist (local)	Local assessment of need for adaptations and activities of living at home and school
Physiotherapist (local)	Assessment of mobility, advice on seating, wheelchair positioning and exercises to maintain posture and mobility
School nurse (local)	Support at school; advice on care provision, medication issues, enteral feeding and continence
Teacher (local)	Educational support
Social worker (local)	Social support, referral for respite, coordination of package of care, joint working with health; advice on benefits, disability living allowance, mobility allowance, carers' allowance
Family health visitor	Support and advice; 2-year-old sibling may need nursery placement to reduce family stress

service which provides a 24 hours and 7 days a week for advice and support with visits as required by the needs of children using the service' (RCPCH, 2015, p. 54). There are several different models of community children's nursing, but the Queens Nursing Institute (QNI, 2018) recommend that:

the role of the community children's nurse is complex requiring skills in nego-tiation, coaching, teaching and supporting children and young people and their families/carers, whilst effectively collaborating with a range of other agencies and services involved in enabling children and young people to remain safely in the community (QNI, 2018, p. 2).

The DoH UK (2011) indicates there are four groups of infants, children and young people who require services of the CCN:

- Those with acute and short-term conditions.
- Those with long-term conditions.
- Those with disabilities and complex conditions including those requiring continuing care.

  Those with life-limiting and life-threatening illness including those requiring palliative and end of life care (DoH UK, 2011).

Reflection

- Reflect on your own area of clinical practice.
- What community children's nursing services are available?
- What care do these nurses provide?

Provision of equipment for home care

Ideally, funding for all aspects of care should be agreed before discharge home. However, obtaining equipment and supplies has been identified as a significant stress factor for families (Thomas & Price, 2012). The provision and maintenance of equipment needs to be formally agreed before discharge. Getting the right equipment early will help in the child's development (Contact, 2019). Supplies are sometimes difficult to obtain in the community or the child's condition may be unpredictable and parents sometimes need to travel long distances to a specialist centre. Parents are often unclear which professional provides which piece of equipment and they often need to collect bulky supplies at short notice. In David's case, this is further complicated by his community care provision being delivered by a different health care trust. This is time consuming and expensive and adds considerably to the stress of caring for a child with complex continuing care needs. The storage of bulky equipment is another issue raised by parents (Thomas & Price, 2012) and it is recommended that the supply of equipment and consumables should be organised to minimise disruption. Table 8.4 outlines an example of responsibilities for provision of equipment.

Reflection

Consider who should provide the equipment that David would require on discharge:

- wheelchair
- bed

- specially adapted eating utensils
- special seating
- enteral feeding pump and supplies
- gastrostomy tubes and extension sets
- medications.

TABLE 8.4   **Example of provision of equipment.**

Provision of community equipment	Professional
Wheelchair	Physiotherapist or occupational therapist
Bed	Health board or trust
Specially adapted eating utensils, for example spoon, fork etc.	Occupational therapist
Special seating	Physiotherapist or occupational therapist
Feeding pump and supplies Gastrostomy tubes	Nutritional nurse specialist or community children's nurse
Medication	Pharmacist

Carers' assessments

The literature highlights the impact and stress on families of living with a child with a long-term condition (Smith *et al.*, 2015). Occasionally, a parent's income often has to be sacrificed so that she/he can be the main carer for their child with complex health needs. This can impact on financial concerns which can cause additional stress to families who may well be experiencing increased costs resulting from their child's condition. For example, these can include special food purchases, travel to hospital, car parking and increased purchases of bed linen and clothing.

Parents who are carers can have an assessment to identify how they might best be supported in their caring role. The Social Services and Well-being (Wales) Act (WG, 2014) changes the way people's needs are assessed and the way services are delivered. The assessment is led by the local authority and might promote a range of support and recommend things such as someone to provide care to allow the parent to take a break from caring, or provide information and advice about benefits and support groups for carers.

◉ Case study 8.7

Six months following diagnosis (aged 4-and-a-half years), during a home visit by the epilepsy outreach nurse, it was noted that David's condition had deteriorated. His seizures had become more difficult to manage and his parents required instruction on how to administer buccal (oromucosal) midazolam. The nurse arranged an appointment for David to be reviewed by the local community paediatrician to avoid the family travelling to the regional centre.

Epilepsy is a common neurological disorder which is characterised by recurring seizures and is a symptom associated with Batten Disease. A seizure is a brief, excessive discharge of electrical activity in the brain that changes how someone feels, senses, thinks, or behaves (Devinsky, 2016). According to the National Institute of Clinical Evidence guidance (NICE, 2019), most children with epilepsy can be managed with anti-epileptic drugs (AEDs). Buccal midazolam or rectal diazepam should only be prescribed when a child or young person has had a previous episode of prolonged or serial convulsive seizures. (NICE, 2019). In the past, rectal diazepam was administered, but many difficulties were experienced in carrying out the procedure at home and at school. The NICE (2019) suggests that buccal midazolam should be administered by trained clinical personnel or, if a specified protocol is drawn up by the specialist, family and carers with appropriate training which the epilepsy nurse can provide.

⊛ Case study 8.8

The major features of Batten Disease are progressive loss of vision, motor and intellectual deterioration and seizures (BDFA, 2014). David's condition has gradually deteriorated over the last year and he is now unable to walk and he requires a wheelchair. He has problems with incontinence and his seizures are controlled by a variety of anti-epileptic drugs (AEDs). He has poor vision, very limited speech and requires 24-hour supervision and care to meet his daily needs due to severe disability and increasing learning difficulties. The community paediatrician reviews David and he is referred to the social worker, who will visit to assess for respite care and provide financial advice and support. David's parents have been finding the continual care exhausting. Mum is the main carer because dad is unable to provide much support as he works long hours on their farm. The key worker is concerned about mum's well-being and the impact that this may be having on the younger child. Respite or short break care has been raised with the family. A referral is also required for an occupational therapist assessment to consider the need for home adaptations as the family are finding it increasingly difficult to carry David upstairs to his bedroom and access for his wheelchair is proving problematic.

The need for respite or short break provision

Over recent years, an improved understanding of the burden of care and the pressures faced by the family of a child with complex health needs has led to an appreciation that these families deserve a break from caring if they are to continue with the demands of the role (Thomas & Price, 2012; Whiting, 2014b). Therefore, it is not surprising to find that the most consistently cited need for the child with complex health needs is short break care or respite, which meets the needs of parents and provides additional opportunities for the child (Thomas & Price, 2012; Whiting, 2014b; Hill, 2016).

There are many types of respite care, for example (Contact, 2019):

- Care at home – includes sitting or care attendant schemes which may have to be provided by a health professional.
- Day care away from home – includes nurseries, playgroups, out of school and weekend clubs and, during school holidays access to play schemes.
- Overnight short breaks; for example, children's hospice.
- Residential breaks – includes residential homes, special units in hospitals and children's hospice.
- Family link schemes – where the child stays with another family on a regular or occasional basis.

Respite or short break provision children with life-limiting conditions can be fraught with difficulties, primarily because of their complex nursing needs, with a recognised shortfall of highly specialised care (Whiting, 2014b). Parents may refuse to accept respite as they have difficulty trusting others in the care of their child or feel that it's their responsibility. Whiting (2014b) suggests 'that a respite /short break can give parents the resilience to continue caring for their child'. The Together for Short Lives study (Hunt *et al.*, 2013) identified that parents felt that more respite care was required.

Research undertaken by Whiting (2014a) states that parents reported that their lives are affected in many ways when caring for a child with complex health care needs. These included their employment, finances, mental and physical health, relationships in the family and loss of social opportunity and time pressures. A qualitative research study undertaken by Thomas and Price (2012) found that of the seven mothers included in the study, all described the demands of constant care and the challenge of enabling the child to undertake routine activities which results in a physical overburden and social isolation. This had a negative impact on the mothers' ability to work and family income. A more recent study (Hill, 2016) agrees and finds the effect on the family including siblings can be overwhelming. Malcolm *et al.* (2014) found that there was a need for breaks to allow the sibling to cope with the family situation. Holiday times were also difficult and even though there were play schemes available for the child, most had issues around access. Even though parents attempt to protect the siblings, the literature generally acknowledges that having a child with complex health needs within the family will have a detrimental effect on siblings, citing behavioural changes, increased responsibility beyond years and feelings of neglect as issues of concern (Thomas & Price, 2012). Parents are also required to learn complex nursing skills and they may feel physically exhausted from constant caring (Thomas & Price, 2012). Equipment is often cumbersome, which has a negative impact on social outings, and family activities can be severely restricted as social plans can be altered at very short notice as a result of the child's health status. The family home often requires adaptation, which jeopardises home comforts, and there is a lack of privacy attributed to the input of health professionals (Thomas and Price, 2012).

Respite care should be tailored to meet the needs of the child and family, and respite care should be part of the continuing care plan.

Home adaptations

Joint assessment with social services for adaptations to the family home for wheel-chair access and activities of living requirements need accurate assessment by an occupational therapist. Although not applicable to England, in some areas adaptations can cause financial difficulties if major adaptations and building works are means tested, resulting in some parents only receiving part funding. Support and advice can be gained from Contact, an organisiation previously known as Contact a Family (Contact, 2017; 2018), that provides support and information; for example, factsheets for families on short breaks and aids and equipment. The rights of children are paramount and the Children and Families Act (2014) Special Educational Needs and Disability Code of Practice states that local authorities need to take into account the views of parents, children and young people so that services like short breaks meet their needs (Contact, 2018).

◉ Case study 8.9

David is now 6 years old and his condition is stable. He is now receiving respite care two days a month at the children's hospice, which is 50 miles from his home. David is awaiting an assessment to identify what support is available to enable him to attend school. The community children's nurse visits on a weekly basis to assess David's condition and provide support to the family. His younger sibling now has a placement in a local nursery three days a week.

Reflection

Reflect on what support you think David might require at school.

Education and support at school

The way children and young people's special educational needs are identified, assessed and met has been under review over recent years. For example, the SEND Code of Practice (Department for Education and Department of Health, 2015), the Major Review into Support for Children with Special Educational Needs (Department for Education, 2019) and the Additional Learning Needs and Educational Tribunal (Wales) Act (WG, 2018).

Children with degenerative medical conditions require special consideration when educational support is being organised. As David has a health condition that restricts or hinders his access school, he will have an Individual Development Plan (IDP) that will identify and focus on his needs at school in order for him to reach his educational potential. The IDP is a legal document and will look at the health and social care support, but only where this affects the child's learning. The special education needs reforms are underway in Wales, where David lives, aiming for services to work together to receive well-coordinated support which helps achieve positive outcomes (WG, 2018).

For David to attend school, he is likely to need support from a classroom assistant who is trained to care for his needs. The support provision is likely to include transport to school, support with mobility around school, gastrostomy feeding, continence and hygiene, and observation for deterioration in condition. The specialist nurse or community children's nurse will be involved in training David's support worker. Consideration should be given to the risk assessment of the school environment to ensure David is safely and competently cared for. A risk assessment will also need to be undertaken for transport to school and the school environment in relation to equipment and emergency procedures.

Support for families

As already discussed, caring for a child with complex health needs on a daily basis can be a fatiguing process both psychologically and physically for parents (Carter & Bray, 2017). Health professionals and voluntary organisations should provide the necessary support. In response to the demand for caring for children and young people with complex care needs in the community (DoH UK, 2011), a number of community children's nursing teams have been set up across the UK. These teams have demonstrated different models of working with children with complex needs in a variety of environments, such as the home, school, respite and hospice setting. Palliative care pathways, for example the Together for Short Lives Core Care Pathway (2013), should be commenced at 'diagnosis to provide support for the child and family throughout their care journey, from diagnosis to end of life care and bereavement support'. As David's condition deteriorates, the multidisciplinary team and key worker will need to support the family by providing a regular review and assessment of David's condition, parental coping and services he and his family will require.

Conclusion

This chapter has explored the issues surrounding the requirements for a child with complex care needs in the community. The emphasis of care has been on collaborative working and the support and empowerment of families to enable them to care for their child safely. The contemporary issue of blended diets via gastrostomy has also been explored.

The roles of the community children's nurse, the multidisciplinary team and the essential role of the professional working in partnership with families has been considered in relation to the provision of a coordinated, seamless service. Continuing care needs of a child with complex health requirements have been described and the important role of parents in this process has been explored.

> **🔑 Key points**
>
> - Effective multiagency and interprofessional working and communication is paramount to enable a coordinated package of care to be delivered to minimise the burden of caring for a child with a life-limiting condition.
> - Follow the Core Care Pathway developed by Together for Short Lives (2013). To support the child and family in the home, school or respite, resources need to be provided and coordinated.
> - It is essential that packages of care spanning health, social care and education are implemented in negotiation with the child and family.
> - Care provision should include the holistic needs of the child and family; this includes direct care at home and in school education programmes, respite provision and financial support.
> - The role of the community children's nurse is important as the key worker for children and families.

Useful websites

Batten Disease Family Association http://www.bdfa-uk.org.uk/
Contact for families with Disabled children https://www.contact.org.uk
Caudwell Children https://www.caudwellchildren.com/
Disabled living foundation https://www.dlf.org.uk/
Family Fund https://www.familyfund.org.uk/
National Institute of Clinical Evidence http://www.nice.org
Scope https://www.scope.org.uk/
Whizz-Kidz http://www.whizz-kidz.org.uk

References

Batten Disease Family Association (BDFA) (2014) What is Batten Disease? www.bdfa-uk.org.uk/what-is-batten-disease/ Accessed 28/01/20.

British Dietetic Association (BDA) (2013) *Policy Statement use of Liquidised Food with Enteral Feeding Tubes*. Birmingham, British Dietetic Association

British Dietetic Association (2019) The Use of Liquidised Food with Enteral Feeding Tubes. Position Statement, 14/11/19. Birmingham, British Dietetic Association. https://www.bda.uk.com/resource/the-use-of-blended-diet-with-enteral-feeding-tubes.html Accessed 26/06/20.

Carter, B., Coad, J., Bray, L., *et al.* (2012) Home-based care for special healthcare needs: community children's nursing services. *Nursing Research*, **61** (4), 260–268.

Carter, B. & Bray, L. (2017) Parenting a child with complex health care needs: a stressful and imposed "clinical career". *Comprehensive Child and Adolescent Nursing*, **40** (4), 219–222.

Children and Family Act (2014) http://www.legislation.gov.uk/ukpga/2014/6/contents/enacted Accessed 28/01/20.

Contact for Families with Disabled Children (Contact) (2017) *Aids, Equipment and Adaptations. A Guide for Families in England, Northern Ireland, Scotland and Wales.* London, Contact.

Contact for Families with Disabled Children (Contact) (2018) *Short Breaks - Help for You and Your Child to Take a Break.* London, Contact.

Contact for Families with disabled children (Contact) (2019) London: Contact. http:// www. contact.org.uk/ Accessed 28/01/20.

Council for Disabled Children (2010) *Guidelines on the Discharge from Hospital of Children and Young People with High Support Needs.* London, National Children's Bureau.

Craig, G. (2013) Psychosocial aspects of feeding children with neurodisability. *European Journal of Clinical Nutrition,* **67**, 17–20.

Department for Education (2019) https://www.gov.uk/government/news/major-review-into-support-for-children-with-special-educational-needs Accessed 28/01/20.

Department for Education and Department of Health (2015) Special educational needs and disability code of practice: 0 to 25 years. https://www.gov.uk/government/publications/send-code-of-practice-0-to-25 Accessed 28/01/20.

Department for Work and Pensions (2014) *Family Resources Survey: United Kingdom 2011/2012.* London, HMSO.

Department of Health, UK (2009) *Reference Guide to Consent for Examination or Treatment.* London, HMSO.

Department of Health, UK (2011) *NHS at Home: Community Children's Nurse.* London, HMSO.

Department of Health, UK (2016) *National Framework for Children and Young People's Continuing Care.* London, HMSO.

Devinsky, O. (2016) *Epilepsy in Children: What Every Parent Needs to Know.* New York, Demos Medical Publishing.

Dunlop, S. & Maunder, E. (2019) Developing and nurturing a community practice network for community children's nurses in Wales. *British Journal of Nursing,* **28** (12), 782–785.

Durnan, S. (2018) 'It's just food, blended': exploring parents' experiences of choosing blended diet for their tube-fed child. PhD Thesis. Coventry University.

Gallagher, K., Flint, A., Mouzaki, M., *et al.* (2018) Blenderized enteral nutrition diet study: feasibility, clinical, and microbiome outcomes of providing blenderized feeds through a gastric tube in a medically complex pediatric population. *Journal of Parenteral and Enteral Nutrition,* **42** (6), 1046–1060.

Groce, N., Challenger, E., Berman-Bieler, R., *et al.* (2014) Malnutrition and disability: unexplored opportunities for collaboration. *Paediatrics and International Child Health,* **34** (4), 308–314.

Hartnett, L. (2019) Batten Disease. *Learning Disability in Practice,* **22** (5), 22.

Hewitt-Taylor, J. (2005) Caring for children with complex and continuing health needs. *Nursing Standard,* **19** (42), 41–47.

Hewitt-Taylor, J. (2012) Planning the transition of children with complex needs from hospital to home. *Nursing Children and Young People,* **24** (10), 28–35.

Hill, K. (2016) Respite services for children with life-limiting conditions and their families in Ireland. *Nursing Children and Young People,* **28** (10), 30–36.

Hillis, R., Brenner, M., Larkin, P.J., *et al.* (2016) The role of care coordinator for children with complex care needs: a systematic review. *International Journal of Integrated Care,* **16** (2), 12.

Holden, C. & MacDonald, A. (2000) *Nutrition and Child Health.* London, Baillière Tindall.

Hunt, A., Coad, J., West, E *et al.* (2013) *The Big Study for Life-Limited Children.* Bristol, Together for Short Lives.

Malcolm, C., Gibson, F., Adams, S., *et al.* (2014) A relational understanding of sibling experiences of children with rare life-limiting conditions: Findings from a qualitative study. *Journal of Child Health Care,* **18** (3), 230–240.

Mink, J., Augustine, E., Adams, H., *et al.* (2013) Classification and natural history of the neuronal ceroid lipofuscinoses. *Journal of Child Neurology,* **28** (9), 1101–1105.

Mole, S.R., Anderson, G., Band, H.A., *et al.* (2018) Clinical challenges and future therapeutic approaches for neuronal ceroid lipofuscinosis. *The Lancet*, **18** (1), 107–116.

National Institute for Health and Care Excellence (2016) Gastro-oesophageal reflux in children and young people (NICE Quality Standard QS112). https://www.nice.org.uk/guidance/qs112 Accessed 28/01/20.

National Institute of Clinical Evidence (2019) *Clinical Guideline (CG137) Epilepsy: Diagnosis and Management* (original publication 2012). London, NICE.

National Institute of Neurological Disorders and Stroke (2019) Batten Disease Fact Sheet. https://www.ninds.nih.gov/Disorders/Patient-Caregiver-Education/Fact-Sheets/Batten-Disease-Fact-Sheet Accessed 28/01/20.

NHS England (2019) Life-changing treatment on the NHS for children with rare, deadly disease. www.england.nhs.uk/2019/09/life-changing-treatment-on-the-nhs-for-children-with-rare-deadly-disease Accessed 28/1/20.

Perrin, J.M., Anderson, L.E. & Van Cleave, J. (2014) The rise in chronic conditions among infants, children, and youth can be met with continued health system innovations. *Health Affairs*, **33** (12), 2099–2105.

Phillips, G. (2018) Patient and carer experience of blended diet via gastrostomy: a qualitative study. *Journal of Human Nutrition and Dietetics*, **32** (3), 391–399.

Queen's Nursing Institute (2018) *The QNI/QNIS Voluntary Standards for Community Children's Nurse Education and Practice*. London, The Queen's Nursing Institute.

Rosen, R., Vandenplas, Y., Singendonk, M., *et al.* (2018) Pediatric gastroesophageal reflux clinical practice guidelines. *Journal of Pediatric Gastroenterology and Nutrition*, **66** (3), 516–554.

Rosenberg, J.B., Chenm A., Kaminsky, S.M., *et al.* (2019) Advances in the treatment of neuronal ceroid lipofuscinosis. *Journal of Expert Opinion on Orphan Drugs*, **7** (11), 473–500.

Royal College of Paediatrics and Child Health (2015) Facing the Future: Together for Child Health. https://www.rcpch.ac.uk/togetherforchildhealth Accessed 28/01/20.

Smith, J., Cheater, F. & Bekker, H. (2015) Parents' experience of living with a child with a long-term condition: a rapid structured review of the literature. *Health Expectations*, **18**, 452–474.

Thomas, S. & Price, C.M. (2012) Respite care in seven families with children with complex needs. *Nursing Children and Young People*, **24** (8), 24–27.

Together for Short Lives (2013) *A Core Pathway for Children with Life Limiting and Life Threatening Conditions* (third edition). Bristol, Together for Short Lives.

WellChild (2018a) Principles for Better Training. htpp//www.wellchild,.org.uk/training principles Accessed 28/01/20.

WellChild (2018b) Our strategy for giving children and young people with serious health needs the chance to thrive 2018–2023. http//www.wellchild.org.uk/about-us/strategy/ Accessed 28/01/20.

Welsh Government (2011) *Welsh Language (Wales) Measure 2011*. Cardiff, Welsh Government.

Welsh Government (2012) *Children and Young People's Continuing Care Guidance*. Cardiff, Welsh Government.

Welsh Government (2014) *Social Services and Well-being (Wales) Act*. Cardiff, Welsh Government.

Welsh Government (2016) *The Welsh Language Standards (No. 2) Regulations*. Cardiff, Welsh Government.

Welsh Government (2018) *Additional Learning Needs and Education Tribunal (Wales) Act*. Cardiff, Welsh Government.

Welsh Government (2019) *Consultation Document: Children and Young People's Continuing Care*. Cardiff, Welsh Government.

Whiting, M. (2014a) Children with disability and complex health needs: the impact on family life. *Nursing Children and Young People*, **26** (3), 26–30.

Whiting, M. (2014b) Support requirements of parents caring for a child with a disability and complex needs. *Nursing Children and Young People*, **26** (4), 24–27.

Whiting, M. (2019) Caring for children '24-7'. The experience of the WellChild Nurses and the families whom they are providing care and support. *Journal of Child Health Care*, **23** (1), 35–44.

CHAPTER 9

Acute Emergencies

Martina Nathan, Peter McNee, and Jane Davies

Introduction

The purpose of this chapter is to explore some of the key factors that need to be considered for the assessment and management of children and young people with long-term illness who have an acute emergency either as a result of their chronic illness or an unrelated health problem. To illustrate these issues, a case study will be used to explore current care practices and organisation for a child with an oncology condition. It is expected that readers of this chapter will have a knowledge and understanding of the normal cell cycle, types of white cells, normal cell properties and blood cell production.

Aim of the chapter

This chapter aims to raise awareness of the problems facing children and young people with chronic illness and their families when an acute emergency occurs. Issues raised, such as the care environment and multidisciplinary care, will be relevant and transferable to a range of chronic conditions and should be able to be considered in the context of most acute emergencies.

Intended learning outcomes

- To critically examine the impact of acute emergencies on the child/young person with a pre-existing chronic illness and their family
- To explore the factors that may lead to acute emergencies in children and young people with long-term illness and the relevant treatment and management requirements; a case study examining the care of a child with an oncology condition will be used to exemplify these factors

Nursing Care of Children and Young People with Long-Term Conditions, Second Edition.
Edited by Mandy Brimble and Peter McNee.
© 2021 John Wiley & Sons Ltd. Published 2021 by John Wiley & Sons Ltd.

- To analyse the role of the children's nurse and the multidisciplinary team in supporting children, young people and their families during an acute phase of their long-term illness
- To explore the context of care in relation to the environment in which care is delivered and its impact on ongoing medical and nursing care

Acute emergencies

Children with a pre-existing long-term condition are at high risk of acute deterioration or suffering complications as a result of their illness. Due to this risk, clinical services have to be provided in acute and community settings that are responsive to the needs of this vulnerable population. The fact that the level of clinical dependency of children and young people nursed in general ward areas has increased over several years mirrors the changes in service provision in the community sector, where more dependent children with chronic and complex health care issues are now cared for at home or in care environments closer to home (RCPCH, 2014). Complications such as diabetic ketoacidosis, sickle cell crisis, status epilepticus, acute renal failure, circulatory instability, acute exacerbation of asthma and severe febrile neutropenia all require rapid access to skilled clinicians and appropriate environments to deliver the initial care required (Department of Health UK (DoH UK), 2001a). To facilitate this rapid access, a number of children are covered by an open-door policy where they can access the services they require when necessary. This flexibility and approach to treatment allows for care to be delivered around the needs of the individual child and young person rather than that of the organisation. This marks a cultural shift from organisational to person-centred care, particularly when continuing care is required (DoH UK, 2010). However, some centres prefer children to be assessed via a GP or an accident and emergency department before admission or transfer to the appropriate care environment. Other centres prefer children to be assessed in their assessment unit, as general wards may not have the staff available with the appropriate level of knowledge and skills to deal with an unexpected emergency admission. This is an important issue that needs to be discussed with parents at discharge, as some parents in the stress of an emergency may take their child inappropriately to their usual admission ward.

⊕ Case study 9.1

Katie is a 3-year-old girl who was diagnosed with acute lymphoblastic leukaemia (ALL) five months ago. She had a two-week history of lethargy, pallor, enlarged abdomen and poor appetite when she presented at the local GP surgery. A full blood count (FBC) was taken which showed a white cell count (WCC) = 12 cells/L, haemoglobin (Hb) = 82 g/L, platelets = 90 X 10^9/L. She was referred to the local children's oncology/haematology unit where, following a bone marrow aspirate, she was diagnosed with ALL.

Katie is an only child who lives with her mother Claire, who is 18 years old, in a two-bedroomed council owned flat. She has no contact with her father, who lives abroad. Before Katie's illness, Claire worked part time in a local shop and Katie attended preschool. Claire's parents, Tom and Sarah, care for Katie sometimes but both have work commitments.

Initially, Katie found it difficult to adapt to the hospital environment but is now less frightened as she has become familiar with the nursing staff and other children who attend the unit. As the treatment for ALL is essentially based on a randomised controlled trial, it was important to gain informed consent from her mother. Informed consent in this case involved an examination of the decision to be made, whether care and treatment would be in the best interests of Katie; with information and support tailored to Claire to aid in the decision-making process (McKenna *et al.*, 2010).

Time out

- Identify and document the childhood leukaemias you are aware of and their presenting signs and symptoms.

Childhood cancer is rare, accounting for 0.5% of all cancers in the UK. Only 1 in every 650 children under the age of 15 years develops a cancer, with 1600 new cases of childhood cancer in this age group in the UK each year (Children with Cancer, 2019).

Leukaemia is the most common childhood malignancy, accounting for 30% of total childhood cancer diagnoses (National Registry of Childhood Tumours UK, 2012). The most prevalent type of leukaemia is acute leukaemia, with acute lymphoblastic leukaemia (ALL) comprising four-fifths of all leukaemias. The peak incidence of ALL occurs between the ages of 2 and 5 years. Acute myeloid leukaemia is the next most common, also known as acute non-lymphoblastic leukaemia (ANLL). Chronic myeloid leukaemia (CML) accounts for only a small percentage, which differs from the adult population where it is much more common.

The above incidence relates to children under the age of 15 years. The incidence differs for young people and adults. As illustrated in Table 9.1, in England, leukaemia is far less common in this population, with carcinomas and lymphomas being the

TABLE 9.1   **Annual average number of cases 13–24 years, 2013–2015.**

Types of cancer	Total
Total leukaemia	199
Lymphomas	461
Central Nervous System	329
Carcinomas	576
Skin	298
Germ cell	278

Source: Modified from Teenage Cancer Trust (TCT) (2018). Summary; 13–24-year-olds with cancer in England; incidence, mortality and survival. https://www. teenagecancertrust.org/sites/default/files/Teenage%20 Cancer%20Trust%20PHE%20Report%202019%20-%20 Summary.pdf (Accessed 6/7/19).

most common cancers. For both age groups, leukaemia rates are higher in males than females, with a ratio of males to females 1.3:1, in the under 15-year age group. ALL is more common among white children than black children, with ALL being rare in North Africa and the Middle East.

Aetiology

When children and young people are diagnosed with cancer, parents often question if it is something they have done or failed to do that has caused the cancer. The aetiology of childhood cancer, including leukemia, is still not fully explained. It is suggested that it is probably due to two events occurring, one pre-birth and the other post-birth (Wiemels, 2012). Therefore, the main factors thought to play a role in the cause of ALL are:

- genetic
- environmental.

Genetic factors are presumed to play a significant role in the cause of acute leukaemia, due to the association between various chromosomal abnormalities and ALL, for example children with Trisomy 21 (Down syndrome) aged 5 years or under are up to 40 times more likely to develop leukaemia than the unaffected population of children in this age range (Hasle *et al.*, 2000).

Other pre-existing chromosomal abnormalities that increase the risk of ALL are:

- Fanconi's anaemia
- ataxia telangiectasia
- neurofibromatosis
- Schwachmann syndrome
- Klinefelter syndrome
- Bloom syndrome.

Environmental factors

Wiemels (2012) believes that ALL is probably the result of genetic susceptibility and exposure to external risk factors at a time when the child is vulnerable. The high incidence of leukaemia following atomic bomb incidents in Japan demonstrated that ionising radiation is a cause of leukaemia. It is widely accepted, also, that if mothers are exposed to radiation during pregnancy, the baby's risk of developing cancer is increased (Grufferman *et al.*, 2009). In a pooled analysis from 11 record-based studies, Amoon *et al.* (2018) found that the risk of childhood leukaemia slightly increased in children living in close proximity to high-voltage power lines.

The issue of nuclear installations where 'clusters' of children nearby have been diagnosed with ALL has given rise to concern. Kinlen (1995) explains that 'clusters' may be due to 'population mixing', where families have moved into new areas, bringing an epidemic of common infections. It is the abnormal responses to these common infectious agents that may increase the risk of ALL. However, Berrie *et al.* (2019)

stress that studies using non-random selection to investigate the association between childhood leukemia and population mixing are likely to have generated biased findings and future studies should use a region wide analytical strategy. Marcotte *et al.*'s. (2014) study results support the hypothesis that a 'delayed' exposure to infection in infancy gives rise to an increased risk of developing leukemia. Therefore, the exposure to other infants and children during the first few months of life can protect against the risk of developing ALL. Day care and crèches are promoted, as they will bring infants into contact with common infections.

Greaves (2018) stresses that childhood ALL can be considered a paradoxical consequence of progression in modern societies, where behavioural changes have confined early microbial exposure. Other possible factors considered in the aetiology of childhood leukaemia are infants born to mothers over the age of 35 years, infants not breastfed and parental occupation. Chapter 1 examines the influence of environmental factors upon a range of chronic diseases.

Pathophysiology

Cancer is a genetic condition (refer to Chapter 1) and is a Latin term meaning 'crab', which is probably linked to the erratic movement of cells, similar to that of crabs (Skuse, 2015). The properties of malignant cells are:

- same chemical structure as normal cells;
- lack control mechanisms – apoptosis;
- critical change in growth;
- lack adhesiveness;
- reduced normal inhibition.

Leukaemia is a Greek term meaning 'white blood'. It is a clonal disease and is the result of the malignant transformation of bone marrow progenitor cells during haematopoiesis. The classification of different leukaemias depends upon the cell lineage in which the mutation occurs. Malignant transformation along the lymphoid cell lineage is known as lymphocytic leukaemia.

The growth of immature white blood cells, called 'blasts', is characteristic of leukaemia. By failing to mature, the cells cannot function as normal white blood cells. The increased cell division (cell production greater than cell loss) results in blast cells overcrowding the bone marrow space and therefore failing to allow production of normal cells.

Presentation

The child or young person with ALL, as in Katie's situation, often presents with non-specific symptoms, which are insidious and subtle (Zupanec & Tomlinson, 2010) and can include:

- bone/joint pain
- limpness

- fever
- weight loss
- bruising
- headache
- weakness
- enlarged lymph nodes.

ALL, however, can present as an acute illness with a short onset, for example flu-like symptoms. Katie's presentation with pallor and lethargy was due to her anaemia, as the normal haemoglobin for a child of this age should be 110–130 g/L. Due to the overcrowding of blast cells in the bone marrow, normal red blood cells cannot be produced. An elevated leukocyte count (greater than 10 000 per mm^3) is commonly associated with leukaemia. Katie's enlarged abdomen is a result of hepatosplenomegaly (enlarged liver and spleen), which arises from extra-medullary disease spread. Hepatosplenomegaly occurs in over 50% of patients and is usually asymptomatic (Clarke *et al.*, 2016). Her poor appetite may have been due to lethargy and the disease process.

⏱ Time out

- Referring to the above list, provide a rationale for these presenting signs and symptoms for a child with ALL.

As clinical features of ALL can be non-specific, other diagnoses are often considered; for example, viral illness or aplastic anaemia. For a definite diagnosis of ALL, a bone marrow aspirate (BMA) is required even though blast cells are usually present in peripheral blood counts. The aspirate site is usually the iliac crest. In children's oncology care, this procedure is usually carried out under a general anaesthetic (GA), but if the patient is respiratory compromised or has a mediastinal mass, it would need to be done under local anaesthetic (LA). The need for a chest X-ray on admission is therefore necessary. A lumbar puncture (LP) is usually performed at the same time, involving a sample of cerebrospinal fluid (CSF) being taken to examine whether the leukaemia cells have spread to the central nervous system (CNS). A count of more than 25% blast cells in the bone marrow will confirm a diagnosis of leukaemia. The BMA or trephine will be further examined to establish the type of leukaemia.

Prognosis

The following factors are examined to determine prognosis and stratify treatment:

- cell morphology
- immunophenotyping
- cytogenetics
- Minimal Residual Disease.

Cell morphology

This examines the appearance and structure of the cell.

Immunophenotyping

This is an essential component of the diagnostic workup that confirms or establishes the lineage of the leukemia and its stage of differentiation (Behm, 2012).

Cytogenetics

Cytogenetics has determined the incidence and prognostic significance of chromosomal abnormalities in ALL. It plays an important role in the risk stratification of patients in treatment. There are essentially two types of chromosomal aberrations

- changes in chromosome number;
- structural abnormalities (Harrison, 2009).

Children and young people with higher ploidy (number of sets of chromosomes in a cell) have the best prognosis. The Philadelphia chromosome translocation t (9:22) remains the translocation of poor prognosis, evident in 1–3% of childhood ALL (Mrozek *et al.*, 2009).

Analysis of patients treated on MRC UKALL X protocol exposed other recognised risk factors such as age, gender and presenting WCC. Esparza and Sakamoto (2005) note that girls have a better prognosis than boys, and that there is a poorer prognosis associated with increasing age (excluding infantile ALL) and increased WCC.

Minimal Residual Disease (MRD)

The UKALL 2011 protocol assesses and monitors Minimal Residual Disease (MRD) at diagnosis and next at Day 29. MRD refers to submicroscopic disease – disease that remains occult within the patient but eventually leads to relapse (Trent, 2005). It has become an important component of modern therapy for leukemia.

◉ Case study 9.2

Katie is being treated with cytotoxic chemotherapy. A central line, namely a Hickman line, was inserted on week five of her treatment.

During the next five months, Katie received treatment that included:

- induction
- consolidation
- standard interim maintenance.

Delayed intensification started at week eighteen. While in hospital, Katie was given cytotoxic agents, vincristine, steroids (dexamethasone) and L'asparaginase as part of her induction treatment for ALL. This drug regime usually produces remission in 95% of children (Zupanec & Tomlinson, 2010). Intrathecal methotrexate was also given for CNS prophylaxis. For the first week of treatment, Katie was given an uricolytic agent and intravenous fluids to prevent tumour lysis syndrome (TLS), although Katie's risk of this was low due to WCC =15 000 per mm^3. She was also commenced on prophylactic co-trimoxazole at the weekends to prevent the development of Pneumocystis jiroveci pneumonia (PCP).

🕐 **Time out**

- Make a list of the potential side effects of chemotherapy and a rationale for their causes.

Tumour lysis syndrome (TLS) occurs as a result of the excretory capacity of the kidneys' inability to cope with the large quantities of uric acid, potassium and phosphate that are emitted due to cancer cell death. Patients with bulky tumours, lymphomas and high WCCs are considered at high risk of developing TLS. Prophylactic measures include identification of risk factors, hydration, monitoring serum U/Es and uricolytic agents (allopurinol, rasburicase).

Pneumocystis jiroveci pneumonia (PCP) is caused by the pathogen *Pneumocystis jiroveci*. It can occur in immuno-compromised individuals, including children and young people, undergoing treatment for cancer (Truong & Ashurst, 2019). Sulphamethox-azole-trimethoprim (co-trimoxazole) is administered as a prophylactic measure while cytotoxic chemotherapy is administered.

Treatment

In the 1940s, cytotoxic chemotherapy was introduced as part of standard treatment for childhood cancer. Before this, surgery and radiation treatment were the only therapies available. Following the discovery of nitrogen mustard after World War 1, rapid drug development occurred in this area.

Cytotoxic chemotherapy means chemical therapy that is toxic to cells. Examples of cytotoxic agents and their actions are given in Table 9.2. These agents kill malignant and non-malignant cells as they move through the five phases of the cell cycle. Cytostatic agents hold cells in a specific phase of the cell cycle and arrest cell development (Lipp & Hartmann, 2009). Cytotoxic agents appear to be most effective in the proliferative phase of the cell cycle. They are classified according to their action within the cell cycle.

- Cell cycle phase specific: agents that act specifically during one phase of the cell cycle. These agents are most effective in tumours with high growth fractions.
- Cell cycle non-phase specific: agents that are effective during all phases of the cell cycle, including the G0 (resting phase). These agents are most effective with tumours of low growth fraction.
- Cell cycle specific: agents that are effective while cells are actively in cycle but not dependent on cells being in a particular phase.

TABLE 9.2 Type and action of cytotoxic agents.

Type of cytotoxic agent	Action	Example
Alkylating agents	Disrupt DNA synthesis Reacts with DNA base forming cross-linking	Cyclophosphamide
Antimetabolites	Mimic metabolites that are essential for formation of nucleic acids	Methotrexate
Antitumour antibiotics	Prevent DNA synthesis by causing single or double strand breaks	Doxorubicin
Plant alkaloids	Interfere with normal microtubule formation and function in mitosis phase	Vincristine
Miscellaneous agents; for example, asparaginase	L'asparaginase is an enzyme that acts by converting asparagines into aspartic acid and ammonia, inhibiting tumour cell protein synthesis	Asparaginase

The efficacy of combinations of chemotherapy agents was first recognised over 40 years ago in the treatment of acute lymphatic leukaemia (Pui *et al.*, 2008). The increase in patients achieving remission was significant, but there was a more remarkable increase in the duration of remission.

The benefits of combination chemotherapy include:

- Prevention of multidrug resistance.
- Maximum cell kill within the range of toxicities.
- No overlapping toxicities.
- It can be administered at regular intervals.
- The dosage of the agents can be maximised.

Key point

- Chemotherapy destroys not only cancerous cells but healthy cells as well. This causes certain common side effects such as alopecia, nausea and vomiting, and mouth ulcers, as well as more acute emergencies such as PCP and TLS.

Administration of chemotherapy

Cytotoxic chemotherapy is given by many different routes. The most common in childhood cancer are intravenous, oral, intrathecal and subcutaneous. Only staff with specific training and education should be involved in the preparation (pharmacists), checking and administration of cytotoxic chemotherapy (qualified registered nurses and for intrathecal (IT): doctors). Administrators of chemotherapy need to be aware of treatment protocols, patient issues and that the basis of good practice in administration of chemotherapy is safety and patient comfort (DOH UK, 2011). The importance of this is clearly demonstrated by the following case example.

In the UK in February 2001, a teenager died following the administration of vincristine by the intrathecal route (IT), rather than the intended intravenous route. The Department of Health UK (2001b) subsequently issued the circular *National Guidance on the Safe Administration of Intrathecal Chemotherapy*, with most of the circular focusing on ensuring the safe administration of IT chemotherapy.

Most anti-cancer drugs are potentially hazardous substances, since they are mutagenic, teratogenic and carcinogenic. Health care personnel who are involved in the preparation and handling of anti-cancer drugs can, if not adequately protected, absorb potentially harmful quantities of such compounds (Murff, 2012). Protective clothing should be worn at all times when handling cytotoxic drugs. There is evidence to suggest that handling excreta (urine, faeces, sweat, saliva and vomit) from patients having or who have just completed cytotoxic chemotherapy, or laundry contaminated with excreta, puts handlers at risk of exposure to cytotoxic drugs (Murff, 2012). Therefore, protective precautions should be taken and carers similarly advised.

◉ Case study 9.3

A decision was made for Katie to have a central venous access device inserted to administer the necessary intravenous therapies. As Katie is needle phobic, thorough preparation and psychological support for this was essential. Katie had her central line inserted on week five of treatment as, during induction treatment, the administration of asparaginase interferes with the clotting mechanism, and insertion of a central venous catheter (CVC) at this stage would predispose the patient to thrombus formation. However, due to her phobia and Katie getting extremely distressed with venepunctures, the decision was made with Claire and the multidisciplinary team that a Hickman line would be more suitable than a port-a-cath, as an implanted device would need to be accessed with a needle for use. Due to the risk of infection, Katie cannot continue swimming with the Hickman line in situ. It also may have an impact on body image, as Katie gets older.

Central venous access devices

To administer intensive cytotoxic chemotherapy, withdraw blood samples and deliver supportive products, children with leukaemia usually have a CVC inserted (Vierboom *et al.*, 2018) which, which reduces the physical and psychological trauma that can be associated with venepuncture (Rauch *et al.*, 2009).

Central venous access devices (CVADs) have been in use since the early 1970s and have had a great influence on the care and management of children with cancer. However, they are not without risk. Potential complications include septicaemia, catheter occlusion, air embolism, catheter displacement/dislodgement and phlebitis.

Katie had a Hickman line inserted, which is an external silicone tunnelled catheter, made of radio-opaque medical grade silicone. The devices can consist of single, double or triple lumens. Hickman lines are usually inserted for patients receiving aggressive chemotherapy regimens. Patients on ALL protocols usually have the implanted subcutaneous device inserted, due to the lower infection risk with this device (Johansson *et al.*, 2009). Besides the risk of infection, psychosocial issues can also arise. Johansson *et al.* (2009) state that a child's response to a CVC could be affected by his/her understanding of the illness, fear of medical procedures, limited coping strategies and impact on body image. Chapter 5 offers a detailed discussion of the psychosocial issues affecting children and young people with a chronic illness.

⊛ Case study 9.4

Katie is currently on week twenty of her treatment undergoing delayed intensification. Since week eighteen, she has received asparaginase and high oral dexamethasone (a corticosteroid) alongside weekly doses of doxorubicin and vincristine. Up to this time, she has coped well with her treatment, only being admitted once to the unit since diagnosis, with a temperature of 38.1 °C. She recovered from this after 48 hours on intravenous antibiotics, with no focus of infection found.

Katie has come to the outpatient department (OPD) this morning for a planned FBC. According to her treatment protocol, she is due to commence a block of cytarabine chemotherapy. Her neutrophil count needs to be 750 cells/mm³ or above to continue with her treatment.

Claire mentions on arrival at the department that Katie has been complaining of a sore mouth and that she has been lethargic for the past few days. Jess, a senior staff nurse who is familiar with Katie, assesses Katie's oral cavity, which she feels is slightly inflamed, and notices a mouth ulcer developing under her tongue. Claire states that she has commenced Katie on the chlorohexidine mouthwash since the beginning of her intensification treatment as per unit policy. Jess informs Claire that she will get a doctor to assess Katie's mouth and get pain relief prescribed.

Mouth care is an important aspect within children's cancer nursing as the mucous membrane is affected by cytotoxic chemotherapy treatment. Mucositis is a general term that refers to an inflammation of the mucous membranes; when it occurs in the oral cavity, is known as stomatitis (Nashwan, 2011). Chemotherapy agents differ in the degree they cause mucositis and the dose also needs to be taken into consideration (Quinn *et al.*, 2015). Katie received doxorubicin, an anti-tumour antibiotic that is considered to be a highly stomatoxic agent. Other risk factors include pre-existing oral disease and poor oral hygiene. Stomatitis usually occurs 5–10 days post-treatment, commencing with a dry mucosa, tongue and lips and may lead to taste alteration and oral ulceration, which predisposes the patient to infection (types of infection are outlined in Table 9.3). Management is symptom related, the main one being pain. Appropriate care includes ensuring that mouth care is performed and that the patient eats

TABLE 9.3 **Types and treatment of mouth infections.**

Infections in the mouth	Most common type	Treatment
Fungal	*Candida albicans*	Amphotericin (ambisome) Fluconazole
Viral	*Herpes simplex*	Acyclovir
Bacterial	*Streptococcus*	Broad spectrum antibiotics Metronidazole

and drinks, to help prevent infection. During times of neutropenia, the mouth is in an ideal condition for microbial growth.

The most common side effect and dose-limiting side effect of cytotoxic chemotherapy is myelo-suppression, which is also potentially the most lethal. Myelo-suppression, also known as bone marrow suppression, consists of neutropenia, thrombocytopenia and anaemia.

⏲ Time out

- What do you understand by the terms neutropenia, thrombocytopenia and anaemia? Jot your thoughts down.

Bone marrow is the principle haematopoietic tissue, where the continual process of production of blood cells occurs in accordance with the body's requirements. The colony stimulating factors and hormone-like glycoproteins mediate haematopoiesis for all blood cell lines, governing production, cell differentiation and maturation. The granulocyte colony stimulating factor is effective on the white cell lineage. All haematopoietic cells divide rapidly and are vulnerable to cytotoxic chemotherapy. The nadir (decline) is 7–10 days post-chemotherapy, with cell cycle non-specific agents causing the most severe myelo-suppression.

Thrombocytopenia occurs when a platelet count is less than 150×10^9/L. The lifespan of a platelet is 7–10 days and its function is haemostasis and fibrinolysis. Claire was given information regarding the signs and symptoms of a low platelet count: fresh bruising, bleeding gums and epistaxis. She was told to avoid administering aspirin and non-steroidal anti-inflammatory drugs to Katie, which may increase the chance of bleeding. When Katie's platelet count dropped below 10×10^9/L or she was actively bleeding, she received a transfusion of platelets in the OPD.

Claire may have already been familiar with the term 'anaemia' from pregnancy, and the associated signs and symptoms of pallor, lethargy and dizziness. As most oxygen is carried by the red blood cells (RBCs) to the body's tissues, a reduction in the red cell mass causes reduced oxygen supply to body cells (Liumbruno *et al.*, 2009). The normal haemoglobin (Hb) of a child is 110–130 g/L with the lifespan of a RBC being 120 days. According to the policy at Katie's centre, Katie will receive a red blood cell transfusion when her Hb drops below 80 g/L.

Although all white blood cells are important, the most significant in patients undergoing treatment for cancer are neutrophils. Neutropenia is a deficiency of circulating neutrophils. The function of a neutrophil is phagocytosis. With reduced neutrophils, the normal process of controlling gram positive and negative infections is therefore diminished.

At the commencement of treatment, Claire had been given advice and information regarding how chemotherapy would cause Katie to be susceptible to infection, and the possible signs and symptoms. The family were advised how to protect Katie from infection, including careful handwashing, keeping Katie away from people who have infections, keeping Katie away from crowded areas when she is severely neutropenic and ensuring food is cooked thoroughly. Katie was discharged following her last admission with pyrexia, after it was ensured that Claire had a thermometer at home, and she understood that she could contact the unit at any time.

> **Key points**
>
> - Myelo-suppression consists of neutropenia, thrombocytopenia and anaemia.
> - The nurse must advise and educate the family on the signs and symptoms of these side effects and how to minimise the possibility of complications arising by undertaking preventative measures.

Case study 9.5

During Katie's visit to OPD (case study 9.4) Jess accesses Katie's Hickman line, known as 'wiggly' to Katie, using the large lumen to obtain the FBC. Katie usually helps to open and close the clamps of her line, but is not interested today. Jess takes blood for an FBC and U/E and sends the sample to the laboratory. As Jess is flushing the line with normal saline, Katie begins to rigor. Jess quickly assesses Katie clinically. Her peripheries are cool and her capillary refill time (CRT) centrally is 2–3 seconds. Her vital signs are taken; temperature 37.6 °C, BP 95/45, HR 110 beats per minute, RR 35 breaths per minute, oxygen saturations 98%.

Jess informs the medical staff about Katie's condition and the registrar and house officer come to review her. They commence her on intravenous fluids via both lumens of her Hickman line and initially prescribe a fluid bolus of 20 ml/kg of 0.9% sodium chloride (NACL). As Katie continues to rigor and her CRT is now 3 seconds centrally, Jess is asked to take blood cultures from both lumens of the Hickman line before IV antibiotics are commenced: a broad-spectrum antibiotic, meropenem, and one to cover gram negative organisms, gentamicin.

Katie's temperature is now 38.1 °C, BP 88/40, HR 140 beats per minute and her respiratory status is stable. A swab is taken from Katie's mouth ulcer and her Hickman line insertion site is examined but shows no obvious inflammation. A creatinine reactive protein test is requested from the U/E sample, which is elevated to 90, suggesting infection. The FBC proves Katie to be neutropenic, with her neutrophils at 600 cells/mm^3, Hb 86 g/L and platelets at 40×10^9/L

Claire is understandably concerned and anxious and Katie says she is frightened. Jess tries to explain to both of them what is happening and tells Claire that Katie probably has an infection in her Hickman line. Katie is commenced on strict fluid balance monitoring with all her urine measured. Due to her current instability, Katie is transferred to the children's high dependency unit for initial management and observation. Katie responds well to her fluid bolus and, after a period of observation, is transferred back to the oncology ward for ongoing care and management prior to discharge.

Sepsis

Sepsis is a reasonably common complication of intensive therapies and is a serious systemic response to infection. Sepsis is a serious complication that can lead to ongoing morbidity and ultimately mortality. The improvement in survivability of childhood cancers over a number of years has been attributable to an escalation in the intensity of therapy (Davies, 2018). Shaw (2002) found that infection was the primary cause of death in eleven non-bone marrow transplant patients; five died due to fungal infection and one due to bacterial infection. Early recognition and commencement of treatment are essential in attempting to reduce mortality and morbidity. If children and young people presenting with sepsis deteriorate to such an extent that paediatric intensive care unit (PIC) admission is required, mortality rates are high at around 48% (Davies & McDougall, 2019). The goal of PIC treatment is the management of complications, the continuance of commenced therapies and the use of appropriate antibiotic therapy to ensure successful outcomes. If a child or young person requires high dependency or PIC care, a range of issues can have an impact on the family, including possible transfer to lead centres, which may be some distance away from the child's normal in-patient or clinic facility. Issues surrounding family-focused care and multidisciplinary working across clinical boundaries can have a major impact on the ongoing treatment and management of the child's underlying condition

Children's critical care

Across the UK, children's critical care is organised through a series of lead centres supporting local trusts. The decision to transfer a child to a high dependency unit or PIC is dependent on a number of factors, the key factor usually being dependency. Between 2015–2017 there were approximately 20,000 admissions per year to PIC across the UK and Republic of Ireland (Paediatric Intensive Care Audit Network For The UK (PICANet), 2018). Paediatric intensive care units have been described as being low volume, high cost facilities that cannot be provided in all localities but to which all children should have access. Children may present in the emergency department or children's assessment unit and then require admission to a ward with escalation of treatment in high dependency and ultimately within a paediatric intensive care unit. In the scenario described, escalation of treatment and admission to PIC is due to increasing clinical need and dependency. Originally the NHSE (1997) identified levels of care as being level 1 equivalent to high dependency care and levels 2 and 3 being PIC. The Paediatric Intensive Care Society (PICS, 2015) have refined the levels of care and associated descriptors over time, also providing further detail on the interventions that would be required at each level. Most paediatric intensive care units will care for children at level 2/3 dependencies, whereas high dependency units will care for children at level 1 (PICANet, 2018). Level 1 has been described as delivering closer observation and monitoring than is usually available in a ward environment, level 2 as children who require continuous nursing supervision and are usually ventilated and level 3 as children and young people with two or more body systems requiring support; for example, a child suffering from multiple trauma (PICS, 2015). Between 5 and 15% of all district general hospital admissions will require paediatric high dependency care and of these 0.5–1% will require a PICU admission (PICS, 2015). As with Katie, most of these children will start and finish their care in clinical environments other than PICU.

 Time out

Think about the children and young people that you have nursed with long-term illness:

- How was their level of dependency assessed clinically?
- What care environments are available on a local and tertiary level to nurse them?
- If they require more intensive nursing, how do the children, young people and their families feel when they are moved from their normal ward environment?

Family-focused care

Admission or transfer from acute general or specialist children's areas to a PIC can cause an inordinate amount of stress to parents (Rodriguez-Rey & Alonso-Tapia, 2016). Children with a range of chronic conditions will spend protracted periods of time in critical care areas; for example, children and young people who require long-term assisted ventilation. A number of these children will experience delays in discharge to their referring hospitals or to their own homes (Hazinski, 2013). (See Chapter 8 for a detailed discussion of this issue.) This situation can have a serious impact on family relationships, and on parental ability and confidence to manage ongoing care at home. Parents of children and young people with chronic illness need to develop and sustain trusting relationships with the health professionals caring for their child, but this is often dependent on the attitudes and values of the professionals concerned.

A number of authors have studied the impact on families of admission to PIC (Colville & Pierce, 2012; Nelson & Gold, 2012; Oxley, 2015). Post-traumatic stress symptoms (PTSS) have been commonly reported. Nelson and Gold (2012) identified that 84% of parents experienced such symptoms, which may persist long after discharge. Oxley (2015) studied the experiences of parents within PIC: the child's deterioration, transfer and admission to PIC were the times of the most significant stress. The nature of the PIC environment with its sights, sounds and interventions contributes significantly to the pressures faced by already stressed parents (Rodriguez-Rey & Alonso-Tapia, 2016).

Parents of children with long-term illness are usually experts in the ongoing treatment and care of their child and this often requires some facilitation in critical care areas. It has been found that nurses in critical care areas are technologically proficient but do not always meet the needs and expectations of families, with parents reporting a reduction in their participation in care and a diminished parenting role. (McAlvin *et al.*, 2014; Oxley, 2015). Parents rely very much on established coping mechanisms in order to fulfil the primary care-giver role and this can be compromised in critical care environments. In family-centred care, it is important that the needs of parents and siblings are identified in addition to those of the child to ensure that a partnership approach is initiated to facilitate continued parental input into care delivery (Oxley, 2015). It is essential that parents are able to establish meaning and understanding to the experience of their child being transferred to high dependency and critical care areas. For care to be successful, it is also important that staff communicate well across clinical environments, sharing both knowledge and expertise, while maintaining ongoing therapeutic relationships with the child and family in their care. Raising staff awareness of the potential for PTSS in parents and providing support resources is essential if the impact of admission to PIC is to be mitigated (Bedford & Bench, 2018).

🕐 **Time out**

- Think about the context of the family situation with reference to Katie and note down areas for key consideration.
- Claire is a young single mum with limited support. What might be some of the psychosocial issues faced by Claire and how might these be exacerbated by her current situation?
- List some of the support mechanisms that could be put in place to help Claire and Katie at this time.

Setting aside the importance of prioritising care directly required by the patient, there are some important considerations in terms of providing support for Katie's mother, Claire. Claire's own stage of development needs consideration as she makes the transition to adulthood. In recent decades it has been suggested that the road to adulthood is a much longer one with young adults not marrying, settling on a long-term career or becoming parents until they are late in their 20s. The capacity to take their time in such matters affords them what is usually and exciting and optimistic time where they can begin to achieve their goals and reach their aspirations (Arnett, 2015). However, in this case the opposite is true. Becoming a parent brings significant responsibilities and it is likely that family and peer relationships could change during this time, which may mean that support can increase but equally could also diminish. It could be the case that where peer relationships have become stronger and more central to the young person (in this case, Katie's mum) that these suddenly have to take second place and family will resume their place as the primary support. Young *et al.* (2002) suggest that while mothers are not unwell themselves, long-term illness and its consequences can have effects on them too. These authors further add that at the point of diagnosis of a long-term condition, the parental self and sense of identity can alter as they have to take on unexpected new roles and responsibilities which are required. Additionally, at this time parents are expected to undertake several tasks for their children which include acting as an advocate where information giving is concerned and helping to manage treatment. For this young parent, Claire, considerations will be twofold: the need of the parent to protect their child, set against their own developmental trajectory. Another central factor in this case is the need for the parent to manage their own emotions when adverse events occur. A lack of life experience might make this a different scenario for someone who is younger and has not had to cope with crises previously. Moreover, the ability of a young parent to be financially stable, particularly in a situation where they may have no income because of their child's illness, could compromise both their well-being and their independence. This could potentially have negative consequences for self-esteem. It will be important for clinicians to recognise the potential need for extra support given the circumstances and life stage of a parent. Different strategies may need to be employed which are tailored to the needs of a younger person in this type of situation. A multidisciplinary approach to support may be required, which would include different personnel; for example, a youth support coordinator will have the relevant skills to be able to provide help and information for a young parent – something that would not be required where parents are older. The 'triple whammy' of young parenthood, serious illness and personal development requires a careful and well-planned approach if the needs of the child and mother are to be appropriately met.

Multidisciplinary working across different organisations

Professional collaboration is a key issue in ensuring that effective outcomes are achieved in the care, treatment and management of children and young people with a chronic illness. A number of children will be nursed in tertiary centres, particularly during the diagnostic period and when specific interventions are required; for example, during Hickman line or port-a-cath insertions. Professional collaboration and access to ongoing support has proved effective in the management of disease processes (Eilertsen *et al.*, 2004). Smith *et al.* (2015) found that to support parents with children with long-term conditions effectively required the development of a culture of engagement and collaboration, which in turn leads to empowerment. (Please see Chapter 6 for more discussion on empowerment.) Parents then have the ability to engage fully with the wider MDT in negotiating care and ongoing management for their children.

Due to ongoing changes in the organisation and delivery of both acute and community services, care is often delivered by a range of professionals who may represent a number of health and social care institutions. Children and young people with a chronic illness need to receive care that is integrated and coordinated around their individual needs. The development of shared, managed clinical networks has allowed care to be provided in a number of localities and closer to the child's home. Some specialities, such as cardiac, renal and oncology, are unable to provide services in all locations, but access to these services needs to be facilitated. This has been achieved by a number of services providing outreach services and clinics. The coordination of health care disciplines from the primary, secondary and tertiary level is intended to provide closer multiagency cooperation and closer integration of care environments (DoH UK, 2016). Care provision should be seamless and based upon the latest evidence.

Parents have recognised the importance of the key worker role in the coordination and facilitation of care (Smith *et al.*, 2015). This is particularly relevant across professional and geographical boundaries (DOH UK, 2016). Cross-boundary working is a key policy objective for the foundation of high-quality care across child health services (While *et al.*, 2006). Chapters 2 and 8 discuss the role of the key worker in coordinating the care process. Examples of cross-boundary working can be seen in the provision of nurse specialists in a range of conditions and in the role of the nurse consultant. These roles are often intended to span both primary and secondary environments and can play an important part in the continuation of care, particularly when children experience deterioration in their condition or a complication due to a subsequent pathology. These roles are particularly important to facilitate information sharing and maintenance of already established treatment protocols. A number of these roles require flexibility in the commissioning process to ensure that their roles are able to span a range of health care and multiagency sectors. Although primarily nursing roles, the RCN (2013) found that these could also be undertaken by general practitioners, occupational therapists or social workers.

Conclusion

Children and young people with a long-term illness may experience rapid changes in the treatment and management of their condition. Within the case study, we have examined a little girl's journey from diagnosis, through the first phase of treatment to the point of an acute deterioration, which may reflect the illness trajectory experienced by children with a range of conditions. It is important that parents and families are provided with effective, skilled and evidence-based care in each of the care environments, whether that be their own homes or tertiary centres. If the aims of treatment are to be achieved, close cooperation and collaboration across professional and geographical boundaries will need to be achieved, which will ensure that the holistic needs of the individual child, young person and family are met. It is essential that children with existing and long-term medical disorders have a clear plan of action in the event of acute deterioration (RCPCH, 2014). This should ensure access to appropriately skilled professionals and care facilities.

Key points

- A range of acute emergencies may affect the child and young person with a long-term illness.
- Patterns of service delivery are continually evolving to meet the needs of children and Young people with a chronic illness.
- Children and young people with long-term illness are nursed and often transferred through a range of care environments.
- Effective intervention by the multidisciplinary team is essential in supporting children, young people and their families through an acute phase of their chronic illness.

Useful websites

Department of Health, UK https://www.doh.gov.uk
Lymphoma Research Foundation https://www.lrf.org.uk/en/1/information.html
Government Research and Statistics https://www.statistics.gov.uk
Children's Cancer and Leukemia Group https://www.cclg.org.uk/

References

Amoon, A.T., Crespi, C.M., Ahlbom, A., *et al.* (2018) Proximity to overhead powerlines and childhood leukemia: an international pooled analysis. *British Journal of Cancer*, **119** (3), 364–373.

Arnett, J.J. (2015) *Emerging Adulthood* (second edition). Oxford, Oxford University Press.

Bedford, Z. & Bench, S. (2018) A review of interventions supporting parent's psychological well-being after a child's intensive care unit discharge. *Nursing in Critical Care*, **24** (3), 153–161.

Behm, F.G. (2012) Immunophenotyping. In: *Childhood Leukemias* (third edition) (ed. C.H. Pui) pp. 71–112. Cambridge, Cambridge University Press.

Berrie, L., Ellison, G., Norman, P., *et al.* (2019) The association between childhood leukemia and population mixing. An artifact of focusing on clusters. *Epidemiology*, **30** (1), 75–82.

Children with Cancer UK (2019) https://www.childrenwithcancer.org.uk/childhood-cancer-info/childhood-cancer-facts-figures/ Accessed 18/8/19.

Clarke, R., Van den Bruel, A., Bankhead, C., *et al.* (2016) Clinical presentation of childhood leukemia: a systematic review and meta-analysis. *Archives of Disease in Childhood*, **101**, 894–901.

Colville, G. & Pierce, C. (2012) Patterns of post traumatic stress symptoms in families after pediatric intensive care. *Intensive Care Medicine*, **38**, 1523–1531.

Davies, J. (2018) *Children in Intensive Care*. London, Elsevier Health Sciences.

Davies, J. & McDougall, M. (2019) *Children in Intensive Care. A Survival Guide*. London, Elsevier.

Department of Health (2001a) *High Dependency Care for Children – Expert Advisory Group Report for the Department of Health*. London, Department of Health.

Department of Health (2001b) *National Guidance on the Safe Administration of Intrathecal Chemotherapy*. London, Department of Health.

Department of Health (2010) *National Framework for Children and Young People's Continuing Care*. London, Department of Health.

Department of Health (2011) Improving outcomes: a strategy for cancer. https://www.gov.uk/government/publications/the-national-cancer-strategy Accessed 18/6/19.

Department of Health (2016) *National Framework for Children's Continuing Care*. London, Department of Health.

Eilertsen, M.E.B., Reinfjell, T. & Vik, T. (2004) Value of professional collaboration in the care of children with cancer and their families. *European Journal of Cancer Care*, **13**, 349–355.

Esparza, S.D. & Sakamoto, K. (2005) Topics in pediatric leukemia - acute lymphoblastic leukemia. *Medscape General Medicine*, **7** (1), 23.

Greaves, M.F. (2018) A causal mechanism for childhood acute lymphoblastic leukemia. *Nature Reviews Cancer*, **18**, 471–484.

Grufferman, S., Ruymann, F., Ognjanovic, S., *et al.* (2009) Prenatal x-ray exposure and rhabdomyosarcoma in children: a report from the children's oncology group (COG). *Cancer Epidemiology Biomarkers and Prevention*, **18** (4), 1271–1276.

Harrison, C.J. (2009) Cytogenetics of paediatric and adolescent acute lymphoblastic leukemia. *British Journal of Haematology*, **144** (2), 147–156.

Hasle, H., Clemmensen, I.H., & Mikkelsen, M. (2000) Risks of leukemia and solid tumours in individuals with Down Syndrome. *Lancet, 15*: **355** (9199), 165–169.

Hazinski, M.F. (2013) *Nursing Care of the Critically Ill Child* (third edition). New York, Elsevier.

Johansson, E., Engervall, P., Bjorvell, H., *et al.* (2009) Patients perceptions of having a central venous catheter or a totally implantable subcutaneous port system – results from a randomized study in acute leukemia. *Supportive Care in Cancer*, **17** (1), 137–143.

Kinlen, L.J. (1995) Epidemiological evidence for an infective basis in childhood leukaemia. *British Journal of Cancer*, **71** (1), 1–5.

Lipp, H.P. & Hartman, J.T. (2009) Cytostatic and cytotoxic drugs. In: *Side Effects of Drugs Annual 31* (ed. J.K. Aronson), pp. 721–729. Amsterdam, Elsevier.

Liumbruno, G., Bennardello, F., Lattanzio, A., *et al.* (2009) Recommendations for the transfusion of red blood cells. *Blood Transfusion*, **7** (1), 49–64.

Marcotte, E.L., Ritz, B., Cockburn, M., *et al.* (2014) Exposure to infections and risk of leukemia in young children. *Cancer Epidemiology, Biomarkers, and Prevention*, **23** (7), 1195–1203.

McAlvin, S. & Carew-Lyons, A. (2014) Family presence during resuscitation and invasive procedures in pediatric critical care: a systematic review. *American Journal of Critical Care*, **23** (6), 477–485.

McKenna, K., Collier, J., Hewitt, M. & Blake H. (2010) Parental Involvement in Paediatric cancer treatment decisions. *European Journal of Cancer Care*, **19**, 621–630.

Mrozek, K., Harper, D.P. & Aplan, P.D. (2009) Cytogenetics and molecular genetics of Acute Lymphoblastic Leukemia. *Haematology/Oncology Clinics of North America*, **23** (5), 991–1010.

Murff, S.J. (2012) *Safety and Health Handbook for Cytotoxic Drugs*. Lanham, Maryland, USA, US Government Institutes Inc.

Nelson, L.P. & Gold J.L. (2012) Posttraumatic stress disorder in children and their parents following admission to the pediatric intensive care unit: a review. *Pediatric Critical Care Medicine*, **13**, 338–347.

Nashwan, A.J. (2011) Use of chlorhexidine mouthcare in children receiving chemotherapy - a review of literature. *Journal of Pediatric Oncology Nursing*, **28**, 295–299.

National Health Service Executive (1997) *Paediatric Intensive Care: A Framework for the Future-National Coordinating Group on Paediatric Intensive Care – Report to the Chief Executive of the NHS Executive*. London, Department of Health.

National Registry of Childhood Tumours Progress Report UK (2012) http://www.ncin.org.uk Accessed 4/7/19.

Oxley, R. (2015) Parents' experiences of their child's admission to paediatric intensive care. *Nursing Children and Young People*, **27** (4), 16–21.

Paediatric Intensive Care Audit Network for the UK (PICANet): Annual Report 2018. (2018) Universities of Leeds and Leicester, PICANet.

Paediatric Intensive Care Society (2015) *Quality Standards for the Care of Critically Ill Children*. London, PICS.

Pui, C.H., Robinson, L.C. & Look, A.T. (2008) Acute lymphoblastic leukemia. *The Lancet*, **371** (9617), 1030–1043.

Quinn, B., Thompson, M. & Treleavan, J. (2015) UK Oral Care in Cancer Guidance. (second edition). http://www.ukomic.co.uk Accessed 21/8/19.

Rauch, D., Dowd, D., Eldridge, D., *et al.* (2009) Peripheral difficult venous access in children. *Clinical Pediatrics*, **48** (9), 895–901.

Rodriguez-Rey, R. & Alonso-Tapia, J. (2016) Development of a screening measure of stress for parents of children hospitalised in a paediatric intensive care unit. *Australian Critical Care*, **29**, 151–157.

Royal College of Nursing (2013) *Specialist and Advanced Children's and Young People's Nursing Practice in Contemporary Health Care: Guidance for Nurses and Commissioners*. London. RCN.

Royal College of Paediatrics and Child Health (2014) *High Dependency Care for Children - Time to Move On*. London, RCPCH.

Shaw, P.J. (2002) Suspected infection in children with cancer. *Journal of Antimicrobial Chemotherapy. Ambisone: An International Workshop*, **49** (1), 63–67.

Skuse, A. (2015) *Constructions of Cancer in Early Modern England: Ravenous Natures*. Basingstoke, Palgrave MacMillan.

Smith, J., Swallow, V. & Coyne, I. (2015) Involving parents in managing their child's long-term condition—a concept synthesis of family-centered care and partnership-in-care. *Journal of Pediatric Nursing*, **30**, 143–158.

Teenage Cancer Trust (TCT) (2018) Summary; 13–24 year olds with cancer in England; incidence, mortality and survival (2018). https://www.teenagecancertrust.org/sites/default/files/Teenage%20Cancer%20Trust%20PHE%20Report%202019%20-%20Summary.pdf Accessed 6/7/19.

Trent, R.J. (2005) Complex genetic traits. In: *Molecular Medicine - An Introductory Text* third edition (ed. R.J. Trent), pp. 77–118. Amsterdam, Elsevier.

Truong, J. & Ashurst, J.V. (2019) Pneumocystis (Carinii) Jivoveci Pneumonia. https://www.ncbi.nlm.nih.gov/books/NBK482370/ Accessed 16/8/19.

Vierboom, L., Darani, A., Langusch, C., *et al.* (2018) Tunnelled central venous access devices in small children; A comparison of open versus ultrasound guided percutaneous insertion in children weighing ten kilograms or less. *Journal of Paediatric Surgery*, **53** (9), 1832–1838.

While, A., Murgatroyd, B., Ullman, R. & Forbes, A. (2006) Nurses', midwives' and health visitors' involvement in cross-boundary working within child health services. *Child: Care, Health and Development*, **32** (1), 87–89.

Wiemels, J. (2012) Perspectives on the causes of childhood leukemia. *Chemico-Biological Interactions*, **196** (3), 59–67.

Young, B., Dixon-Wood, M., Findlay, M., *et al.* (2002) Parenting in a crisis: Conceptualising mothers of children with cancer. *Social Science and Medicine*, **55**, 1835–1847.

Zupanec, S. & Tomlinson, D. (2010) Leukemia In: *Paediatric Oncology Nursing – Advanced Handbook* (second edition). (eds D. Tomlinson & M. Kline) pp. 2–29. Berlin, Springer-Verlag.

CHAPTER 10

Adolescence

Siân Bill and Taryn Eccleston

Introduction

Adolescence is a time of rapid growth, development and change and this can be a difficult period for some young people. Any potential difficulties experienced during adolescence can be compounded by the presence of a long-term condition. As advances in medical technology have improved life expectancy, young people with a long-term condition and their families are faced with new challenges. Additionally, health care professionals need to revisit the way in which young people with long-term conditions are managed, to ensure that their care meets the holistic needs of the individual.

Aim of the chapter

The purpose of this chapter is to critically examine the issues relating to adolescents with a long-term condition. To examine the pertinent issues, a case study focusing on a young person with chronic renal failure will be used throughout the chapter. However, issues that are raised within this scenario could be applied to young people with different types of long-term conditions.

This chapter will not provide an in-depth exploration of adolescent physical or psychosocial development. Neither does this chapter provide an in-depth physiological account of renal failure or the breadth of psychosocial issues that can evolve from this condition. There are a number of available texts that provide comprehensive coverage of adolescent development and paediatric nephrology, and references for these are provided at the end of the chapter. Readers not familiar with these topics, and particularly adolescent growth and development in the context of this chapter, are advised to access these texts (see Recommended reading) to help them understand and apply the information covered in this chapter.

Nursing Care of Children and Young People with Long-Term Conditions, Second Edition.
Edited by Mandy Brimble and Peter McNee.
© 2021 John Wiley & Sons Ltd. Published 2021 by John Wiley & Sons Ltd.

Intended learning outcomes

- To critically examine the impact of having a long-term condition on adolescent physical and psychosocial development
- To develop an understanding of the associated health risk factors relating to long-term conditions and the consequences of these, with particular regard to compliance/non-compliance
- To examine the psychosocial and physical developmental needs of the hospitalised adolescent
- To explore the role of the nurse in facilitating the empowerment of adolescents within the health care setting

Existing knowledge

This chapter is written on the assumption that the reader has some prior knowledge and understanding of adolescent physical and psychosocial development. This includes the stages of adolescent development, physical growth patterns, physiological and hormonal changes, sexual development, development of cognition and the 'conception of self'. As physical and psychosocial development is closely linked with adolescent behaviour, without an understanding of these concepts it will be difficult for the reader to develop an understanding of the way in which young people respond to and cope with a long-term condition. Take some time to try and answer the following questions.

⏱ Time out

- What hormones are responsible for triggering adolescent development?
- How many phases of adolescent development are there?
- What tool is used to monitor adolescent physical development?
- Who leads the way in adolescent developmental milestones: boys or girls?
- What are the first signs of sexual maturation in girls?
- What is the mean age of menarche?
- When does puberty occur?
- At what stage does the peer group become important to adolescents?
- When are adolescents most concerned with their body image?
- At what stage of development is the adolescent capable of abstract thought?

Why nurses need knowledge of adolescence

It is estimated that there are currently approximately 11.6 million young people between the ages of 10 and 24 years living in the UK (Hagel & Shah, 2019). This has clear implications for policy development and the provision of appropriate services for this age group (Hagel & Shah, 2019). It also highlights that as nurses we need to become more aware of, and develop strategies to meet, the health care needs of young people.

There is still no clear consensus regarding definitions of adolescence (Santrock, 2018) with a variety of terms used in practice to depict this age range, including youth, teenager, young people and adolescents. Since 1993, the World Health Organization (WHO) has suggested that the following definitions should be used: adolescents for individuals aged 10–19 years, youth for those aged 15–24 years and young people when they are between 10–24 years of age (WHO, 1993). However, this is in itself slightly confusing, as these definitions overlap considerably.

The word adolescent is derived from the Latin word *adolescere*, meaning 'to grow to maturity' (Rice & Dolgin, 2008) and it is important to keep this translation in mind. Adolescence, therefore, is a transitional period between childhood and adulthood, which involves a great deal of physical, cognitive and psychosocial change (Santrock, 2018).

Since the early 1900s, developmental theorists such as Hall (1844–1924), Gesell (1880–1961), Sigmund Freud (1856–1939), Anna Freud (1895–1982), Piaget (1896–1980) and Erikson (1902–1994) have all provided a range of opinions on the development of adolescents.

However, the most influential person in the development of adolescence as a construct, was the psychologist G. Stanley Hall (1844–1924), who is considered to be the 'father of adolescence'. Hall's two-volume work *Adolescence*, published in 1904, was the first publication of its kind, and at the time, was widely credited as being ground breaking (Arnett, 2006).

Hall identified issues that are as relevant to contemporary adolescents as they were to adolescents in 1904. For example, the tendency towards fluctuating moods, thrill seeking behaviour, the importance of peers and the influence of the media were all described in some detail by Hall (Arnett, 2006). However, as it was Hall who first described adolescence as a period of 'storm and stress' (Casey *et al.*, 2010) it could also be suggested that Hall in some ways has done adolescents a disservice, particularly as some subsequent theorists made this a focus of their work.

Although certain developmental milestones can be followed, adolescent development is unique for each individual. It is difficult, therefore, to categorise adolescents into specific age groups. Also, different cultures have varied markers for determining when adolescence ends and adulthood begins, for example rites of passage, marriage and employment. For the purpose of this chapter, the terms adolescent and young person will be used interchangeably and, unless otherwise stated, will refer to individuals between the ages of 10 and 24 years.

Brief overview of adolescent development

Traditionally, adolescent development has been divided into three stages: early, middle and late adolescence (Rice & Dolgin, 2008). More recently, however, some developmentalists have divided adolescence into two main periods: early adolescence and late adolescence (Santrock, 2018). The main points of development that occur during the stages of adolescence are briefly outlined in Table 10.1. This is only an overview of the topic and further reading in this area is recommended.

TABLE 10.1 Stages of adolescence.

	Early (11–14 yrs)	Middle (14–17 yrs)	Late (17–20/5 yrs)
Physical growth	Rapid growth Secondary sex characteristics appear	Decelerating growth in girls Reach 95% adult height	Physically mature Reproductive growth almost complete
Cognition	Limited abstract thought Comparisons of 'normal' with same sex peers	Abstract thinking developing Still idealistic in thoughts Concerned with political and social issues	Abstract thought established Can perceive and act on long-term issues Established functional and intellectual identity
Identity	Preoccupied with body changes Conforms to group 'norms' Attractiveness measured by rejection/ acceptance by peers	Body image modified Self-centred Idealistic Variable ability to perceive future implications of behaviour	Gender role/body image almost secured Mature sexual identity Self-esteem – stable Definition and articulation of social roles
Parental relationships	Defining boundaries for independence Self-conflict – need to remain dependent on parents/desire for more freedom Conflicts with parental control	Conflict-control/ independence Difficulties in parent/ adolescent relationship Significant struggle for emancipation/ disengagement with final detachment from parents; period of 'loss' for parents	Emotional/physical separation from family complete Independent with less conflict Emancipation almost secured
Peer relationships	Start of peer identification Mainly same sex friendships Dating and intimacy limited	Stronger peer identification Standards of behaviour set by peer group Acceptance by peers very important/fearful of rejection	Increase in individual relationships Development of intimate relationships Relationships more reciprocal Gender role defined

Source: From Bill, S. and Knight, Y. (2007) Adolescence. In: *Nursing Care of Children with Chronic Illness* (eds F. Valentine and L. Lowes), pp. 203–230. © 2007. Reproduced with permission of John Wiley & Sons.

Understanding long-term conditions from a young person's perspective

The case study referred to in this chapter explores some of the experiences of a young person with kidney disease.

🕐 **Time out**

- Write down what you know regarding the normal function of the kidney.

🌐 Case study 10.1

Thomas is a 15-year-old boy, who has chronic kidney disease (CKD). He lives at home in a supportive family, with both his parents and his younger brother, Sam. Thomas' father is a lorry driver and works away from home a great deal. Thomas' mother works part time as a cleaner in the local school. At the age of 9 years Thomas was investigated for being small for his age, which led to the discovery of his kidney disease. Since this time, Thomas has been managed conservatively. This entails having regular blood tests, such as biochemistry and full blood counts, along with dietary interventions, taking medication and the careful monitoring and managing of symptoms that may further progress the deterioration of his renal function; for example, high blood pressure and urinary tract infections (Blyton & Jepson, 2019).

The management of kidney disease is complex, leading to a range of health care professionals being involved with Thomas' care. These include a paediatric nephrologist, children's renal nurse specialist, dietitian, psychologist, social worker, general practitioner (GP) and school nurse. Since being diagnosed, Thomas has regularly visited the outpatient department of his regional specialist centre. During one of his recent appointments, the specialist paediatric nephrologist informed Thomas and his family that his condition had further deteriorated and that he would soon require dialysis or a renal transplant. Understandably, Thomas' family are anxious but Thomas himself appears to be unconcerned and refuses to discuss this with his parents or younger brother.

Thomas has always been very close to his parents, but they are becoming concerned that he seems to be spending more and more time with his friends. They believe that this is the reason he refuses to discuss his condition with them and that his friends may be influencing his behaviour. Thomas believes there is no problem with his behaviour or his friends, and he is upset about his parents' negative views towards them.

Chronic kidney disease

CKD is an insidious condition, which can present in children and young people at any age. Some superseded literature refers to CKD as chronic renal failure (Rigden, 2003). Schnaper's (2014) definition of CKD describes a glomerular filtration rate (GFR) of less than 60 ml/min/1.73 m² surface area (SA). CKD is irreversible, usually progressive, associated with metabolic abnormalities and can adversely affect a child's growth (Blyton & Jepson, 2019). Blyton and Jepson (2019) highlight that presenting symptoms of CKD may trigger families to access medical advice and alert health care professionals to refer and investigate the underlying causation. In Thomas' case, his kidney disease lay undetected until he was 9 years old, when he presented as small for his age. Potential presentation features of CKD (Blyton & Jepson, 2019) include:

- nausea and vomiting
- faltering growth

- short stature
- urinary tract infections
- enuresis
- haematuria
- hypertension
- seizures
- lethargy and pallor.

Occasionally, the underlying cause of kidney failure is unknown, but the main causative factors of CKD in children and young people in the UK are congenital abnormalities (Blyton & Jepson, 2019; Li & Chu, 2018; Department of Health UK (DoH), 2006).

As Thomas' renal function continues to deteriorate and progress towards established renal failure, careful consideration is required regarding the choice of renal replacement therapies, such as peritoneal dialysis, haemodialysis or a pre-emptive renal transplant.

⏱ Time out

- What do you understand by the terms peritoneal dialysis, haemodialysis and pre-emptive renal transplant?

Peritoneal dialysis (PD) involves instilling dialysis fluid via a PD catheter into the peritoneal cavity. The peritoneal membrane has a good blood supply, large surface area and is semi-permeable. Waste products and excess fluids are filtered from the blood via the semi-permeable membrane by osmosis, diffusion and convection (Worsey, 2019).

Haemodialysis (HD) requires venous access, specialist equipment, specialist staff and technical support, so that the patient's blood can be mechanically circulated to a haemodialyser (artificial kidney). The haemodialyser consists of synthetic semi-permeable membranes that separate the patient's blood from the dialysis fluid. The movement of fluid and solutes across the membrane takes place by the processes of diffusion, ultrafiltration and convection (Fielding, 2019).

Pre-emptive renal transplant is a renal transplant that can be performed for children and young people with chronic kidney disease before the necessity of dialysis. Compared to dialysis, renal transplantation may be viewed as the treatment of choice and optimal regarding quality of life. However, it is indicated that having a pre-emptive renal transplant is dependent upon the status of the patient's health, as well as donor organ availability (Blyton & Jepson, 2019).

In the UK, the incidence of renal failure and those receiving renal replacement therapy in the adolescent population is difficult to ascertain, as there is a potential that those who are over the age of 16 years, could be managed within adult renal services. This is recognised by Hamilton et al. (2017), who suggest that although over 90% of 16–18-year-olds receiving care related to renal transplantation are managed within children's services, more than 70% of 18–25-year-olds are managed within adult services. However, the actual numbers of these combined age groups are not identified.

What is known, though, is that improvements in diagnosis and medical care have seen the survival rates in children and adolescents with a long-term condition improve dramatically (Becherucci *et al.*, 2016). It is estimated that during the past 50 years, the number of young people with a long-term condition surviving to their 20th birthday has risen considerably (Fegran *et al.*, 2014). Now, almost 90% of young people with a long-term condition survive to adulthood (Mazzucato *et al.*, 2018). While this can be viewed as a considerable improvement in health care overall, it does create some challenges and have lasting implications for adolescents.

Adolescence can be a difficult period for some young people, and this is compounded in the presence of a long-term condition. In addition to their age-related developmental tasks, young people with a long-term condition have to deal with the demands and challenges of their condition (Blyton & Jepson, 2019). They need to consider the limitations their condition places upon them (Badawy *et al.*, 2017) the uncertainty of their condition (Sharkey *et al.*, 2018; Suris *et al.*, 2004) and sometimes even need to confront their own mortality. Many young people with a long-term condition need to comply with medication regimes, special diets, exercise programmes (or are faced with immobility problems), regular testing/monitoring and frequent visits to health care providers (Badawy *et al.*, 2017). In cases such as Thomas', nutritional therapy is central to CKD management, requiring the input of a children's dietitian with specialist renal knowledge and experience (Blyton & Jepson, 2019). Conservative management can potentially prolong renal function, thereby extending the opportunity for normal growth and development and delaying the necessity of dialysis (Blyton & Jepson, 2019). These demands are invasive and affect almost every aspect of the young person's life, including school, recreation, employment, family life, and personal and social life (Badawy *et al.*, 2017).

The psychological implications of having a long-term condition on children and young people has been well documented over a long period of time (Eiser, 1990; Madden *et al.*, 2002; Schmidt *et al.*, 2003; Olsson *et al.*, 2005; Blyton & Jepson, 2019) and these issues will be discussed later in this chapter. It is not surprising, therefore, that there are times when some adolescents have difficulty communicating their feelings and concerns, or communicating with others in general, including their parents, as highlighted by the case study.

🔑 Key point

- Adolescence can be a difficult period for some young people, and this is compounded when they have a long-term condition.

🕐 Time out

- Reflect on the young people that you have cared for. What potential psychosocial implications could having a long-term condition have on young people? Write your thoughts down.

Communicating with young people

Good communication is generally viewed as an important aspect of cohesive family functioning (Towle *et al.*, 2006). Communication within families where an adolescent is part of the family is vitally important (Xiao *et al.*, 2011). If communication is breaking down in Thomas' family, it is understandable that his parents will be concerned. Communication is key to making adolescents feel 'connected' with their families (or peers) and connectedness can be a key factor in building resiliency strategies.

Although there is limited research into adolescent–parental communication, it is known to be complex with some apparent difference in the communication patterns between males and females (Rudi *et al.*, 2015). Although at times it can be challenging, communication between adolescents and their parents is vital as limited communication has the potential to impact on a range of issues for young people including their overall well-being (Rudi *et al.*, 2015).

In relation to the health care setting, it is important that the opinions of young people are valued and that they are listened to when they voice their opinions or raise any issues. As with any other age group, adolescents want to be shown respect and viewed as valued participants in conversations and discussions related to their own care (Royal College of Paediatrics and Child Health (RCPCH), 2012).

Renal failure can be life-threatening, and in order to provide appropriate interventional therapies, communication pathways and information sharing between patients, their families and specialist paediatric renal health care professionals is crucial. The *NSF for Renal Services. Working for Children and Young People* (DoH UK, 2006) promotes delivery of patient-centred services, identifying access to information as one method of achieving this goal. In 2003, Watson suggested a range of strategies could assist in sharing information with young people, including verbal, written, video, CD-ROMs and audio taping consultations. However, the advent of smartphones has enabled another layer of effective communication with adolescents (Garabedian *et al.*, 2015). Providing information has the potential to reduce anxiety, assisting in the development of coping strategies that improve treatment compliance.

> ### 🔑 Key point
>
> - The ability to employ effective communication strategies is important in all nurse/client relationships and this is particularly important with young people. If a good rapport is not developed between health care workers and young people, open channels of communication will not be maintained, and a trusting relationship will not be formed.

In 1995, Sanci and Young developed some guidelines for communication with young people. Although at the time this was primarily aimed at GPs, the principles within this paper are equally applicable to nurses and other health care providers. They are also as relevant today as they were in 1995.

🕐 **Time out**

Before reading the next section, try this short exercise to help you develop an understanding of your current communication skills.

- Think about the way in which you currently communicate with young people – you may want to make some notes.
- Write a list of the strategies you think would be important when communicating with young people.

The communication strategies outlined in Table 10.2 are predominantly based on the work of Sanci and Young (1995) and the experience of the authors of this chapter, and are provided to help you develop your communication skills with young people.

How do they match with your notes?

Since the development of the Sanci and Young (1995) communication strategies, a number of other authors have also highlighted the importance of communicating effectively with young people (e.g. Wheal, 1999; Beresford & Sloper, 2002; Christie & Viner, 2005; Towle *et al.*, 2006; Xiao *et al.*, 2011; Sawyer *et al.*, 2014; Garabedian *et al.*, 2015) and you may want to source some of these articles to expand your reading in this area.

🔑 **Key point**

- The ability to employ effective communication strategies is particularly important with young people.

Communication issues for Thomas

It would be important to encourage Thomas to discuss his concerns with his parents and try to reach some agreement regarding his friends and his association with them. Parents and adolescents often have disagreements about friendships, with parents frequently suggesting that friends are a 'bad influence' or blaming the friendship on the changing relationships at home. In some situations, parents can be right and certain friends may be an undesirable influence. It has even been suggested that some parents will manipulate their adolescents towards certain friendships and away from others, by organising their social activities (Steinberg, 2001). However, in many situations, disagreements occur because adolescents are passing through the developmental stage where they are testing boundaries, have the desire for more freedom and are expanding their social circle.

Peer groups

During early adolescence, young people usually begin to develop a wider circle of friends. Although some young people attend the same school from preparatory to senior level, many will change schools at the commencement of secondary education. Young people

TABLE 10.2   Useful communication strategies.

	Useful communication strategies
Be yourself	When attempting to develop communication channels with young people, above all you should be yourself. Be friendly, relaxed and responsive but do not try to be something you are not. Adolescents have an ability to 'see through' people and will quickly establish whether the person they are dealing with is the 'real you'. You do not need to try to talk or dress like an adolescent (unless you do normally) and this type of behaviour can actually hamper your ability to communicate effectively with young people.
Be flexible	Although adolescents value consistency, there is also a need to be flexible in your approach to communication. A rigid approach could be viewed as being confrontational and can often make young people 'dig in their heels' and be reluctant to respond to your efforts. This again has the potential to impede effective communication.
Establish confidentiality	Confidentiality is a very important issue for young people and this has been discussed in depth in Chapter 9. It is, however, important to remember that unconditional, complete confidence should not be promised to adolescents, and guidelines should be established before they disclose anything to you. Therefore, if the adolescent wishes to disclose something, it is better to suggest at the outset that any conversation will be kept confidential providing their (or anyone else's) safety is currently, or potentially, not compromised.
Listen	Always listen to what young people tell you, be attentive and look as if you are listening and interested in what they have to say. As adolescents belong to a group that generally have little attention paid to what they have to say, being listened to is important to them. During your conversation, you may find that the adolescent deviates from the topic or your particular line of questioning. If the adolescent is inclined to talk, it is important to let them identify what is important to them and you can always bring the conversation back to where you would like it to be at a later time.
Be informed	As with all patients/clients, it is vitally important that any information you provide is factual and accurate. However, whether we are clinical nurses or educators, we are not endless vaults of knowledge and there will be times when you may not know the answer to a question the young person may ask. If you do not know the answer, admit it, but ensure that you find out the answer and convey this to the adolescent as soon as you can.
Be consistent	Adolescents value consistency. Therefore, within any area of practice, providing there are no specific contraindications (e.g. changes in medical management or safety issues), what is appropriate today should be appropriate tomorrow and the next day. Any rules and guidelines need to be consistent to enable the young person to establish her/his boundaries. Inconsistent guidelines and rules become confusing and can sometimes lead to confrontational behaviour where the young person may be viewed as being disruptive or non-compliant.

TABLE 10.2   (Continued)

Useful communication strategies	
Use understandable language	When you need to provide information to adolescents, make sure that it is in easy to follow terms that are free of medical/nursing jargon and presented in a way that is easy for them to follow. Try to present the information in blocks of no more than two sentences at a time, and allow time for the adolescent to ask questions. Patience may be required because, if there is something they are not able to understand, you may need to provide the information a few times and in easier to follow language. This is acceptable practice when dealing with parents and adult patients, and providing information to adolescents should not be any different.
Remember, you are not indispensable	Establishing a good relationship with a young person is not the same as being indispensable. Establishing relationships with adolescents where they/you believe that you are the best person to deliver their care or understand their needs is not conducive to their overall well-being. The management and care of a young person with a long-term condition, regardless of the setting, is continuous and generally undertaken using a multidisciplinary team approach. Although there will always be times when we are able to relate to one person better than another, it is important to remember that the provision of care is a team effort and no 'player' is more important than another.

Source: From Bill, S. and Knight, Y. (2007) Adolescence. In: *Nursing Care of Children with Chronic Illness* (eds F. Valentine and L. Lowes), pp. 203–230. © 2007. Reproduced with permission of John Wiley & Sons.

are exposed to individuals who come from a larger geographical area and as a consequence new friendships and peer groups are formed. Peer group formation is an important developmental phase, when young people develop their ability to interact socially. During this phase, young people can also learn to interact with individuals from different regional, societal, religious and ethnic backgrounds. As adolescents are still maturing, they have not fully developed their identities and personalities (Rice & Dolgin, 2008), and this can lead to adolescents becoming anxious and insecure about themselves as individuals. Socialising with a close-knit group of peers allows adolescents to learn from each other, form their own identity, increase their self-esteem and develop the social and societal skills that are necessary for them to become part of an adult society (Rice & Dolgin, 2008).

Developing solid and supportive peer relationships has a positive effect on the overall well-being and mental health of adolescents (Mundt & Zakletskaia, 2014). This is of particular relevance to young people who have a long-term condition, as some may spend varying amounts of time away from school and/or in hospital, and have difficulty maintaining contact with their peer group. This, in conjunction with the presence of a long-term condition, can have a detrimental effect on the young person's overall psychological, social and physical well-being.

Key point

- Socialising with a close-knit group of peers allows adolescents to learn from each other, form their own identity, increase their self-esteem and develop the social and societal skills that are necessary to enable them to become part of an adult society.

To gain a deeper understanding of the importance of the peer group, you may wish to read Mundt and Zakletskaia (2014).

The impact of having a long-term condition on growth and development

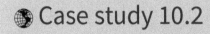

Case study 10.2

Developmental issues

Until recently, Thomas has had a good relationship with his peers. However, as an adolescent with a long-term condition, Thomas is not developing physically at the same rate as his peers. As his condition deteriorates, his short stature and small physique is becoming more obvious to his friends and he is unable to keep up with them psychosocially and educationally. It has been noticed that even when in warm environments Thomas, unfashionably, prefers to wear bulky clothes. This coupled with his moody behaviour and his reluctance to engage in group activities, has led his parents to question whether he is developing poor body image and low self-esteem.

Time out

It is recognised that having a long-term condition has a considerable overall impact on the individual. Take some time out to consider the following questions.

- How do you think a long-term health condition impacts on the physical growth and development of young people?
- In what way does this have the potential to affect their psychosocial development?

Delayed growth and puberty

Most young people with long-term condition have some degree of delayed growth and puberty (including delayed menstruation in girls), although the actual extent of the delay is unclear and varies with individuals and conditions (Martinez *et al.*, 2010). Delayed growth and puberty can result in adolescents being smaller than their peers in height and overall physique (Wiehe & Amdt, 2010). In some situations, the delay may be temporary, and the adolescent will 'catch up' with her/his peers over time. However, in adolescents with CKD, this does not always occur, and the administration of a growth hormone would be carefully considered (Drube *et al.*, 2019).

Inconsistencies between physical and psychological development

As physical and psychosocial development are significantly interrelated, any alteration in the timing of one can have a detrimental effect on the other (Rice & Dolgin, 2008). It is important, therefore, that the effects of delayed puberty on the adolescent's psychosocial development are not underestimated. Although delayed pubertal development can affect both boys and girls, it has the potential to have a particularly adverse effect on boys due to the importance that boys place on their physical (muscular) development. Therefore, in boys, it is not uncommon for delayed puberty to result in low levels of self-esteem and varying degrees of depression.

People's attitudes towards young people who are smaller than their peers can be an issue. It is not uncommon for adolescents with delayed growth/puberty to be treated as less mature than their age, and they may experience difficulty gaining autonomy and independence from their parents, as their outward appearance may suggest immaturity. For older adolescents, this can pose a problem when they try to gain employment as they are frequently viewed as being younger than their chronological age (Suris *et al.*, 2004). It is demeaning for young people to continue to be thought of as children, particularly when they have a far greater level of understanding than children. It is understandable, therefore, that delayed growth/puberty can have an adverse effect on adolescents' overall well-being, particularly regarding body image and self-esteem, which can lead to mental health and behavioural problems. It is not unusual for young people with a long-term condition to be depressed and have suicidal thoughts (Pinquart & Shen, 2011).

Reflection

Reflect on your own adolescence and young people you have cared for.

- What do you understand by body image?
- What can influence people's perceptions of body image?
- What can be the consequences of having a poor body image?

Body image and self-esteem

Body image is defined as the way in which we perceive ourselves and the way in which we believe others perceive us. Individuals can view this in both a positive and a negative way. The importance of body image to adolescents has long been established. With regard to bodily perception, there are certain differences noted between genders, with girls being more dissatisfied than boys, particularly during puberty. This is probably because girls experience a redistribution and increase of fat deposits. Boys, however, tend to be more satisfied with their body image due to an increase in muscle mass as they move through puberty (Santrock, 2018). As we have already noted, this is in direct contrast to the perceptions of adolescent boys who have a long-term condition that is associated with pubertal/growth delay.

During adolescence, young people become preoccupied with their bodies and develop individual perceptions of what their bodies are actually like (Santrock, 2018) and the way they would like them to be. These expectations are often unrealistic, and it could be argued that young people's perceptions of what is 'normal' are heavily swayed by the influence of the media (Vries *et al.*, 2019). Although adolescents' preoccupation with their body continues throughout adolescence, it is at its strongest point during puberty when, generally due to physical changes in bodily shape, they are more dissatisfied with their bodies than towards the end of adolescence (Santrock, 2018).

Any condition that may affect growth, or a disfigurement (e.g. burns, amputations, scarring), which has the potential to alter adolescents' perception of their body image, or how they believe others perceive them, can have an overall detrimental effect on adolescents (Bill & Knight, 2007; Pinquart, 2015). Being attractive to others is important to adolescents, as they believe this will make them more accepted by their peers. Adolescents believe that if they are viewed as attractive, their peers will think of them in more positive terms, for example friendly, successful and intelligent (Bill & Knight, 2007). Although this may seem to be an unrealistic belief, evidence does suggest that there is a direct link between the way adolescents look and the way they are treated by their peers (Koff *et al.*, 1990).

The concept of the perception of attractiveness in adolescence is supported in the seminal work undertaken by Koff *et al.* (1990), who found that 'attractive' adolescents are generally more popular than their 'less attractive' peers. Although the work by Koff *et al.* was undertaken a number of years ago, there is no evidence to suggest that adolescents' feelings and beliefs have altered in any way. To the contrary, studies undertaken since Koff *et al.* have continued to demonstrate the damaging effect of having a long-term condition on adolescents' body image and self-esteem (Sawyer *et al.*, 1995; Pinquart, 2013).

Adolescents who are thought of in more positive terms are also found to have higher levels of self-esteem, healthier personalities and achieve a wider variety of social and interpersonal skills. Conversely, adolescents who are thought of in less positive terms and do not enjoy the same level of popularity can experience negative effects on their personality and self-esteem. These include lack of connectedness, social exclusion and depression.

In Thomas' situation, as he is already less physically developed than his peers, it is possible that he has developed a negative body image and low self-esteem. If he is no longer able to keep up with his peers, he may begin to feel socially isolated and depressed. Young people are preoccupied with their 'ideal' body image and if this is altered in any way it can easily lead to feelings of inadequacy. Health adjustment can be difficult, and some young people and their families may experience periods of depression or behavioural changes (Blyton & Jepson, 2019). To meet the psychological and social needs of children and adolescents with renal problems and their families, the British Association for Paediatric Nephrology (BAPN) (2008) identified the need for psychosocial services to be available within paediatric renal teams. Maintaining a cohesive and supportive family relationship is vitally important as evidence suggests that a supportive relationship with one or more parents (or other caregiver) is crucial to adolescents, as this promotes resilience and an increased ability to cope with their illness (Traub & Boynton, 2017).

⊶ Key point

- During adolescence, young people become preoccupied with their bodies and develop individual perceptions concerning what their bodies are actually like.

Compliance and non-compliance, concordance and co-production

It has already been established that young people experience significant physical and psychosocial changes during adolescence. The presence of a long-term condition is an added pressure that challenges adolescents' ability to eat what they should, take the medication they need, attend medical appointments and adhere to demanding management programmes. At the same time, they are expected to juggle their home, school and social life and be a 'normal' adolescent. It is not surprising, therefore, that some young people are unable to meet the expectations of health care professionals, their families and even themselves regarding the management of their condition.

Reflection

Reflect on young people with long-term conditions that you have cared for. Can you consider reasons why they may not be compliant with their care management plans?

Without using a general dictionary definition, which suggests that to be 'compliant' is to be 'obedient' (*Oxford Dictionary and Thesaurus*, 2019), it is difficult to establish an accepted definition of compliance within a health care setting. As a consequence, for some time, terms such as 'adherence', 'cooperation' and 'mutuality' have been used as alternatives (Kyngäs, 2000). In 1995, Blair and Bowes suggested that compliance within the health care setting could be defined as 'the extent to which behaviour coincides with advice' (p. 2037). Then in 2000, Kyngäs viewed adolescents who are compliant with their management as those who demonstrate an active and responsible approach to managing their care while working in collaboration with health care professionals. However, although it is important for young people to adhere to management programmes, there is more to compliance within adolescent health care, than just simply following the 'rules'. Therefore, more recently, the terms concordance (Chapman, 2018) and co-production, which imply a more negotiated approach (Batalden *et al.*, 2016) have been introduced into health care vocabulary.

By definition, this means that adolescents who are non-compliant are not able or willing to achieve this level of approach to managing their care. Although the Kyngäs (2000) view would probably be the preferred definition, it is still probably Blair and Bowes (1995) who more realistically describe the achievement of compliance within adolescent health. Young people are not always compliant with their management (Dean *et al.*, 2010) and this viewpoint provides a more flexible approach with regard to addressing the issues.

Non-compliance is an issue to consider when discussing the management of young people who have a long-term condition. It is difficult to ascertain the exact numbers of adolescents who do not comply with their management programmes as the collection of this sort of data is heavily reliant on self-reporting. However, there are some conditions where compliance can be estimated based on blood test results or lung function tests, which provide an indication of the level of compliance.

Young people with a long-term condition do not set out to be non-compliant. Coping with adolescence as well as a long-term condition is not easy, and it could be suggested that sometimes it is just too difficult for them to be compliant. As Ahmad and

Sorensen (2016) note, there are a range of reasons why young people are not compliant. Attitudes towards health, their understanding of what is expected of them, relationships with health care providers, family and peers all have an effect on individuals' level of compliance (Ahmad & Sorensen, 2016). Although Ahmad and Sorensen (2016) discuss adolescent compliance within the context of asthma management, there is no evidence to suggest that these reasons could not be transferred to young people with other conditions. Additionally, it is recognised (Rice & Dolgin, 2008) that young people do not want to be different to their peers and striving not to 'be different' sometimes results in non-compliance. For example, drinking alcohol, which can have adverse effects overall and in some conditions can cause side effects. Young people desire peer acceptance, which we know is sometimes difficult to achieve for young people with a long-term condition (as noted by Koff *et al.*, 1990), and the importance of the peer group to adolescents is potentially a significant influencing factor in relation to compliance. Therefore, in some situations, involving peers during an adolescent's hospital admission can improve their acceptance of restrictions.

Just as there are factors that influence non-compliance, there are factors that influence compliance. Family support and cohesion have a positive impact and can enhance the adolescent's level of compliance (Gabr & Shams, 2015). It is also suggested that developing an awareness that non-compliance, particularly with medication, can cause the individuals condition to deteriorate (De Simoni *et al.*, 2017) is another motivator for compliance.

Even when an adolescent is generally well managed and compliant, the potential for non-compliance always exists. Increased stress at school, changes in medical management or an alteration in the adolescent's developmental phase can influence the level of compliance. Although adolescents should be encouraged and trusted to manage their condition, it is important to keep the potential problem of non-compliance in mind when managing their health care needs. Being alert to the issue of potential non-compliance in adolescent health care will help ensure that young people are provided with the support and encouragement they need to assist them in the decision-making process (Mehta *et al.*, 2017).

Key point

- The issue of non-compliance needs to be kept in mind when discussing the management of young people who have a long-term condition.

The social aspects of having a long-term condition

Case study 10.3

Currently, Thomas is at a crucial stage in his schooling. Despite his past hospital admissions and numerous visits to the outpatient department, he has been maintaining an average level of academic attainment. A contributing factor to his education has been his parents' diligence in ensuring that he attends school, as Thomas dislikes school and would not attend if he were given the choice.

As Thomas' renal function continued to deteriorate, he presented with some of the clinical symptoms of uraemia, which include nausea and vomiting. As a result, Thomas' renal disease has not only impacted on his time away from school for clinic appointments, but also on his ability to concentrate on academic studies. Lethargy is also a symptom of Thomas' condition, which can adversely affect his ability to participate in his favourite sporting activities.

🕐 Time out

- Before reading the next section, take some time out to consider some of the wider social implications of having a long-term condition for young people and their families. You may want to make some notes and then compare them with the content of the next section.

Young people, long-term conditions and school

School plays an important part in adolescent development both academically and socially (Hamre & Cappella, 2015). Peer groups are formed and extended during the school years and it is important for all young people to be a part of this. However, not all young people adjust well to school and truancy is a widespread problem throughout the UK (Attwood & Croll, 2014). For some young people trying to cope with a long-term condition, school can be an added 'stress'. It can be an equally stressful issue for adolescents who have a newly diagnosed illness (e.g. epilepsy/diabetes) when they return to school for the first time, or for young people who have an existing condition.

It is important for young people with a long-term condition to be treated as 'normally' as possible. This includes attending school regularly, but many adolescents with long-term conditions do miss varying amounts of school, which disrupts their peer group contact and results in them missing vital educational activities. This potentially impacts on their long-term career goals and financial independence as adults (Ferro et al., 2017). In some situations, adolescents with long-term conditions are unable to attend school (Ferro et al., 2017), which can mean they have additional issues of loneliness and isolation to contend with, which can in turn lead to depression.

Some adolescents with long-term conditions miss so much school that they constantly need to play 'catch up' with missed work and have difficulty grasping the new work being taught when they return to school. Where the volume of work needed to 'catch up' is deemed too great, it may be recommended that they repeat a school year. When this occurs, it is understandable that adolescents feel left out, insecure, have low self-esteem and, given the opportunity, would not attend school, so that 'school avoidance' becomes a problem. In Thomas' case, striving to provide educational opportunities for him is challenging. The work of Collier and Watson (1994), further explored by Jayaraman and Van der Voort (2010) and Wong et al. (2014) offers practical measures to assist adolescents with renal problems maintain their schooling. They suggest that, where possible, hospitalisation is minimised to limit disruption of schooling, there is promotion of continuity of schoolwork through educational liaison between hospital and community school and, where appropriate, the provision of home tutoring services.

Although most hospitals employ teachers, many of these may be primary school teachers (Steinke *et al.*, 2016), which emphasises the importance of adolescents maintaining contact with their own schools. In today's technological society, email and facsimile facilities can be used during extended periods of time in hospital (condition permitting) so that young people do not miss too much schoolwork. To optimise career opportunities later in life, young people should be encouraged to continue with their schooling to maximise their potential.

Having a long-term condition does not mean that young people are unable to succeed in life. As the life expectancy of young people with long-term conditions continue to increase, it is important that all aspects of their lifestyle are promoted in a positive way. The writers have known young people with long-term conditions who have achieved higher degrees and others who have been barely able to read and write. With regard to school and education, young people need support, encouragement and realistic career counselling. The school nurse has an important role to play concerning the care of young people with long-term conditions, and it is vital that nurses caring for adolescents with a long-term condition liaise closely with school nurses in an attempt to provide a well-balanced level of care.

In the case study, Thomas' continued attendance at school was mainly due to his parents' perseverance and encouragement. This is an important point, because it is recognised that parental support and the way parents communicate with adolescents play a significant role in ensuring that they continue at school (Hamre & Cappella, 2015). However, for many adolescents, the decision to stay on in school is often dependent on a variety of factors, including access to amenities and the level of support and services provided by the school, particularly when young people are physically disabled.

Bullying

 Time out

Before reading the next section, answer the following questions.

- What types of bullying can occur?
- What are the possible effects of bullying on the young person?

It would be negligent to review school issues and not discuss bullying. Bullying is a considerable problem throughout schools in the UK. However, this is not a situation unique to UK schools, as both the USA and Australia also have considerable problems with school bullying (Menesini & Salmivalli, 2016). Bullying presents in a variety of forms and can include physical and verbal abuse, teasing, being taunted and threatened, and name-calling. It is more common for boys to experience physical violence than girls, particularly in the lower school years (Silva *et al.*, 2013) but violence by girls appears to be occurring more frequently.

It is not uncommon for young people with a long-term condition, or those with physical or cognitive impairment, to experience bullying in school. The inability to 'fit in' with the peer group and conform to the influence of social media, being different, needing to take medication in school or just not being able to keep up with their peers is a potential 'reason' for bullying. It is important to recognise that bullying is a reality for some young people with a long-term condition, as this can add to the negative issues surrounding body image and self-esteem, in addition to school avoidance.

🔑 Key point

- Bullying is a significant problem throughout schools in the UK and this is a stark reality for some young people with a long-term condition as this can add to the negative issues surrounding body image and self-esteem, in addition to school avoidance.

🌐 Case study 10.4

Recently, Thomas has been admitted to hospital following further deterioration of his renal function. His parents and health care professionals suspect that this is as a direct result of non-adherence to his conservative management regime. Following assessment by the multidisciplinary team, a number of issues have been identified. In relation to Thomas' CKD, he needs more frequent monitoring of his renal function, which involves additional blood analysis, careful adjustment of his conservative management and open discussions regarding his future renal therapy, for example dialysis and/or renal transplantation. From a psychosocial perspective, Thomas needs further support and encouragement to help him through this difficult phase of his development and medical care. While the whole of the MDT are involved, the youth worker, social worker and clinical psychologist play key roles in his psychosocial care.

🕑 Time out

There has been much discussion regarding the appropriate placing of young people within a hospital setting. For this exercise consider:

- The appropriateness of children's and adult wards for adolescent patients.
- The facilities that would be important to hospitalised adolescents.

The hospitalised adolescent

The debate regarding the most suitable place to care for young people in hospital is long-standing, with the general opinion that neither adult nor children's wards are appropriate for young people. On adult wards adolescents may encounter individuals with the same long-term condition as they have, but at a more advanced stage, and on children's wards, the age range can be far too great to be able to accommodate young people appropriately.

If adolescents are viewed as a distinct group for developmental purposes, then it is important that their development is taken into account when we manage them as patients. The need to care for adolescents as a developmentally distinct group within the health care setting was originally identified towards the end of the 1950s in the *Platt Report* (Ministry of Health, 1959) and was again reinforced by the Court Report (1976) and the Kennedy Report (2010). In 2003, when the Royal College of Paediatricians and Child Health (RCPCH) produced the document: *Bridging the Gaps: Health Care for Adolescents*, it was suggested that, despite the many adolescents who use health care services and the recognition of the need to manage them as a distinct group, services for young people were limited. However, although services for young people have improved in some areas, since this document was published, it could be argued that inpatient services for young people in the UK, still trail behind countries such as Australia, Scandinavia and North America (James *et al.*, 2014).

The effect of hospitalisation on adolescents has been well documented over many years (Stevens, 1987; MacKenzie, 1988; Gillies & Parry-Jones, 1992; Taylor & Müller, 1995; Kelly & Hewson, 2000; Hutton, 2002; 2007; 2010). Ultimately, the evidence suggests that adolescents need to be managed within a specialised age-appropriate adolescent unit by staff specifically educated in the care of young people (Payne *et al.*, 2011). In some parts of the UK and the Republic of Ireland, where new hospitals have been built, consideration has been given to the development of adolescent specific wards (Payne *et al.*, 2011). However, this is not consistent throughout all regions of the UK, as the anticipated adolescent ward at the Children's Hospital for Wales was not incorporated into the final design.

Issues for young people in hospital

Where young people are managed outside specialised adolescent wards, many of the issues are purely logistical, particularly when they are cared for on children's wards that are more appropriately targeted towards young children. Children's wards are not always able to provide the facilities that adolescents need and some of the issues raised by young people concerning children's wards (outlined below) have been recognised for some time:

- Small beds and other furniture items.
- Décor aimed at children.
- Poorly fitting bed curtains that inhibit privacy.
- Lack of privacy overall.
- Afternoon 'rest' times.
- Inflexible rules and regulations.
- Being located near small children and crying babies.
- Lack of quiet area for young people to study.

- Recreation facilities aimed at small children.
- Limited opportunity to talk with people of their own age.
- Small bathroom facilities, with no locks on doors (Taylor & Muller 1995; Hutton, 2005).

From a child's perspective, it could be suggested that it is also inappropriate for children to be located in close proximity to older adolescents, even on wards where there are separate bays for adolescents. For example, adolescents, by definition of their age, can watch television programmes and movies that are not suitable for children. Likewise, not all contemporary music enjoyed by adolescents is appropriate for children. Additionally, many adolescents are as physically developed as adults, and as we would not place children and adults on a ward together, careful consideration should also be given to accommodating children and adolescents on the same wards.

In addition to the physical needs of young people, thought also needs to be given to the psychosocial needs of hospitalised adolescents. The importance of the peer group has already been discussed and maintaining peer group contact while in hospital is vitally important. Hospitalised adolescents who are unable to maintain contact with their peer group can develop the perception of having lost their status within their peer group and this can be very worrying for them (Mundt & Zakletskaia, 2014). It should be noted, however, that not all young people with a long-term condition want to be visited by their peers; therefore, it is important to assess each situation individually.

Young people who are admitted to children's wards frequently complain about a lack of privacy. Adolescent males who may already have facial hair and need to shave do not necessarily want to share a bathroom with a 5-year-old. Lack of privacy raises another important issue – sexuality.

Sexual development is an integral part of adolescent development (Santrock, 2018) and young people with long-term conditions are no different. Although puberty and sexual development may sometimes be delayed, having a long-term condition does not preclude young people from having an interest in sexual matters. In 2005, Horseman described her 'excruciating embarrassment' (p. 27) when, on two separate occasions on a children's ward, she accidentally encountered adolescent boys masturbating, and cites this issue alone as a reason for adolescents needing extra privacy. Although this article is now dated, Horseman appears to be the only person to have recognised such a sensitive topic in relation to the management of young people in hospital. It is also worthy of noting, that although the Taylor and Muller (1995) reference is also dated, they are still the only authors in the UK to have published a book on the care of the hospitalised adolescent. In addition to sexuality issues and privacy, nurses caring for adolescents also need to consider the issues of confidentiality, negotiating care, promoting autonomy, decision making (Lugasi *et al.*, 2011; Wong *et al.*, 2010) and managing more 'adult' behaviour, such as smoking, swearing and on occasion the use of alcohol or 'recreational' drugs.

What this situation does highlight, however, is that adolescents clearly have distinctly different needs to children, and what is normal behaviour for them is not necessarily appropriate in the presence of younger children. Furthermore, it emphasises that young people need to be cared for by health professionals who have an understanding of their development needs, issues surrounding confidentiality and privacy and have an interest in and feel comfortable working with them.

Key point

- It is not appropriate to admit young people to adult wards as this can be a distressing experience for them and lead to altered impressions of illness (Taylor & Müller, 1995). Children's wards are also inappropriate to meet adolescents' psychosocial and physical developmental needs. The ideal situation is to admit young people to wards dedicated to this specific age group, where their individual needs can be recognised and met by appropriately qualified staff.

Specialised adolescent units

Adolescent units are wards where the speciality is 'adolescence' and are specifically designed based on young people's needs. Quite often, adolescents are able to have input into the development of these units and the facilities they provide, which is particularly relevant, because understanding the needs of individuals using such units is vital (Hutton, 2010). Many adolescent units have an underlying focus of general medicine and surgery and are staffed by a combination of Child and Adult qualified nurses (Payne *et al.*, 2011).

Generally, the aims of such units are to assist young people to gain autonomy and start to take some responsibility for and make decisions about their care to support them towards self-management. Based on personal experience, ward rules and guidelines on adolescent units tend to be more flexible than children's wards and are more appropriate to the needs of young people. Additionally, there are usually separate recreation facilities and facilities for adolescents to make themselves drinks or snacks and entertain their friends. The staff would also be well versed in issues surrounding adolescent competency and consent, as well as confidentiality and privacy, which are very important issues for young people (Payne *et al.*, 2011). Health promotion specific to the needs of young people (e.g. smoking and sexual health) can also be undertaken.

Time out

Please review Chapter 6 regarding the principles of health promotion and education before moving on to the next section of this chapter.

How do you think these principles can be adapted when working in partnership with young people?

Dedicated adolescent units are usually staffed by a multidisciplinary team educated in-house by their employing hospital regarding adolescent health issues to ensure they are responsive to young people's needs. Some staff will hold specific qualifications in adolescent health, but finding appropriately qualified staff to work on adolescent units may pose a problem in the UK. Although some opportunities now exist for health care professionals to gain education in the care of adolescents – for example, NHS England and the RCPCH both provide online modules and a London University provides a two day face-to-face programme – in general, education regarding adolescent health as a whole and adolescent health related issues is still limited, particularly in regional areas.

There has been a long-standing requirement that children aged 16 years and under need to be cared for by children's nurses, which is an undisputed issue, as it is vitally important that appropriately qualified staff care for children and young people. What is questionable, though, is whether there is sufficient adolescent health content in current pre-registration Children's Nursing Programmes to provide children's nurses with sufficient knowledge to be able to care for young people appropriately. It could also be questioned whether nurses specialising in condition specific roles (e.g. cystic fibrosis, diabetes) have sufficient opportunity to gain appropriate education in adolescent health. Since 1998, Viner and Keane have promoted the development of an adolescent specialist nurse role and have suggested that health care professionals who work with young people need 'core skills' and additional specialist education. Therefore, increasing the provision of education programmes for nurses, doctors and allied health professionals, across all regions throughout the UK, need to be prioritised to ensure that adolescent health care meets the needs of our young people and keeps pace with other countries in the Western world.

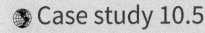 **Case study 10.5**

Conclusion

As part of Thomas' continued management, he will be encouraged to maintain communication and contact with the MDT (multidisciplinary team); this may include the ongoing use of support and counselling services. Thomas will be encouraged to be more proactive in the management of his own health care needs and work closely with his parents to manage his care. A health promotion and education plan is negotiated and agreed with Thomas and his family.

Effective health education for families with children and young people with renal failure is vital to maintain residual renal function and prepare for future health care needs. At Thomas' stage of development, it would be important to ensure that he was provided with appropriate information regarding his condition. Involving Thomas in devising his health management plan should enable him to start taking some responsibility for his care, as well as encourage independence and compliance. However, the complexity of renal disease, coupled with the unique experience of adolescence can prove to be challenging. Therefore, health education should be centralised around the needs of Thomas, but take into account the vital, supportive role of his family, thus ensuring the development of a 'family friendly service' (DoH UK, 2006).

Service delivery and adolescent health

 Time out

For this final exercise:

- Identify the role of the nurse within the MDT specific to the care of young people.
- Consider the role of the children's nurse in facilitating the link between young people and their smooth transition to adult hospital services.

Promoting excellence

Approximately one in four young people aged between 11 and 15 years have a long-term condition or disability (Association for Young People's Health (AYPH), 2019) and use health care services, but despite this there is limited evidence of involvement of this group in service development; this has been discussed in Chapter 2. If we are truly to address the needs of young people, this is a situation that needs significant revision. A good starting point would be to develop the role of adolescent health nurses, which would send a clear message to young people that health care services are actually interested in addressing their needs.

Over a period of time, a range of documents such as the *Guidance for Paediatric Nephrology Nurses* (Royal College of Nursing (RCN), 2000), the *NSF for Renal Services* (DoH UK, 2006) and *Improving the Standards of Care for Children with Kidney Disease* (2011) have all been developed to provide children, young people and their families with quality renal services and to enhance overall standards of care. These are important reference points for children's nurses regarding the management of children with CKD.

The role of the nurse

The role of the nurse working with young people, as with all patients, is multifaceted. Predominantly, though, the adolescent nurse would need to work in the best interest of young people, promoting autonomy and independence, and acting as an advocate by making sure that adolescents' voices are heard within the health care setting. Acting as a liaison between adolescents, their families and the MDT is as important as working comfortably within a MDT setting. The nurse working with young people would need to be committed to and interested in the health of young people, be able to communicate with them effectively and demonstrate a sound knowledge of adolescent physical and psychosocial development. Additionally, the adolescent health nurse would promote adherence to a healthy lifestyle and undertake health promotion specifically addressing the needs of young people. The main health promotion themes important to young people are smoking, the use of alcohol and recreational drugs, contraception, sexual health and safeguarding themselves from harm and abuse, and it is vital that they are provided with the correct information about these issues.

Part of the role of the nurse working with young people should also encompass working towards the development or improvement of transitional services, including developing trust-wide policies and guidance. Disseminating information, networking and the establishment of research pathways within adolescent health would also be important aspects of this role.

MDT working across agencies and organisations is vital to the care of adolescents, to ensure a cohesive, continuing care approach between health, social care and educational settings. Therefore, a considerable aspect of the adolescent health nurse's role is liaison with staff from these areas to facilitate open communication and enable care pathways to be holistic and to span all areas where the adolescent is based, be it at home, school or in hospital. Working within the MDT, adolescent health nurses could coordinate a smooth transition process for the adolescent from children and young people's services to adult services. They would ensure that adolescents and their families are provided with the appropriate education and information and act as advocates in this area to make sure the needs of adolescents and their families are addressed, and their voices heard. Transition of care is reviewed in detail in Chapter 11.

Conclusion

Adolescence is a time of rapid growth and physiological development. Managing a long-term condition during this time is a significant challenge for young people, their family and health care providers. Adolescents are a distinct group of individuals that require their specific health care needs to be addressed and effectively managed by appropriately educated staff.

Thomas and other young people with a long-term condition have to contend with the developmental changes experienced during adolescence and the constraints placed on them by their condition. This is not easy for many adolescents and there is the potential for stress-related conditions and depression to occur. However, with support from families, friends and health care professionals, many young people are generally able to manage their condition, reach their full potential and lead independent and productive lives.

Key points

- Adolescence is a time of rapid growth, development and change, which can be a difficult period for some young people. Any potential difficulties experienced during adolescence can be compounded by the presence of long-term condition.
- Adolescents have distinctly different needs to children, and what is normal behaviour for them is not necessarily appropriate in the presence of children. Therefore, it is inappropriate for them to be cared for on the same ward, and the development of specialised adolescent units is advocated.
- The ability to employ effectivve communication strategies is particularly important when working with young people to help ensure compliance and facilitate health education, in assessment of psychosocial problems and in enabling their independence.
- The role of the nurse working with young people is important and multifaceted and needs to be undertaken by individuals who have an interest in adolescent health and a competent level of skill and knowledge in this area.
- Adolescents are a distinct group of individuals that need to have their specific health care needs addressed and effectively managed by appropriately educated staff.

Acknowledgement

We acknowledge the contribution of Yvonne Knight with whom Sian Bill jointly authored the previous version of this chapter (Bill & Knight, 2007).

Useful websites

Association for Young People's Health www.ayph.org.uk
Royal College of Paediatrics and Child Health (*Bridging the Gaps*) www.rcpch.ac.uk
The UK Renal Association http://www.renal.org/index.html
UK National Kidney Federation Young Person Group https://www.kidney.org.uk/support-for-children-and-young-people

Recommended reading

Blyton, D. & Jepson, S. (2019) Renal care in infancy, childhood and early adulthood. *In: Renal Nursing: Care and Management of People with Kidney Disease* (fifth edition) (ed. N. Thomas), pp. 349–366. Chichester, John Wiley and Sons.

Hockenberry, M. & Wilson, D. (2018) *Wong's Nursing Care of Infants and Children* (eleventh edition). St Louis, Mosby.

Rice, F.P. & Dolgin, K.G. (2008) *The Adolescent: Development, Relationships and Culture* (twelfth edition) Boston, Pearson.

Santrock, J.W. (2018) *Adolescence* (seventeenth edition). Boston, McGraw Hill.

Webb, N. & Postlethwaite, R. (eds) (2003) *Clinical Paediatric Nephrology (third edition).* New York, Oxford University Press.

References

Ahmad, A. & Sorensen, K. (2016) Enabling and hindering factors influencing adherence to asthma treatment among adolescents: a systematic literature review. *Journal of Asthma,* **53** (8), 862–878.

Arnett, J. J. (2006) G. Stanley Hall's Adolescence: brilliance and nonsense. *History of Psychology,* **9** (3), 186–197.

Association for Young People's Health (2019) Key Data on Young People 2019: Latest information and statistics. http://www.youngpeopleshealth.org.uk/wp-content/uploads/2019/09/AYPH_KDYP2019_FullVersion.pdf Accessed 18/6/20.

Attwood, G. & Croll, P. (2014) Truancy and well-being among secondary school pupils in England. *Journal of Educational Studies,* **41** (1–2), 14–28.

Badawy, S., Barrera, L., Sinno, M., *et al.* (2017) Text messaging and mobile phone apps as interventions to improve adherence in adolescents with chronic health conditions: a systematic review. *JMIR mhealth uhealth,* **5** (5), e66.

Batalden, M., Batalden, P., Margolis, P., *et al.* (2016) Coproduction of health care service. *British Medical Journal,* **25** (7), 509–517.

Becherucci, F., Roperto, R.M., Materassi, M., *et al.* (2016) Chronic kidney disease in children. *Clinical Kidney Journal,* **9** (4), 583–591.

Beresford, B.A. & Sloper, P. (2002) Chronically ill adolescents' experiences of communication with doctors: a qualitative study. *Journal of Adolescent Health,* **33** (3), 172–179.

Bill, S. & Knight, Y. (2007) Adolescence. In: *Nursing Care of Children with Chronic Illness* (eds F. Valentine & L. Lowes), pp. 203–230. Oxford, Blackwell Publishing.

Blair, S. & Bowes, G. (1995) Compliance issues in adolescence: practical strategies. *Australian Family Physician*, **24** (11), 2037–2040.

Blyton, D. & Jepson, S. (2019) Renal care in infancy, childhood and early adulthood. In: *Renal Nursing: Care and Management of People with Kidney Disease (fifth edition)* (ed. N. Thomas), pp. 349–366. Chichester, John Wiley and Sons.

British Association for Paediatric Nephrology (2008) *Haemodyalisis Clinical Practice Guidelines for Children and Adolescents*. London, British Association for Paediatric Nephrology.

Casey, B. J., Jones, R. M., Levita, L., *et al.* (2010) The storm and stress of adolescence: insights from human imaging and mouse genetics. *Developmental Psychology*, **52** (3), 225–235.

Chapman, H. (2018) Nursing theories 4: adherence and concordance. *Nursing Times*, **114** (2), 50.

Christie, D. & Viner, R. (2005) ABC of adolescence: adolescent development. *British Medical Journal*, **330** (7486), 301–304.

Collier, J. & Watson, A.R. (1994) Renal failure in children: specific considerations in management. In: *Quality of Life Following Renal Failure* (eds H. McGee & C. Bradley), pp. 225–246. Chur, Switzerland, Harwood Academic Publishers.

Court, S.D.M. (1976) *Fit for the Future: Report of the Committee on Child Health Services* (vols **I and II**). London, Her Majesty's Stationery Office.

Dean, A.J., Walters, J. & Hall, J. (2010) A systematic review of interventions to enhance medication adherence in children and adolescents with chronic illness. *Archives of Disease in Childhood*, **95** (9), 717–723.

Department of Health UK (2006) *The National Service Framework for Renal Services. Working for Children and Young People*. London, Department of Health, UK.

De Simoni, A., Horne, R., Fleming, L., *et al.* (2017) What do adolescents with asthma really think about adherence to inhalers? Insights from a qualitative analysis of a UK online forum. *BMJ Open*, **7**, e015245

Drube, J., Wan, M., Bonthuis, M., *et al.* (2019) Clinical practice recommended for growth hormone treatment in children with chronic kidney disease. *Nature Reviews Nephrology*, **15** (9), 577–589.

Eiser, C. (1990) *Chronic Childhood Disease: An Introduction to Psychological Theory and Research*. Cambridge, Cambridge University Press.

Fegran, L., Hall, E., Uhrenfeldt, L., *et al.* (2014) Adolescents' and young adults' transition experiences when transferring from paediatric to adult care: A quantitative metasynthesis. *International Journal of Nursing Studies*, **51** (1), 123–135.

Fielding, C. (2019) Haemodialysis. *In: Renal Nursing: Care and Management of People with Kidney Disease* (fifth edition) (ed. N. Thomas), pp. 179–233. Chichester, John Wiley and Sons.

Ferro, M., Rhodes, A., Kimber, M., *et al.* (2017) Suicidal behaviour among adolescents and young adults with self-reported chronic illness. *Canadian Journal of Psychiatry*, **62** (12), 845–853.

Gabr, W.M. & Shams, M.E.E (2015) Adherence to medication among outpatient adolescents with epilepsy, *Saudi Pharmaceutical Journal*, **23** (1), 33–40.

Garabedian, L.F., Ross-Degnan, D. & Wharam, J.F. (2015) Mobile phone and smartphone technologies for diabetes care and self-management. *Current Diabetes Reports*, **15** (120), 109–123.

Gillies, M.L. & Parry-Jones, W.L. (1992) Suitability of the hospital setting for hospitalised adolescents. *Archives of Diseases in Childhood*, **67**, 1506–1509.

Hagel, A. & Shah, R. (2019) *Key Data on Young People 2019*. London, Association for Young People's Heath.

Hamilton, A.J., Casula, A., Ben-Shloma, Y., *et al.* (2017) The clinical epidemiology of young adults starting renal replacement therapy in the UK: presentation, management and survival using 15 years of UK Renal Registry data. *Nephrology Dialysis Transplantation*, **33** (2), 356–364.

Hamre, B. & Cappella, E. (2015) Measures of early adolescent development and school contexts: narrowing the research to practice divide. *Journal of Early Adolescence*, **35** (5–6), 586–596.

Hockenberry, M., Wilson, D., Winklestein, M.L., *et al.* (2003) *Wong's Nursing Care of Infants and Children* (seventh edition). St Louis, Mosby.

Horseman, W. (2005) Sexuality in the hospital setting. *Paediatric Nursing*, **17** (8), 27–29.

Hutton, A. (2002) The private adolescent: privacy needs of adolescents in hospital. *International Pediatric Nursing*, **17** (1), 67–72.

Hutton, A. (2005) Consumer perspectives on adolescent ward design. *Journal of Clinical Nursing*, **14** (5), 537–545.

Hutton, A. (2007) An adolescent ward; In name only? *Journal of Clinical Nursing*, **17** (23), 3142–3149.

Hutton, A. (2010) How adolescents use ward space. *Journal of Advanced Nursing*, **66** (8), 1802–1809.

James, D.R., Emedo, M. & Hargreaves D.S. (2014) What are we doing with young people in hospital? As adolescent in-patient survey. *Archives of Disease in Childhood*, **99**, A18–A19.

Jayaraman, R. & Van der Voort, J. (2010) Principles of management of chronic kidney disease. *Paediatrics and Child Health*, **20** (6), 291–296.

Kelly, A.F. & Hewson, P.H. (2000) Factors associated with recurrent hospitalisation in chronically ill children and adolescents. *Journal of Paediatrics and Child Health*, **36** (1), 13–18. https://doi: 10.1046/j.1440-1754.2000.00435.x.

Kennedy, I. (2010) *Getting it Right for Children and Young People: Overcoming Cultural Barriers in the NHS so as to Meet their Needs*. London, Department of Health UK.

Koff, E., Rierden, J. & Stubbs, M.L. (1990) Gender, body image and self-concept in early adolescence. *Journal of Early Adolescence*, **10** (1), 56–68.

Kyngäs, H. (2000) Compliance of adolescents with chronic disease. *Journal of Clinical Nursing*, **9** (4), 549–556.

Li, B. & Chu, D. (2018) Screening for the management of chronic kidney disease for children with congenital abnormalities of kidney and urinary tract. *Current Paediatric Reports*, **6** (3), 237–245.

Lugasi, T., Achille, M. & Stevenson, M. (2011) Parents perspectives on factors that facilitate transitions from child-centred to adult-centred healthcare: a theory integrated metasummary of quantitative and qualitative studies. *Journal of Adolescent Health*, **48** (5), 429–440.

MacKenzie, H. (1988) Teenagers in hospital. *Nursing Times*, **84** (35), 55–58.

Madden, S.J., Hastings, R.P. & V'ant Hoff, W. (2002) Psychological adjustment in children with end stage renal disease: the impact of maternal stress and coping. *Child Care Health and Development*, **28** (4), 323–330.

Martinez, A.E., Allgrove, J. & Brain, C. (2010) Growth and pubertal delay in patients with epidermolysis bullosa. *Dermatalogic Clinics*, **28** (2), 357–359.

Mazzucato, M., Pozza, L.V.D., Minichello, C., *et al.* (2018) The epidemiology of transition into adulthood of rare diseases patients: results from a population-based registry. *International Journal of Environmental Research and Public Health*, **15** (10), E2212.

Mehta, P., Steinberg, E.A., Kelly, S.L., *et al.* (2017) Medication adherence among adolescent solid-organ transplant recipients: A survey of healthcare providers. *Pediatric Transplantation*, **21** (7), e13018. https://doi: 10.1111/petr.13018.

Menesini, E. & Salmivalli, C. (2016) Bullying in schools, the state of knowledge and effective interventions. *Journal of Psychology, Health and Medicine*, **22** (1), 240–253.

Ministry of Health (Central Health Services Council) (1959) *The Welfare of Children in Hospital. Report of the Committee (The Platt Report)*. London, Her Majesty's Stationery Office.

Mundt, M.P. & Zakletskaia, L.I. (2014) That's what friends are for: adolescent peer social status, health related quality of life and healthcare costs. *Applied Healthcare Economics Healthcare Policy*, **12** (2), 191–201.

Olsson, C.A., Boyce, M.F., Toumbourou, J.W., *et al.* (2005) The role of peer support in facilitating psychosocial adjustment to chronic illness in adolescence. *Clinical Child Psychology and Psychiatry*, **10** (1), 78–87.

Oxford Dictionary (2019) *Oxford Dictionary and Thesaurus*. Oxford: Oxford University Press.

Payne, D., Kennedy, A., Kretzer, V., *et al.* (2011) Developing and running an adolescent in patient ward. *Archives of Disease in Childhood*, **99**, A18–A19.

Pinquart, M. (2013) Self-esteem of children and adolescents with chronic illness: a meta-analysis. *Child: Care, Health and Development* **39** (2), 153–161. https://doi: 10.1111/j.1365-2214.2012.01397.x

Pinquart, M. & Shen, Y. (2011) Depressive symptoms in children and adolescents with chronic physical illness: an updated meta-analysis. *Journal of Pediatric Psychology,* **36** (4), 375–384.

Pinquart, M. (2015) Body image of children and adolescents with chronic illness: a meta-analytic comparison with healthy peers. *Body Image,* **10** (2), 141–148.

Rice F P & Dolgin, K.G. (2008) *The Adolescent, Development Relationships and Culture (twelfth edition).* Boston, Pearson.

Rigden, S.P.A. (2003) The management of chronic and end stage renal failure in children: In: *Clinical Paediatric Nephrology* (third edition) (eds N. Webb & R. Postlethwaite), pp. 427–446. New York, Oxford University Press.

Royal College of Nursing (2000) *Guidance for Paediatric Nephrology Nurses.* London, Royal College of Nursing.

Royal College of Paediatrics and Child Health (2003) *Bridging the Gaps: Health Care for Adolescents.* London, Royal College of Paediatrics and Child Health.

Royal College of Paediatrics and Child Health (2011) *Improving the Standards of Care of Children with Kidney Disease through Paediatric Nephrology Networks.* London, Royal College of Paediatrics and Child Health.

Royal College of Paediatrics and Child Health (2012) *Involving Children and Young People in Health Services.* London, Royal College of Paediatrics and Child Health.

Rudi, J.H. Walkner, A. & Dworkin, J. (2015) Adolescent-parent communication in a digital world: differences by family communication patterns *Youth and Society,* **47** (6), 811–828.

Sanci, L. & Young, D. (1995) Engaging the adolescent patient. *Australian Family Physician,* **24** (11), 2031–2127.

Santrock, J.W. (2018) *Adolescence* (seventeenth edition). Boston, McGraw Hill.

Sawyer, S.M., Rosier, M.J., Phelan, P.D., *et al.* (1995) The self-image of adolescents with cystic fibrosis. *Journal of Adolescent Health,* **16** (3), 204–208.

Sawyer, S.M., Ambresin, A.-E., Bennett, K.E., *et al.* (2014) A measurement framework for quality health care for adolescents in hospital. *Journal of Adolescent Health,* **55** (4), 484–490.

Schnaper, H.W. (2014) Remnant nephron physiology and the progression of chronic kidney disease. *Pediatric Nephrology,* **29** (2), 193–202.

Schmidt, S., Petersen, C. & Bullinger, M. (2003) Coping with chronic disease from the perspective of children and adolescents - a conceptual framework and its implications for participation. *Child: Care, Health and Development,* **29** (1), 63–75.

Sharkey, C.M., Perez, M.N., Bakula, D.M., *et al.* (2018). Exploratory factor analysis of the Michel Uncertainty in Illness scale among adolescents and young adults with chronic medical conditions. *Journal of Pediatric Health Care,* **33** (2), 186–194.

Silva, M., Pereira, B., Mendoca, D., *et al.* (2013) The involvement of girls and boys with bullying: An analysis of gender differences. *International Journal of Environmental Research and Public Health,* **10** (2), 6820–6831.

Steinberg, L. (2001) We know some things: parent-adolescent relationships in retrospect and prospect. *Journal of Research on Adolescence,* **11** (1), 1–19.

Steinke, S., Elam, M., Irwin, M., *et al.* (2016) Pediatric hospital school programming: an examination of educational services for children who are hospitalized. *Physical Disabilities: Education and Related Services,* **35** (1), 28–45.

Stevens, M.S. (1987) Which adolescents' breeze through surgery? *American Journal of Nursing,* **87** (12), 1564–1565.

Suris, J.C., Michud, P.A. & Viner, R. (2004) The adolescent with a chronic condition: Part 1 developmental issues. *Archives of Disease in Childhood,* **89** (10), 938–942.

Taylor, J. & Müller, D. (1995) *Nursing Adolescence, Research and Psychological Perspectives.* Oxford, Blackwell Science.

Towle, A., Godolphin, W. & Van Staalduinen, S. (2006) Enhancing the relationship and improving communication between adolescents and their health care providers: A school based intervention by medical students *Patient Education and Counseling*, **62** (2), 189–192.

Traub, F. & Boynton, R. (2017) Modifiable resilience factors to childhood aversity for clinical pediatric practice. *Pediatrics*, **139** (5), e20162569; https://doi.org/10.1542/peds.2016–2569.

Viner, R. & Keane, M. (1998) *Youth Matters: Evidence Based Practice for the Care of Young People in Hospital*. London, Action for Sick Children.

Vries, D., Vossen, H. & Kolk-Van der Boom, P. (2019) Social media and body dissatisfaction: investigating the role of positive parent-adolescent relationships. *Journal of Youth and Adolescence*, **48** (3), 527–536.

Watson, A.R. (2003) Meeting the information needs of children and their families. In: *Clinical Paediatric Nephrology (third edition)* (eds N. Webb & R. Postlethwaite), pp. 465–474. New York, Oxford University Press.

Wheal, A. (1999) *Adolescence: Positive Approaches for Working with Young People*. Lyme Regis, Russel House Publishing.

Wiehe, M. & Arndt, K. (2010) Cystic fibrosis: a systems review. *American Association of Nurse Anaesthetists Journal*, **78** (3), 246–251.

Wong, G., Medway, M., Didsbury, M., *et al.* (2014) Health and wealth in children and adolescents with chronic kidney disease (K-CAD study). *BMC Public Health*, **14**, 307 https://doi: 10.1186/1471-2458-14-307.

Wong. L.H.L., Chan, F.W.K., Wong, F.Y., *et al.* (2010) Transition care for adolescents and families with chronic illness. *Journal of Adolescent Health*, **47** (6), 540–546.

World Health Organization (1993) *The Health of Young People*. Geneva, World Health Organization.

Worsey, L. (2019) Peritoneal dialysis. In: *Renal Nursing: Care and Management of People with Kidney Disease (fifth edition)* (ed. N. Thomas), pp. 235–276. Chichester, John Wiley and Sons.

Xiao, Z., Xiaoming, L. & Stanton, B. (2011) Perceptions of parent-adolescent communication within families: it is a matter of perspective. *Psychology Health and Medicine*, **16** (1), 53–65.

CHAPTER 11

Transitional Care

Siân Bill and Amie Hodges

Introduction

Improvements in health care have seen increased numbers of children and young people with long-term conditions surviving into adulthood. Therefore, the seamless transition between child and adult services should be viewed as a priority for all health care professionals working with children and young people. Currently, there are inequalities in the provision of transitional care, which has the potential to lead to a fragmented provision of services.

Aim of the chapter

The purpose of this chapter is to critically examine the transitional issues faced by young people with long-term conditions and their families. The discussion surrounding these issues will highlight the need for, and the importance of, a seamless transitional service. Although a scenario of a young person with cystic fibrosis will be used to explore the issues raised within this chapter, these will be applicable to many other young people with long-term conditions moving through the transitional phase. As this chapter specifically relates to young people, it is suggested that you first read Chapter 10, which gives an overview of adolescent development. Chapter 10 also explores many of the issues that arise for adolescents with long-term conditions, so it will give you an insight into the topics covered here.

Intended learning outcomes

- To develop an awareness of the issues surrounding adolescents with long-term conditions related to the transitional phase of their health care
- To explore the differences between transitional care and transfer
- To examine the psychosocial and physical developmental needs of the adolescent in the transitional phase of the illness trajectory

Nursing Care of Children and Young People with Long-Term Conditions, Second Edition.
Edited by Mandy Brimble and Peter McNee.
© 2021 John Wiley & Sons Ltd. Published 2021 by John Wiley & Sons Ltd.

- To critically analyse the current evidence to demonstrate the benefits of providing an adolescent transitional service
- To outline the role of the nurse in facilitating the transition process for young people and their families

Overview of cystic fibrosis

Cystic fibrosis (CF) is the most common life-limiting inherited condition in the Caucasian population (Havermans et al., 2011; McCullough & Price, 2011; CF Trust 2020). It can affect 1 in 2500–3000 live births in the UK and 100,000 live births globally (Filbrun et al., 2016; CF Trust, 2019). CF can also occur in other ethnic/mixed heritage populations (Wallis, 2019), with prevalence as follows:

Non-Hispanic white 1 in 32,000 live births, Hispanic 1 in 92,000 live births, African American 1 in 15,000 and Asian American 1 in 31,000 live births (Filbrun et al., 2016).

Most children with CF are diagnosed through newborn screening programmes or by the presence of meconium ileus within the first few days of life (Filbrun et al., 2016; Wallis, 2019), presenting with fatty stools, faltering growth or a recurrent chest infection (Bush et al., 2015). However, even though most children are diagnosed by the age of 1 year, approximately 10% of individuals with CF are not diagnosed until beyond 7 years of age (Wallis, 2019), usually when their condition is caused by one of the more unusual mutations. If a child looks well or appears older, they should not be discounted from having a possible diagnosis if they are presenting with symptoms. Children from non- Caucasian ethnicities can be more susceptible to delays in diagnosis (Wallis, 2019). If both parents have the faulty gene there is a one in four chance of conceiving a child with CF. Therefore, the carrier rate in the Caucasian population is about 1 in 20–30 individuals (Filbrun et al., 2016).

Historically, CF was recognised as a childhood disease, but with advances in newborn screening, the use of the gold standard sweat test, early diagnosis, treatments and technology, the life expectancy now reaches beyond the childhood years. In 2018, the median predicted rate of survival being 41 years old for females and 46 years old for males who have the F508del mutation (Filbrun et al., 2016; CF Trust, 2018). However, the disease is complex and multifaceted and so can affect people in a multitude of ways, hence the age of death can differ from the predicted survival rate. According to Keogh et al. (2018), half of babies born with CF in 2018 are expected to live into their mid 40s.

🌐 Case study 11.1

Background information

Sophie is a 17-year-old girl who has CF and lives at home with her father and younger sister Sally, aged 14 years, who does not have CF. Sally is very supportive of her sister and they get on well together. When Sophie was 6 years old, her mother died in a car accident and, since then, her father has been the main carer for Sophie and Sally, with some support from both sets of grandparents. Sophie's father works full time as a civil engineer and occasionally works away. Sophie recently left school and works in the local supermarket. Although she achieved good results in her end of school exams, Sophie decided that she did not want to stay on at school.

Sophie was diagnosed at birth as she developed a meconium ileus. Sophie has the most common form of CF, which is the ΔF508 deletion (CF Trust, 2019). She has both respiratory and digestive problems and needs to undertake daily physiotherapy and exercise regimes, as well as eating a high fat, high calorie diet. She has recently been diagnosed with CF-related diabetes.

Since starting her new job, Sophie is finding it difficult to maintain her usual physiotherapy and dietary programme. She has acquired a new social circle of friends, but she has not informed them that she has CF, as she is concerned that she will not be able to maintain these friendships if she discloses her diagnosis. Sophie believes that by requesting time off to visit the hospital, her new friends will find out about her condition. Currently, Sophie is losing weight and has developed another chest infection. Her father believes that she needs a hospital admission for reassessment. Sophie is reluctant to visit the hospital and, although her father has made some appointments with Sophie's GP, she has not attended them.

Sophie currently accesses services at the local children's hospital where she attends clinic regularly and is admitted for antibiotic therapy as required. She is managed by a multidisciplinary team (referred to as the CF team), which generally includes a paediatric respiratory consultant, a CF children's nurse specialist, a paediatric physiotherapist and a paediatric dietitian. The suggestion has been made that Sophie needs to be transferred to the adult hospital, which manages patients with CF. However, this is further away from Sophie's home and working environment.

 Time out

This may be a good time to recap what you have learned from this chapter and review your current knowledge regarding CF by answering the following questions.

- What impact does long-term illness have on young people? Consider this from a physical and psychosocial perspective.
- What is the aetiology of CF? (Refer to Chapter 1.)
- How is CF diagnosed?
- What are the main symptoms of CF and their underlying rationale?

Due to a defect on chromosome 7, CF is a genetic autosomal recessive disorder caused by mutations in the gene encoding the CF transmembrane conductance regulator (CFTR) protein, an adenosine triphosphate binding chloride anion channel that functions at the epithelial cell membrane (Kuk & Taylor-Cousar, 2015; Filbrun *et al.*, 2016; Hodges, 2016).

Two mutated copies of the CFTR gene are inherited and they can either be homozygous, meaning that they are both the same, or heterozygous meaning that they are both different (CF Center Stanford, 2019). There are 2000 CFTR mutations that have been identified and it is these mutations that are responsible for the dysfunction in the protein production that regulates salt and water transportation within the mucous membrane lined organs. This causes mucous within the body to thicken and block ducts which prevent the removal/clearance of secretions (Kuk & Taylor-Cousar, 2015; NICE, 2015). This leads to the increased risk of respiratory infection, difficulty digesting food, malabsorption and intestinal obstruction, pancreatic insufficiency, diabetes and liver cirrhosis. This is because CF is a multisystem disorder that affects many organs, including the digestive system, the pancreas, the liver, endocrine and reproductive system as well as the respiratory system (Kuk & Taylor-Cousar, 2015; Hodges, 2016; Filbrun, 2016). It is suggested that these bodily dysfunctions occur where tissues become inflamed or destroyed (Kuk & Taylor-Cousar, 2015; Hodges, 2016). Symptom severity varies between individuals and can change as the condition progresses (Kuk & Taylor-Cousar, 2015; Bush *et al.*, 2015; Filbrun, 2016; Wallis, 2019).

Eventually, most children and young people affected by CF colonise a variety of pathogens in the lungs. The most common being *Pseudomonas aeruginosa* which is a gram negative bacteria which can be very difficult to treat and can be detrimental to the pre-existing condition of CF. Furthermore, it can be influential in survival rate prediction (Normura *et al.*, 2014; Hodges. 2016). *Pseudomonas aeruginosa* can lead to poor morbidity and increased mortality rates. It can be resistant to regular intravenous antibiotics therapy, hence some patients can be colonised with the bacteria for the remainder of their life (Folkesson *et al.*, 2012; Normura *et al.*, 2014; Hodges, 2016). Also, children with CF are susceptible to contracting other detrimental bacterial infections which include *Burkholderia Cepacia, staphylococcus aureus* and *haemophilus influenza*. Therefore, it is important that patients with CF avoid cross-infection by avoiding contact with each other (Hodges, 2016).

Further complications

Due to the nature of the CF disease trajectory, and it no longer being a disease specific to early childhood, further complications can occur. These can include nasal polyps, sinus disease, asthma, liver disease, depression, atypical mycobacteria, CF-related diabetes as well as the need for transplant of the lung, heart and lung or the liver (UK Cystic Fibrosis Registry, 2014; Bush *et al.*, 2015; Hodges, 2016). Further information on diabetes can be viewed in Chapter 3.

Genotype

The most common genotype that affects people with CF in the UK is DF508. It is named as such because the phenylalanine amino acid is missing from position 508 of the gene mutation. DF508 is otherwise known as the F508 DEL or its new name p.Phe508del (the phe representing the missing phenylalanine). Less common is the G551D (new name p.GLY551Asp) mutation which affects 6% of people with the disease (UK Cystic Fibrosis Registry, 2014). The CF Trust (2015) advocates that patients with CF should know their genotype, so that they can access the most appropriate recent advances in treatment (Hodges, 2016).

> 🔑 **Key points**
>
> - Cystic fibrosis is a multisystem disorder caused by a defect on chromosome 7. It is an autosomal recessive disorder and is life-limiting.
> - It is important that patients know their genotype so that they can have access to appropriate information and treatment.

Management

A multidisciplinary team approach is required for the management of children and young people with CF. The key purpose is to maintain their nutritional status as well as healthy lung function in order to minimise previously mentioned symptoms and to maintain as healthy a lifestyle as possible (Hodges, 2016). Promoting airway clearance through a regime of physiotherapy, which aids in expectorating mucus from the lungs, along with the use of antibiotics, aims to prevent repeated lung infections (Williams et al., 2009; Barker et al., 2011; Filbrun et al., 2016). Pancreatic enzymes and nutritional supplements are given to prevent malabsorption, alongside a high protein, high calorie diet to reduce malnutrition and minimise growth delay (Williams et al., 2009; Barker et al., 2011; Filbrun et al., 2016). As the ability to absorb fat-soluble vitamins (A, D, E and K) is inhibited, vitamin supplements are also necessary (Veal et al., 2018). However, it is suggested that most patients with CF will still have some level of malabsorption and faltering growth regardless of their dietary and enzyme intake (Williams et al., 2009; Barker et al., 2011; Filbrun et al., 2016). Additionally, in approximately 2.5–12% of individuals with CF, there is the possibility that diabetes mellitus, caused by pancreatic insufficiency, will also develop (Filbrun et al., 2016). This type of diabetes is known as cystic fibrosis-related diabetes (CFRD).

To gain more information regarding CF and its management, please refer to the Recommended reading section at the end of this chapter.

> 🔑 **Key Points**
>
> - A multidisciplinary team approach is required when caring for children and young people with CF.
> - Maintaining a healthy lung function as well as a healthy nutritional status is essential.

Adolescents with a long-term condition

The effect of a long-term condition on adolescents was discussed at length in Chapter 10 and readers may want to revisit this chapter before continuing further. One of the main issues regarding long-term conditions and young people is that advances in management have increased the overall survival rates for children and young people with life-limiting conditions such as CF (Schwartz *et al.*, 2014; Elborn, 2016). Fifty years ago, most infants born with CF died within the first year of life, and CF was considered to be a condition confined to childhood (Stephenson *et al.*, 2017). However, a considerable number of individuals with CF, now live to over 40 years of age (Stephenson *et al.*, 2017; Bowmer *et al.*, 2018). It is also estimated that by the mid-2000s, survival rates could rise to 50 years or above (Simmonds, 2013; Kerr *et al.*, 2018). Consequently, as many individuals with CF will receive the majority of their care in the adult setting, the focus of care is changing and greater emphasis now needs to be placed on the development of an appropriate, supportive transition process between child and young people's services to more adult-focused services (Lapp & Chase, 2018).

Transitional care

The need for a supportive transition between children and young people's services to more adult-focused services has been a recognised health care need for some time (Department of Health, UK (DoH), 1991; Betz, 2004; While *et al.*, 2004; McDonagh, 2005). Transition services for young people with CF was initially fragmented and unpredictable and although this may have improved over time, transition services remain inconsistent (Glasper, 2018; Kerr *et al.*, 2018) and transition continues to be a potential source of anxiety of young people and their parents (Okumura *et al.*, 2014).

Developing and implementing effective transition programmes can be challenging for health care providers for a range of reasons and where programmes do exist, there is little research into their effectiveness (Crowley *et al.*, 2011). Other challenges include budget and staffing issues (McDonagh, 2005). Although the McDonagh reference is now dated, it remains relevant, particularly as budgeting and staffing within the NHS has not improved since this paper was published. However, improvements are anticipated over time since the implementation of the Nurse Staffing Levels (Wales) Act 2016, as it is highly likely that safe nurse staffing levels will be adopted in the other countries of the UK.

The philosophy of transitional care

Transitional care has been described as a multifaceted active process that attends to the medical, psychosocial and educational/vocational needs of young people as they move from child to adult care services (Blum *et al.*, 1993; Soanes & Timmons, 2004; Crowley *et al.*, 2011). This identifies that the process of transition is far more involved than simply transferring a patient from one hospital/unit to another.

Models of transition

There are several identified models of transitional care; for example, transition based on chronological age or specific conditions. However, there is still little evidence to demonstrate that one transition model is more effective than another (Conway, 1998; Rosen *et al.*, 2003; Crowley *et al.*, 2011) and more research is needed in this area. Regardless of which model is used, it has been recognised over a long period of time that transition needs to be informal and flexible, with young people and their families being involved in any decisions about transferring to adult services (Conway, 1998; Rosen, *et al.*, 2003; Towns & Bell, 2011; Touchman & Schwartz, 2013). What has also been noted is that transition is likely to be more successful when it is coordinated by a designated health care professional who, in conjunction with the needs of young people and their families, is responsible for the transition process.

⌫ Key point

- As more young people with long-term conditions survive into adulthood, the transition from child to adult services becomes a significant issue (Stephenson *et al.*, 2017).

Reflection

Transition is a major step for many young people. Before continuing with the rest of the scenario, pause to think about the issues you consider may be of concern to Sophie as she contemplates moving to adult services.

🌐 Case study 11.2

As Sophie has been attending the children's hospital since birth, she is familiar with both the outpatient and ward multidisciplinary team (MDT), so she is reluctant to transfer to a new service where she may not trust the staff as she currently does. She feels that, at the new hospital, she will have to relate her history all over again, which is often the case. As one of her friends, who also had CF, died not long after being transferred to the adult services, Sophie is concerned about transferring and worries that this only happens 'when the doctors think that you are going to die'. She is also afraid that she will be left with strangers at the 'new hospital' and that it will be full of old and dying people. Although she has not discussed this with the medical staff, she has mentioned it to the CF specialist nurse who recently visited her at home. Additionally, the adult hospital is further away, and it will be difficult for her to get time off work to travel to her clinic appointments, as she cannot drive.

Sophie's father is her sole carer, with help from both sets of grandparents. Since her diagnosis, Sophie's father or one of her grandparents has probably been encouraged to stay with her when she is in hospital. Although parents do not usually tend to stay with hospitalised adolescents within children's services, it is still an option for them. It is issues such as this that help to make young people feel comfortable with their surroundings. Lack of knowledge about what is available for them in the adult setting (Bowmer *et al.*, 2018) is another example of the way in which the adolescent can be made to feel vulnerable.

There are several key issues that are raised within the case study that have implications for nursing practice. This part of the chapter will focus on issues regarding transition for young people, vulnerability, advocacy, managing a long-term condition, support and decision-making.

 Time out

- What are the possible reasons that adolescents may be anxious or concerned about moving to adult services?

Issues regarding transition for adolescents

Transferring from child to adult services can be problematic and stressful for adolescents (Al-Yateem, 2012), particularly when they are not prepared appropriately for the move (Lapp & Chase, 2018). Consequently, young people may be frightened of moving to adult services for a variety of reasons, including:

- Fear of the unknown.
- Moving away from familiar surroundings and staff they have known for many years.
- A lack of confidence and trust in the new service.
- Not feeling ready.
- Need for more preparation.
- Too much change at one time, because it may coincide with other changes that are occurring in their lives; for example, leaving school, starting a new job.
- Negative perceptions given by children's services staff regarding adult services.
- Parental views of the transition process.
- Having to provide information about themselves to the new service providers.
- Being cared for by health care professionals with limited knowledge of their condition.
- Coming into contact with older people with CF who may be more unwell, which increases the adolescent's awareness that CF is a life-limiting condition.
- Facing their own mortality.
- Previous experience of adult services; for example, they may have adult relatives who have been hospitalised.

In children's nursing, where the concept of family-centred care is fostered, parents are encouraged to participate in the care of their child and this may mean staying overnight (Mikkelson & Frederiksen, 2011). In children's health care, the focus is on making the hospital environment more like home, which can be in stark contrast to the services and philosophies of adult care (MacLuskey & Keilty, 2018). Making the transition from familiar children's services, where they feel comfortable and safe, to an adult service that is new and unknown to them, is a particular challenge for some young people and has the potential to cause stress, anxiety and increase their overall vulnerability (Al-Yateem, 2012).

It is not uncommon for young people to be anxious about the new services that they will be offered within adult care and some are concerned that it will be 'impersonal' with 'unfriendly' staff (Viner, 2003; Bill 2019). This is understandable as young people who have had a long-term condition since birth or early childhood are familiar with staff that have been caring for them, as was reinforced in the recent doctoral study by Bill (2019). Moving away from people they trust and respect, towards people they do not know, may mean that they will have difficulty trusting 'new' staff in the adult setting (Towns & Bell, 2011). Some parents and young people are also concerned that they may have a reduced level of service provision in the adult setting (Coyne *et al.*, 2017) and this can lead to a lack of confidence in the service by both adolescents and their families. Almost two decades ago, Viner (2003) suggested that some parents may actually 'sabotage' the transition process if they do not understand the need for transition or are not included in any decisions regarding transition. Although this work is dated, evidence continues to demonstrate that parents are still not always included in the transition process (Towns & Bell, 2011; Coyne *et al.*, 2017, Lapp & Chase, 2018; Coyne *et al.*, 2018). Therefore, transition should be a well-coordinated, planned and unhurried process (Okumura *et al.*, 2014) and although there is no specific fixed time recommended for transition (Viner, 2003; Al-Yateem, 2012; Touchman & Schwartz, 2013) young people and their families need to be ready to move to adult services.

Young people experience significant developmental changes as they move though the life continuum from childhood to adulthood (Santrock, 2018). This is often a difficult time for them as they come to terms with the final years of their education, move to higher education or employment and form new relationships (Santrock, 2018). Adding a long-term condition to this developmental stage increases the factors that adolescents need to cope with, and the stress that young people can experience at this time should not be underestimated. Therefore, it is important that during the transition between services, appropriate and relevant information is shared to ensure that young people and their parents are kept up to date (Towns & Bell, 2011). This also includes the sharing of relevant information between the MDT in both child and adult services, with regard to the young person's past history (Coyne *et al.*, 2018), which as Viner has noted previously, will remove the need for the adolescent to keep providing information about themselves and in some situations having tests and investigations repeated unnecessarily (Viner, 2003; Lapp & Chase, 2018).

Although improvements have been made to potential life expectancy, the trajectory of CF is unpredictable and young people can still die at an early age. Therefore, it is possible that many young people with CF will have had friends within their peer group who have already died (Ernst *et al.*, 2011). When young people move to adult hospitals it is expected that they will come into contact with older people who have CF. Potentially, these individuals could be at a more advanced stage of the disease process and as a consequence of this young people may be forced to confront their own mortality, even if they are not ready to do so. Young people with CF can develop a range of psychological issues, such as depression (Ernst *et al.*, 2011), and confronting their own mortality may cause them additional distress.

Key point

- Adolescents with a long-term condition have much to cope with and this can increase their overall vulnerability.

Gaining autonomy

Autonomy is an important part of adolescent development (Santrock 2018) and excessive dependence on the family, particularly where a long-term condition is present, can result in a lack of autonomy (Ernst *et al.*, 2011). Recently, Sophie has left school and is working part time. It is sometimes difficult for young people with a long-term condition to achieve independence and starting work is one way of trying to achieve this. However, gaining and maintaining employment can be challenging for young people due to overall health and management needs (Hale & Viner, 2018). Taking time off work for hospital appointments may lose Sophie any 'good will' she has with her employer Therefore, transferring to the adult hospital, which is further away from Sophie's home, has the potential to impact on her job and therefore her autonomy.

Managing a long-term condition

Maintaining a physiotherapy and exercise programme while trying to work is difficult, as demonstrated in the case study. It is important that this should be as flexible and manageable as possible to make it easy for the adolescent to comply with their management, including attendance at outpatient appointments. The issue of adolescent compliance and the ability to cope with a long-term condition has been discussed in Chapter 10.

Another issue highlighted in the scenario is Sophie's reluctance to disclose her condition to new friends. This is not unusual because, above all, adolescents want to be the same as their friends, since the peer group is very important to adolescents (Santrock, 2018). While they are still maturing and developing their personalities, adolescents can often feel insecure about themselves (Santrock, 2018). By socialising with their peers, adolescents are learning from each other and developing their ability to interact socially on a wider scale (Santrock, 2018). The presence of a long-term condition has the potential to inhibit this. Where adolescents have a long-standing illness, it is likely that their 'old' schoolfriends were aware of this. However, many young people have concerns about meeting 'new' friends (CF Trust, 2017) either through changing schools or starting work. Understandably, no one would want to say, 'Hi, I'm Sophie and I have CF' (diabetes or any other condition) on first meeting someone, and the issue for many young people is at which point to disclose. Some young people are very concerned that disclosure of a long-term condition will prevent new friendships being made. Publishing information such as the Secondary School Pack is just one way that the Cystic Fibrosis Trust is able to provide advice to young people (CF Trust, 2017).

Support and decision-making

Within the scenario, Sophie has raised concerns regarding her transfer to the adult services. She is feeling frightened, which can be a natural reaction for any young person with a long-term condition facing the prospect of moving from child to adult services. Such a transition is a life-changing event that needs to be managed in a sensitive manner for the transition to be effective (Okumura *et al.*, 2014; Towns & Bell, 2011; Lapp & Chase, 2018).

The move from child to adult services can coincide with a period of developmental transition for young people, a stage where they are maturing and want to be recognised as individuals and accepted by their peer group (Santrock, 2018). Not only are they adapting to growing up with a long-term condition, but they are also confronting the same issues as many other young people, such as finding their independence and discovering where they fit into the wider context of society. This could include exploring their sexuality and being involved in the misuse of alcohol and other substances. It is a stage where young people want to be respected and gain more responsibility. All these issues need to be considered within the transition process, particularly as young people like Sophie, with a long-term condition, may be frightened of moving to adult care (Towns & Bell, 2011).

Key point

- Young people with a long-term condition need to be recognised as individuals. They have the same needs as their peer group but often have additional needs related to living with a long-term condition.

Case study 11.3

Sophie has continued to lose weight and her chest infection has worsened. With much persuasion from her family and the CF team, she has finally agreed to be admitted to the children's hospital for assessment and management. Sophie is really unhappy as she has recently met a new boyfriend and feels she is being 'forced' to tell people about her condition because she has to be admitted to hospital.

During the admission process, Sophie was noted to have diabetes, caused by pancreatic insufficiency, which occurs in approximately, 40–50% of young people who have CF (Bridges, 2013). Understandably, Sophie was shocked and distressed by the new diagnosis as she feels that she has enough to cope with already.

While Sophie has been in hospital, the CF specialist nurse has been visiting her on a daily basis. She has a good rapport with Sophie and has identified a number of issues which are causing Sophie concerns. These include her fear of transfer to adult services, her ability to form relationships, to be accepted as an individual, to cope with the additional diagnosis of CF related diabetes and trying to juggle her home, work and social life within her current management regime. Sophie has met with the diabetes nurse consultant who will now be part of the MDT caring for her.

The CF team has identified a plan of action including the support needed in relation to the issues outlined above.

Time out

- What key factors do you consider ought to be included in a plan of action?
- Provide the rationale to support your choice.

The role of the nurse

It is important to remember that not only do adolescents and their families experience concerns about the transition process, but so too can health care professionals. Many staff will have known the young people in their care for some time and it can be difficult for them to 'let go' (Coyne *et al.*, 2017). It is possible, therefore, that staff could send out non-verbal messages to young people causing them increased anxiety about the transition to adult services, thereby hindering the process (Lapp & Chase, 2018).

The nurse, whether a children's nurse, adult nurse, CF or adolescent specialist nurse, has an important role to play in facilitating transition. It is imperative that nurses build good relationships and maintain open channels of communication with young people and their families. It is important, however, that young people and their families do not become overly dependent on the nurse, and any relationship forged should maintain professional boundaries as set out in *The Code: Professional Standards of Practice and Behaviour for Nurses, Midwives and Nursing Associates* (Nursing and Midwifery Council (NMC), 2018). Further suggestions regarding ways in which nurses can facilitate the transition process are outlined later in the chapter.

As the CF specialist nurse described in the case study has already built up a good rapport with Sophie, she is ideally placed to act as an advocate within the transition process. To ensure a meaningful, involved transition, the CF specialist nurse will need to identify the needs of Sophie and her family through exploration of their views, values and beliefs, and past experiences. It is essential to find out what is important to young people in relation to their long-term condition, as well as exploring their aspirations and goals in life. This will allow options to be considered before the transition, as well as anticipating future needs.

Key point

- To promote a purposeful transition, the children's nurse/CF specialist nurse should identify the needs of young people and their families, through exploration of their views, values and experiences.

It is important to consider the individual needs of the young person, because transition does not occur in a single step (Okumura *et al.*, 2014; Towns & Bell, 2011; Coyne *et al.*, 2017; Lapp & Chase, 2018). Flexibility and the gathering of appropriate information enable effective planning of a supportive network. This includes multidisciplinary and multiagency involvement in the transitional process, as the CF nurse does not work in isolation. An MDT approach will allow thorough preparation, greater continuity of care, a communication network and enhancement of trust within the therapeutic relationship. Facilitation of the transition should aim to meet the expectations of young people and their families, which will help alleviate any apprehension regarding the move to adult services. If expectations are not met, it could impact on the outcomes of transition planning.

To enable a more seamless transition, it is essential that the CF nurse and the MDT involve young people with a long-term condition (like Sophie) and their families in the decision-making process. Involvement in decision-making allows a more 'person-centred' approach to care (Beresford, 2004), which focuses on the young person's preferences, goals and outlook for the future.

> 🔑 **Key point**
>
> ● It is during the transition period that there is a 'locus of control' shift in the amount of involvement in decision-making between the parent/carer and the young person. You may want to review locus of control in Chapter 6.

🕐 **Time out**

● Consider why there may be changes in the amount of involvement in decision-making for young people and their parents and how this may impact on their relationship.

Due to their increasing level of maturity and need for independence, young people will be more involved in decisions about their care and treatment, and the CF team will encourage this process. Some young people may be apprehensive initially regarding their level of involvement in decision-making, but by including them at an early stage, they will begin to understand the relevance of their participation. This will impact on their understanding of their health, well-being and treatment regimen, encouraging them to take responsibility for themselves. Many young people who have been involved in their care and decision-making from an early age become experts in their own condition and its management. This has the potential to influence their ability to adapt to living with their long-term condition, reduce the potential problem of non-compliance, and be comfortable with balancing their lifestyle in terms of education, social relationships, work life and home life (Cronley & Savage, 2019). Consideration of all of these issues is important when planning the transition process with any young person with a long-term condition.

While the young person is establishing independence and having greater involvement in decision-making, the role of the parent/carer cannot be ignored. The parental role in decision-making is now changing. Potentially, this can be a difficult time of adjustment as previously the parent would have worked closely with the CF team, often taking full responsibility for decisions about their child's care and treatment. This may have included involvement in learning about all aspects of care in order to manage their child's CF appropriately. The young person is now seeking independence and will take centre stage in decisions made. Parents' views may be consulted and considered in decision-making, but their role will not be in the forefront as it has been previously. This can leave parents feeling a sense of loss and helplessness. The CF team can help promote this shift in the parental role as parents move to a more supportive/advisory role, enabling them to engage with their adolescents and actively encourage their newfound responsibility.

In the earlier part of the case study, Sophie did not want to go to hospital despite her father's concerns. Conflict can occur during the transitional phase, as the young person and parent may have differences of opinions relating to aspects of changes in care. Some young people may actively rebel against their treatment as they adjust within the period of adolescent development, as well as with their long-term condition, whereas others may embrace this transitional time.

The CF team needs to support parents and young people through this process in a sensitive manner, offering guidance and reassurance throughout to enhance positive outcomes. Such support is demonstrated within the scenario. Members of the CF team will have built up a relationship with young people and their families over several years. They will have become familiar with their patients, building strong attachments along the way. Thus, this can also be a difficult time for the staff involved in the care of young people, because they have protected and nurtured their patients. Having watched young people with a long-term condition grow up, it may not be easy for the health professional to 'let go' of their care (Coyne *et al.*, 2017). Health professionals need to be mindful of their role in supporting young people and involve them in decisions about their care to increase their confidence and their self-esteem. This can promote the development of their identity, allowing them to feel in control, and give them the ability to cope with the transition process and beyond.

Lack of involvement in decision-making and inadequate transitional support can disadvantage the young person. It could create developmental difficulties in terms of self-concept and autonomy (Ernst *et al.*, 2011) and may hinder the evolution of their identity and movement towards adulthood. Additionally, this has the potential to impact on their ability to integrate into the wider social world because, as a consequence, they may lack confidence, feel lonely and have low expectations of their illness and future outlook. This can have a negative influence on their ability to establish new relationships, their career choice and ability to become economically viable and independent.

Lack of involvement in decision-making and inadequate transitional support also has a counter-impact on the family, as the young person with a long-term condition may be more dependent and over-reliant upon them. This can be a worrying, anxious time, putting an added strain on the family emotionally and financially. Parents may need to support the young person for a longer period of time.

🌐 Case study 11.4

While in hospital, Sophie's condition improved, her chest infection subsided and she gained some weight. As she feels better in herself, she is able to think more rationally about her present situation. During her hospital admission, her boyfriend and a few work friends visited her and to her surprise were more accepting than she had expected they would be. This has helped her feel more secure.

During Sophie's hospital admission, the CF team have taken the opportunity to provide her with some education about her overall condition and the process of moving to another hospital. She has been informed that transition is not a sudden process and that she will be transferred via a transition clinic where she will get the opportunity to visit the new hospital and the staff, but still be predominantly under the care of the children's hospital. Due to the structure of the transition protocol, Sophie will be able to choose her own timing for transfer and thus have an element of control in deciding when it is right for her to move on. Consequently, Sophie feels much happier in herself and with the transition process.

Time out

- What are the benefits of involving young people and their families in decision-making?

Promoting the paradigm shift

In 2003, the Royal College of Paediatrics and Child Health (RCPCH) identified that young people had previously been disadvantaged in relation to transitional service provision. They suggested that the specific needs of young people and their families had not been sufficiently met, potentially due to a variety of reasons, including:

- An overall lack of understanding of adolescent transitional care issues.
- Lack of provision of staff training regarding understanding the needs of young people and their families during the transition phase.
- Clinical areas being too focused on children's health care issues and not acknowledging the growing independence of young people.
- Clinical areas too focused on adult issues, valuing autonomy, but not acknowledging concerns of the family and young people's state of readiness in the move towards independence.
- Insufficient specialist staff to offer appropriate support.
- Poor communication and collaboration between children, young people and adult services (RCPCH 2003).

Although transition services can still be inconsistent, changes are being made to address the problems that some young people and their parents encounter. For example, in 2018, the RCPCH published *Facing the Future; Standards for Children with On-going Health Needs*. Standard Six of this document recommends that there should be an identified person within both child and adult services to ensure that a developmentally appropriate transitions service is provided for young people (RCPCH 2018).

 Time out

- Outline the consequences of inadequate transitional support for the young people and their families.

Over time, there has been a growing recognition of the importance of providing an effective transition service (Blum *et al.*, 1993; Conway, 1998; Cowlard, 2003; While *et al.*, 2004; Crowley *et al.*, 2011; Coyne *et al.*, 2017). Developing transitional services was identified in the original National Service Framework (DoH UK, 2004) and the Royal College of Nursing (RCN) developed guidelines for nurses in 2004. More recently, transition has also been addressed by the Care Quality Commission (CQC) (2014) and the National Institute for Health and Care Excellence (NICE) (2016). The overall aim of all interested parties is to promote a paradigm shift that informs, guides and educates health care professionals in the importance of providing an effective and developmentally appropriate transition service. To facilitate a seamless transition, MDT working is essential and continuing education can add to the development of knowledge and skills in this area.

The principles of successful transitional care

 Time out

- What do you think should be included in transitional care training programmes?

The RCPCH have developed online resources regarding transitional services and you may want to review their webpage for further information: www.rcpch.ac.uk/sites/default/files/generated-pdf/document/Health-transition-resources.pdf.

The main focus for any transition programme, however, is that it should be person focused and developmentally appropriate.

> **Key point**
>
> • It is essential that health care professionals collaborate and share their expertise to ensure a smooth transition between child and adult services.

Once staff have enhanced their knowledge by undertaking further training, they need to bridge the gap between child and adult services by ensuring a multiagency approach to care, whereby expertise is shared and appropriate resources are provided to support the young person and their family. Out-of-hours clinics and collaborative joint clinics can be more suitable for the young person in the transition phase. Young people may or may not wish to have their parents present at their clinic consultation. As they become more involved in their own decision-making and geared towards self-care they should be supported in their preference. While the multidisciplinary approach is essential, the role of the children's nurse is paramount.

> **Key points**
>
> • Young people need to be allocated a key worker to coordinate, involve, guide and educate them and their families through the process of transition. The CF nurse may take on this role.
> • The transition from child to adult services does not need to occur during a fixed timeframe but can take place when it is felt that the adult hospital would be more appropriate in meeting the young person's needs (Rutishauser *et al.*, 2014).

Transition should be planned and purposeful; therefore, it is important to highlight as early as possible that transition will need to happen at some point, particularly for children with a long-term condition. Discussion may begin when the child is 12 years of age and should continue until such time that the young person actually makes the transition to adult services. The complex issues surrounding adolescent development determine that adolescents of the same age are not all at the same level of physical and cognitive development (Santrock, 2018). Consequently, it would not be appropriate to suggest that chronological age alone should be the major determining factor in adolescent transition. The transition from child to adult services does, however, need to be planned and well coordinated.

In 2004, the RCN identified the need for three stages of transition. These stages are outlined in Table 11.1. The RCN makes further recommendations about the ways in which nurses can facilitate the transition process. It is recommended that at each transitional stage, the children's nurse or allocated key worker can assist the young person in six key areas. These are outlined in Table 11.2.

It is interesting to note that, although transition remains on the agenda within health care as a whole, the RCN has offered no updated information or guidance for nurses on facilitating the transition of young people from child to adult services. However, the RCN website does signpost individuals to the NICE (2016) guidelines regarding transition.

In the main, the RCN (2004) stages of transition, are still relevant as young people do need to become more aware of their own condition and management regime, start participating in their own care and become increasingly involved within the decision-making process. At what age the subject of transition should be raised with adolescents and their families is still questionable, but in a recent study, parents and young people all identified they always knew that transition would be inevitable, it was the way it was managed was the important factor (Bill, 2019).

TABLE 11.1   Stages of transition.

Early stage (12–14 years)

At this stage, the young people can be introduced to the idea of transition and move towards independence with support from their family. The young people should be encouraged to develop an awareness of their long-term condition and care needs, and future implications of their condition. Assessment of their understanding of their illness at this stage is essential to support them.

Middle stage (14–15 years)

Young people and their families should be introduced to the process of transition. They should be informed about what they can expect from adult-led services. The children's nurse can encourage the young person to participate in goal setting.

Late stage (15–16 years)

At this stage, young people may feel more confident regarding their move to adult care. Young people may have adopted a self-caring approach to dealing with their long-term condition.

Source: Modified from Royal College of Nursing (2004) *Adolescent Transition Care. Guidance for Nursing Staff*. London: Royal College of Nursing.

TABLE 11.2   Guidelines for nurses in facilitating the transition process.

Self-advocacy

The nurse can:

- Provide education regarding the condition
- Encourage them to ask questions
- Ensure they know how and where to access health care information

Independent health care behaviour

The nurse can:

- Provide them with a personal health care record book
- Assess their level of understanding regarding their medication
- Discuss the principles of confidentiality

Sexual health

The nurse should be able to discuss:

- Changes associated with puberty
- Safe sex practices and general sexual well-being
- Issues regarding fertility and provide basic genetic counselling
- Their concerns and allow them to ask questions

Psychosocial support

The nurse will encourage:

- The adolescent to talk about their friends and supportive relationships
- The adolescent to join social groups
- The adolescent to set positive and realistic goals
- Autonomy and decision-making

Education and vocational planning

The nurse should:

- Discuss the responsibilities and restrictions affecting education and recreational activities
- Have an awareness of health care entitlements and benefits and guide the adolescent appropriately

Health and lifestyle

The nurse should be able to discuss and advise young people on:

- Smoking, alcohol consumption, drug use and overall general well-being
- Weight gain and weight loss related to their condition
- Issues related to body image

Source: Modified from Royal College of Nursing (2004) *Adolescent Transition Care. Guidance for Nursing Staff*. London: Royal College of Nursing.

While the main focus of adolescent health is to promote autonomy and decision-making, it is important to maintain a close relationship with parents throughout the transition process so that they still feel involved. Therefore, it is recommended that young people are encouraged to include their parents in the information-sharing process. This will ensure that the health and lifestyle needs of young people are addressed, helping them to develop and feel respected as individuals.

It is important to remember that parents are also going through a transition process. In most cases, parents have been involved in their child's care since infancy and during the transition process, not only are they expected to step back from managing their young person's care, but they must also recognise that they will not have as much involvement in adult services as they had within children's services (Bill, 2019).

> ⬛━🔑   **Key point**
>
> ● Children's nurses/specialist nurses should start talking about the move to adult services at least one year prior to transfer. This will allow time for questions and discussion with young people and their families.

To enable a seamless transition, the role of the children's nurse/specialist nurse during this time will involve:

- The coordination of joint clinics.
- Provision of adequate information and support.

Again, much of the above remains relevant. However, one issue that has not been addressed and that parents and young people can find challenging is the considerable difference between child and adult health care. The philosophies of family-centred care and adult-focused care are polar opposites and it is not easy to move from one to the other in the space of one admission. This is something that needs to be given serious consideration with regard to the care of young people, particularly with regard to the model of care that is used within the management of adolescents (Bill, 2019).

Although many young people enjoy the additional 'freedom' they feel they have within the adult setting, some are unhappy that they are unable to have a parent stay with them overnight. Parents can feel excluded and that their input is not wanted; conversely, some adolescents complain that they are not listened to and that their views are not heard (Bill, 2019). However, in a recent study, the overwhelming concerns for parents of young people with CF, was that their son/daughter would come into contact with other individuals who had CF and increase their risk of acquiring an infection such as *pseudomonas aeruginosa, burkholderia cepacia, staphylococcus aureus* and *haemophilus influenza* (Bill, 2019).

It is recommended that care is audited to monitor its effectiveness. It has already been noted that the transition from child to adult services does not always occur in a seamless manner, although every effort should be made to ensure that it does. The children's nurse has a vital role to play with regard to evaluating the progress of the transitional process. If children's nurses are able to monitor the progress of transition, they will be able to address any identified problems early and renegotiate goals and timescales where appropriate.

🕐   **Time out**

You can now use these next questions to test your knowledge on the content of this chapter:

- What is the most common gene mutation in CF?
- What is the philosophy of transitional care?
- Why is it important for young people to be involved in decision-making?
- Outline the role of the nurse in the transition process.

Conclusion

This chapter has clearly identified that there are ongoing needs for young people and their families as they move through the transition process. However, transition is currently often a neglected dimension of health care provision, which clearly needs to be addressed. An MDT and multiagency approach is required to accomplish this, and further education for health care providers is required if they are to deliver an enhanced level of care and a seamless transition between child and adult services. Nurses working with young people with a long-term condition play a key role in the transition process, promoting autonomy and self-actualisation, which will enable adolescents to make a successful transition between service providers.

Key points

- As more young people with long-term conditions survive into adulthood, the transition from child to adult services becomes a significant issue (Bowmer *et al.*, 2018) and poor transitional support can have a detrimental effect on young people.
- Transitional care is a multifaceted active process that attends to the medical, social and educational/vocational needs of young people as they move from child- to adult-centred care (Rutishauser *et al.*, 2014). However, research in this area is limited.
- The nurse working with young people has an important role to play in facilitating the transition process.
- During the transition period, there is a 'locus of control' shift in the amount of involvement in decision-making between the parent/carer and the young person. With increased autonomy, the young person will have greater involvement in the decision-making process.
- Regardless of the evidence to support the importance of a smooth and coordinated transition process, transition remains a frequently neglected area of health care provision.

Useful websites

Cystic Fibrosis Trust http://www.cf.org.uk
Association for Young People's Health http://www.ayph.org.uk
Young Minds http://www.youngminds.org.uk

Recommended reading

Glasper, E.A. & Richardson, J. (2010) *A Textbook of Children's and Young People's Nursing*. Edinburgh, Churchill Livingstone.
Glasper, E.A., Richardson, J. & Randall, D. (2021) *A Textbook of Children's and Young People's Nursing*. Edinburgh, Churchill Livingstone. (In Press.)

Hockenberry, M. & Wilson, D. (2018) *Wong's Nursing Care of Infants and Children (eleventh edition)*. St Louis, USA, Mosby.

Price, J. & McAlinden, O. (2018) *Essentials of Nursing Children and Young People*. Sage, London.

References

Al-Yateem, N. (2012) Child to adult: transitional care for young adults with cystic fibrosis. *British Journal of Nursing*, **21** (14), 850–854.

Barker, E.T., Hartley, S.L., Seltzer, M.M., *et al.* (2011) Trajectories of emotional wellbeing in mothers of adolescents and adults with autism. *Developmental Psychology*, **47** (2), 551–561.

Beresford, B. (2004) On the road to nowhere? Young disabled people and transition. *Child: Care, Health and Development*, **30** (6), 581–587.

Betz, C.L. (2004) Transition of adolescents with special health care needs: review and analysis of the literature. *Issues in Comprehensive Pediatric Nursing*, **27** (3), 179–241.

Bill, S. (2019) An interpretative phenomenological analysis of the transition from child to adult services for young people with cystic fibrosis and their families in Wales. Doctoral Thesis. Cardiff University.

Blum, R., Garrell, D. & Hodgman, C. (1993) Transition from child-centred to adult health care systems for adolescents with chronic conditions: a position paper of the Society for Adolescent Medicine. *Journal of Adolescent Health*, **14** (7), 570–576.

Bowmer, G., Sowerby, C. & Duff, A. (2018) Transition and transfer of young people with cystic fibrosis to adult care. *Nursing Children and Young People*, **30** (5), 34–39.

Bridges, N. (2013) Diabetes in cystic fibrosis. *Paediatric Respiratory Reviews*, **14** (1), 16–18.

Bush, A. Bilson, D. & Hodson, M. (2015*) Hodson and Geddes Cystic Fibrosis* (fourth edition). New York, CRC Press.

Care Quality Commission (2014) *From Pond to Sea: Children's Transition to Adult Health Services*. London, Care Quality Commission.

Conway, S.P. (1998) Transition from paediatric to adult-oriented care for adolescents with cystic fibrosis. *Disability and Rehabilitation*, **20** (6–7), 209–216.

Cowlard, J. (2003) Cystic fibrosis: transition from paediatric to adult care. *Nursing Standard*, **18** (4), 39–41.

Cronley, J. & Savage, E. (2019) Developing agency in the transition to self-management of cystic fibrosis in young people. *Journal of Adolescence*, **75**, 130–137.

Crowley, R., Wolfe, I., Lock, K., *et al.* (2011) Improving the transition between paediatric and adult healthcare: a systematic review. *Archives of Disease in Childhood*, **96** (6), 548–533.

Coyne, I., Sheehan, A.M., Heery, E., *et al.* (2017) Improving transition to adult healthcare for young people with cystic fibrosis: a systematic review. *Journal of Child Healthcare*, **21** (3), 312–330.

Coyne, I., Malone, H., Chubb, E., *et al.* (2018) Transition from paediatric to adult healthcare for young people with cystic fibrosis: parents' information needs. *Journal of Child Healthcare*, **22** (4), 646–657.

Cystic Fibrosis Center at Stanford (2019) The Basics of CF. https://med.stanford.edu/cfcenter/education/english/BasicsOfCF.html Accessed 28/01/20.

Cystic Fibrosis Registry (2014) Cystic Fibrosis Strength in Numbers: UK Cystic Fibrosis Registry 2014 Annual Data Report. London, Cystic Fibrosis Trust

Cystic Fibrosis Trust (2015) Cystic Fibrosis strength in numbers: UK CF Registry Survey Report. London, Cystic Fibrosis Trust.

Cystic Fibrosis Trust (2017) Starting Secondary School. London, Cystic Fibrosis Trust. https://www.cysticfibrosis.org.uk/life-with-cystic-fibrosis/secondary-school Accessed 22/01/20.

Cystic Fibrosis Trust (2018) Annual Data Report 2018. London, Cystic Fibrosis Trust.

Cystic Fibrosis Trust (2020) What is CF? https://www.cysticfibrosis.org.uk/what-is-cystic-fibrosis Accessed 28/01/20.

Department of Health, UK (1991) *Welfare of Children and Young People in Hospital.* London, Her Majesty's Stationery Office.

Department of Health, UK (2004) *National Service Framework for Children, Young People and Maternity Services. Core Standards. Change for Children - Every Child Matters.* London, Department of Health.

Elborn, J.S. (2016) Cystic fibrosis. *Lancet,* **388** (10059), 2519–2531.

Ernst, M.M., Johnson, M.C. & Stark L.J. (2011) Developmental and psychological issues in cystic fibrosis. *Pediatric Clinics of North America,* **58** (4), 865–885.

Filbrun, A., Lahiri, T. & Ren, L.C. (2016) *Handbook of Cystic Fibrosis.* Basel, Springer International Publishing.

Folkesson, A., Jelsbak, L., Yang, L., *et al.* (2012) Adaptation of pseudomonas aeruginosa to the cystic fibrosis airway: an evolutionary perspective. *National Review Microbiology,* **10** (12), 841–851.

Glasper, A. (2018) Enhancing the experience of transition from child to adult health services. *British Journal of Nursing,* **27** (16), 958–959.

Hale, D.R. & Viner, R.M. (2018) How adolescent health influences education and employment: investigating longitudinal and associations and mechanisms. *Journal of Epidemiological and Community Health* **72** (6), 465–470.

Havermans, T., Wuytack, L., Deboel, J., *et al.* (2011) Siblings of children with cystic fibrosis: quality of life and the impact of illness. *Child: Care, Health and Development,* **37** (2), 252–260.

Hodges, A.S. (2016) The family centred experiences of siblings living in the context of cystic fibrosis: A dramaturgical exploration. PhD Thesis. Cardiff University.

Kerr, H., Price, J., Nicholl, H., *et al.* (2018) Facilitating transition from children's to adult services for young adults with life limiting conditions (TASYL): programme theory developed from a mixed method realist evaluation. *International Journal of Nursing Studies,* **86**, 125–138.

Keogh, R.H., Szczesniak, R., Taylor-Robinson, D., *et al.* (2018) Up to date and projected estimates of survival for people with cystic fibrosis using baseline characteristics: a longitudinal study using UK patient registry data. *Journal of Cystic Fibrosis,* **17** (2), 133–134.

Kuk, K. & Taylor-Cousar, J.L. (2015) Lumacaftor and ivacaftor in the management of patients with cystic fibrosis: current evidence and future prospects. *Therapy Advances in Respiratory Disease,* **9** (6), 313–26.

Lapp, V. & Chase, S.K. (2018) How do youth with cystic fibrosis perceive their readiness to transition to adult healthcare compared to their caregivers views? *Journal of Pediatric Nursing,* **43**, 104–110.

MacLuskey, I. & Keilty, K. (2018) Transition from pediatric to adult care. *Canadian Journal of Respiratory, Critical Care and Sleep Medicine,* **2** (1), 83–87.

McCullough, C. & Price, J. (2011) Caring for a child with cystic fibrosis: The children's nurse's role. *British Journal of Nursing,* **20** (3), 164–167.

McDonagh, J.E. (2005) Growing up and moving on: transition from pediatric to adult care. *Pediatric Transplantation,* **9** (3), 364–372.

Mikkelson, G. & Frederiksen, K. (2011) Family-centred care of children in hospital: a concept analysis. *Journal of Advanced Nursing,* **67** (5), 1152–1162.

National Institute for Health and Care Excellence (2015) Guideline scope. Cystic Fibrosis: Diagnosis and management of cystic fibrosis. https://www.nice.org.uk/guidance/ng78/documents/final-scope Accessed 28/01/20.

National Institute for Health and Care Excellence (2016) *Transition from Children's to Adults' Services.* London, National Institute for Health and Care Excellence.

Normura, K., Obatoto, K., Keira, T., *et al.* (2014) Pseudomonas aeruginosa elastase causes transient disruption of tight junctions and downregulation of PAR-2 in human nasal epithelial cells. *Respiratory Research,* **15** (21), 1–13.

Nurse Staffing Levels (Wales) Act 2016. www.legislation.gov.uk/anaw/2016/5/contents/enacted Accessed 28/01/20.

Nursing and Midwifery Council (2018) *The Code: Professional Standards of Practice and Behaviour for Nurses, Midwives and Nursing Associates.* London, Nursing and Midwifery Council.

Okumura, M.J., Ong, T., Dawson, D., *et al.* (2014) Improving transition from paediatric to adult cystic fibrosis care, programme implementation and evaluation. *British Medical Journal: Quality Safety.* doi:10.1136/bmjqs-2013-002364.

Rosen, S.D., Blum, R.W., Britto, M., *et al.* (2003) Transition to adult health care for adolescents and young adults with chronic conditions. *Journal of Adolescent Health* **33**, 309–311.

Royal College of Nursing (2004) *Adolescent Transition Care. Guidance for Nursing Staff.* London, Royal College of Nursing.

Royal College of Paediatrics and Child Health (2003) *Bridging the Gaps: Health Care for Adolescents.* London, Royal College of Paediatrics and Child Health.

Royal College of Paediatrics and Child Health (2018) *Facing the Future: Standards for Children with On-going Health Needs.* London, Royal College of Paediatrics and Child Health.

Rutishauser, C., Sawyer, S. & Ambresin, A.E. (2014) Transition of young people with chronic conditions: a cross-sectional study of patient perceptions before and after transfer from pediatric to adult health care. *European Journal of Pediatrics,* **173** (8), 1067–1074.

Santrock, J.W. (2018) *Adolescence* (seventeenth edition). Boston, McGraw Hill.

Schwartz, L.A., Daniel, L.C., Brumley, L.D., *et al.* (2014) Measures of readiness to transition to adult health care for youth with chronic physical health conditions: a systematic review of recommendations for measurement testing and development. *Journal of Pediatric Psychology,* **39** (6), 588–601.

Simmonds, N.J. (2013) Ageing in cystic fibrosis and long-term survival. *Pediatric Respiratory Reviews,* **14** (1), 6–9.

Soanes, C. & Timmons, S. (2004) Improving transition: a qualitative study examining the attitudes of young people with chronic illness transferring to adult care. *Journal of Child Health Care,* **8** (2), 102–112.

Stephenson, A.L., Stanojevic, S., Sykes, J., *et al.* (2017) The changing epidemiology and demography of cystic fibrosis. *La Presse Medicale,* **46**, e87–95.

Touchman, L. & Schwartz, M. (2013) Health outcomes associated with transition from pediatric to adult cystic fibrosis care. *Pediatrics,* **132** (5), 847–853.

Towns, S.J. & Bell, S.C. (2011) Transition of adolescents with cystic fibrosis from paediatric to adult care. *The Clinical Respiratory Journal,* **5** (2), 64–75.

Veal, Z., McAlinden, O. & Crawford. D. (2018) Care of children and young people with respiratory problems. In: *Essentials of Nursing Children and Young People* (eds J. Price & O. Mc Alinden), pp. 270–284. London, Sage Publications.

Viner, R. (2003) Bridging the gaps: transition for young people with cancer. *European Journal of Cancer,* **39** (18), 2684–2687.

Wallis, C. (2019) Diagnosis and presentation of cystic fibrosis. In: *Kendig's Disorders of the Respiratory Tract in Children* (ninth edition) (eds R.W. Wilmott, A. Bush, R. Deterding, *et al.*), pp. 769–776. Amsterdam, Elsevier.

While, A., Forbes, A., Ullman, R., *et al.* (2004) Good practices that address continuity during transition from child to adult care: synthesis of the evidence. *Child: Care, Health and Development,* **30** (5), 439–452.

Williams, P.D., Ridder, E.L., Setter, R.K., *et al.* (2009) Pediatric chronic illness (cancer, cystic fibrosis) effects on well siblings: parents' voices. *Issues in Comprehensive Paediatric Nursing,* **32** (2), 94–113.

Index

Nursing Care of Children and Young People with Long-Term Conditions, Second Edition.
Edited by Mandy Brimble and Peter McNee.
© 2021 John Wiley & Sons Ltd. Published 2021 by John Wiley & Sons Ltd.